Breast MRI

Breast MRI

Virginia M. Molleran

Mary C. Mahoney

ELSEVIER
SAUNDERS

ELSEVIER
SAUNDERS

1600 John F. Kennedy Blvd.
Ste. 800
Philadelphia, PA 19103-2899

BREAST MRI ISBN: 978-1-4557-4061-1

ISBN: 978-1-4557-4061-1

Senior Content Strategist: Don Scholz
Content Development Specialist: Julia Roberts
Publishing Services Manager: Julie Eddy
Senior Project Manager: Andrea Campbell
Design Direction: Steven Stave

Printed in China

Last digit is the print number: 9 8 7 6 5 4 3 2 1

This book is dedicated to Kevin, Ellie, and Sam.
Thanks for your incredible patience and support!
—Virginia M. Molleran

For my children—Jane, Sarah, Will, and Jack.
You are the center of everything I do.
—Mary C. Mahoney

Contributors

AMY ARGUS, MD
Assistant Professor of Radiology
University of Cincinnati Medical Center
Cincinnati, Ohio

CHRISTOPHER E. COMSTOCK, MD
Attending Radiologist
Director of Breast Imaging Education
Memorial Sloan-Kettering Cancer Center
New York, New York

STAMATIA DESTOUNIS, MD, FACR
Elizabeth Wende Breast Care, LLC
Clinical Associate Professor, University of Rochester School of Medicine & Dentistry
Rochester, New York

SAMANTHA L. HELLER, MD, PhD
Consultant
St. George's Hospital
London, United Kingdom

ANNE E. KLEIMEYER, MD
Kettering Network Radiologists, Inc.
Kettering, Ohio

CAROL H. LEE, MD, FACR
Attending Radiologist
Memorial Sloan-Kettering Cancer Center
Professor, Department of Radiology
Weill Medical College, Cornell University
Cornell, New York

SU-JU LEE, MD, FACR
Assistant Professor of Radiology
Barrett Breast Center
University of Cincinnati Medical Center
Cincinnati, Ohio

MARY C. MAHONEY
Professor of Radiology and Vice Chair of Research
Eugene L. and Sue R. Saenger Chair of Radiological Sciences
University of Cincinnati Medical Center
Director of Breast Imaging
Barrett Cancer Center
Cincinnati, Ohio

VIRGINIA M. MOLLERAN, MD
Assistant Professor of Radiology
UC Health/University Hospital
Breast Imaging Department
Cincinnati, Ohio

LINDA MOY, MD
Assistant Professor of Radiology
New York University Langone Medical Center
New York University Cancer Institute
New York, New York

HAYDEE OJEDA-FOURNIER, MD
Assistant Professor of Clinical Radiology
Medical Director, Breast Imaging Section
Moores Cancer Center
University of California San Diego
San Diego, California

ROBERT A. POOLEY, PhD
Consultant in Radiologic Physics
Department of Diagnostic Radiology
Mayo Clinic
Jacksonville, Florida
Assistant Professor of Radiologic Physics
Mayo Medical School
College of Medicine
Rochester, Minnesota

JANICE S. SUNG, MD
Assistant Attending Radiologist
Memorial Sloan-Kettering Cancer Center
New York, New York

PATRICIA POOLE, MD
Resident–Department of Radiology
UC San Diego Health System
San Diego, California

Preface

For many radiologists, the continual development and application of new and improved technologies and imaging modalities is part of the allure of the specialty, but it can also be one of its greatest challenges. As radiologists, we take pride in providing the highest quality care to our patients and excellent service to our referring physicians. Patients and referring physicians expect us to provide emerging, "cutting edge" imaging of the same excellence with which we provide the conventional imaging modalities. This entails a diligent lifelong learning process. The wealth of available educational resources in radiology is a testament to this.

MRI has emerged as an important component of breast care. The care of patients with newly diagnosed breast cancer is no longer complete without breast MRI, nor can a breast radiology practice adequately care for high-risk patients without offering breast MRI. Furthermore, a prerequisite to performing breast MRI is the capability of performing an MRI-guided breast biopsy. Today's radiologists need to be proficient in interpreting breast MRI and performing MRI-guided breast biopsies. He or she also needs to accurately communicate with patients and their physicians regarding breast MRI indications, results, and limitations.

In our busy lives as radiologists, spouses, parents, and so on, there is a need for concise, easy-to-use educational material. Texts need to be comprehensive, yet easy to use, a go-to source when there is a clinical question. Our goal was to make this text a clear, readable reference for breast MRI. We have made the chapters image-rich, somewhat in the style of an atlas. We have also tried to be very comprehensive in coverage of all aspects of breast MRI, from breast cancer screening to tips and techniques for MRI-guided breast biopsy. We thoroughly describe imaging features of both benign and malignant breast disease, as well as the role of breast MRI in determining extent of disease in patients with newly diagnosed cancers. Our book also discusses MRI features of the postoperative breast, including a chapter on implant evaluation. For those who are new to breast MRI, we have included chapters on setting up a breast MRI practice, breast MRI physics, and breast MRI CAD.

Virginia M. Molleran
Mary C. Mahoney

Contents

CHAPTER 1

Setting Up and Optimizing a Breast MRI Practice

Stamatia Destounis

Breast magnetic resonance imaging (MRI) was introduced into the breast imaging community in the 1990s. A considerable number of research studies were conducted, with findings revealing promising results[1-3] Breast MRI provided a novel approach to detecting breast cancer and diagnosing additional unsuspected breast lesions alongside the standard mammography technique. Implementation of breast MRI now was being considered by facilities as an additional imaging modality.

Published breast MRI research has shown 94% to 100% sensitivity in diagnosing invasive cancer, with a lower sensitivity of 40% to 100% for ductal carcinoma in situ (DCIS).[4] A study by Zakhireh and colleagues showed a sensitivity of 95% in detecting breast cancer when mammography and breast MRI were combined for screening women at high risk of developing cancer.[5] Such literature supports implementing breast MRI into a practice because it has the ability to enhance services provided to patients. However, adding breast MRI is a major undertaking. This chapter will be based on our experience of implementing breast MRI in our practice, which is located in western New York in the city of Rochester. We are an outpatient breast imaging center founded in 1976 that currently staffs approximately 130 employees. We offer a wide range of services to our patients: mammography, bone densitometry, ultrasonography, ductography, needle biopsy, and breast MRI. We see approximately 80,000 patients and diagnose approximately 650 cancers annually. Our facility has evolved over the years to continue to provide the latest technology and offer the best care to our patients. This chapter will discuss our experience and the importance of adequate planning and education to optimize and minimize the challenges that may occur when incorporating breast MRI into your practice.

Existing Practice Needs

Initially, when breast MRI is added, the needs of the facility must be considered. This section will discuss many of the topics that should be addressed before purchase.

Once the decision is made to incorporate breast MRI into the practice, it is beneficial to assign either an individual or a group of staff members to perform the initial research. A search should be conducted of equipment (magnets and coils) available on the market: What is out there? What are the costs? Many options are available, including purchasing equipment that is new or refurbished, as well as leasing the equipment. Based on a facility's particular practice setting, one of these options will be the most optimal. Vendors can present various choices that meet the needs and specifications of the site. The vendor may also provide beneficial business information, such as the number of imaging procedures needed to pay for the equipment. This information will give a site's manager the ability to compare vendors and help make purchasing decisions that will best fit the practice.

Community Research

Some medical communities have boards that have been created to ensure that patients have access to beneficial technology while minimizing increasing community costs. In our community of Rochester, located in western New York, this board is called the Community Technology Assessment Advisory Board (CTAAB). Such boards are made up of individuals representing the business and insurance community, consumers, physician groups, health systems, and other community groups. Initially, a site's officials may have to plead their case as to why a particular modality is essential to their practice. An application providing all information regarding equipment (proposed use, staffing, projected costs, and revenue) and an oral presentation of the proposal are usually required. This process can be lengthy and time intensive, but it is essential for a positive outcome that due diligence are given. To provide evidence for the proposal, published research on using breast MRI will need to be incorporated in the application and presentation. If the board grants approval, the site will be able to move forward with implementation.

Patient Referral Base

Concerns that should be addressed to help assess the initial patient needs of the practice include the following:

- How large is the breast imaging practice? What percentage of the practice's work is for breast imaging?
- What type of patients will be referred to breast MRI: newly diagnosed breast cancer patients, high-risk patients, patients with an inconclusive work-up?

- How many cases of breast cancer are diagnosed at the facility?
- Does the practice serve a high-risk population? If so, what services have been put into place to identify those at risk? Is there a genetic counseling program with risk assessment available?
- Will the magnet be used for breast imaging only or will it be used for whole body imaging as well?
- How will the practice communicate with and educate referring physicians about the new breast MRI program?

Initial Investigation

Before a purchasing decision is made, the benefits and shortcomings of the available options must be diligently explored. Conversations with experienced breast MRI personnel and visits to their practices will be very beneficial to the decision-making process (as it was in our experience), especially if MRI is new to the physicians and staff. These actions will help site officials make the best decisions for the facility and for its patients.

Facility Limitations

Personnel at breast centers that have no MRI experience should take the opportunity to learn all they can about MRI safety. A good place to begin is to consult the American College of Radiology's (ACR) guidance document on MRI safety.[6] This document provides guidance and sample diagrams for the design of a safe MRI suite; it is crucial that safety be incorporated into its infrastructure. The ACR recommends four safe zones, with zones three and four having the strictest access. These zones are restricted and controlled by MR personnel and are physically restricted by passkey locking systems, key locks, and so on. Our facility uses a passkey locking system, which we have found has elevated the level of security. This system provides a much more secure environment because only key personnel know the passkey, ensuring that those who are not authorized cannot gain access. When designing a suite, a project manager from the MRI vendor familiar with executing an MRI safe design will most likely be involved.

Space is a big consideration in the installation plan for an MRI suite. It must be determined whether the facility has existing space available, will need an addition to the building, or will need to acquire additional department space. Each MRI unit on the market will have its own room specifications. Other important areas associated with the MRI examination that need to be created are as follows: patient changing rooms, nurse station for IV access, technologist control room, patient reception and waiting area, storage room, and bathrooms. If a facility has to build an addition to an existing structure, building codes will need to be addressed and an architect hired. If space is limited, a dedicated breast MRI magnet may be an option to explore because this type of unit is smaller than a whole body magnet. Another option if space is limited is to lease a mobile unit. This is especially beneficial if the referral base is unknown or if a low number of referrals is expected initially.

Our first experience with breast MRI was with a leased 1.5 Tesla (T) General Electric mobile unit, staffed with a

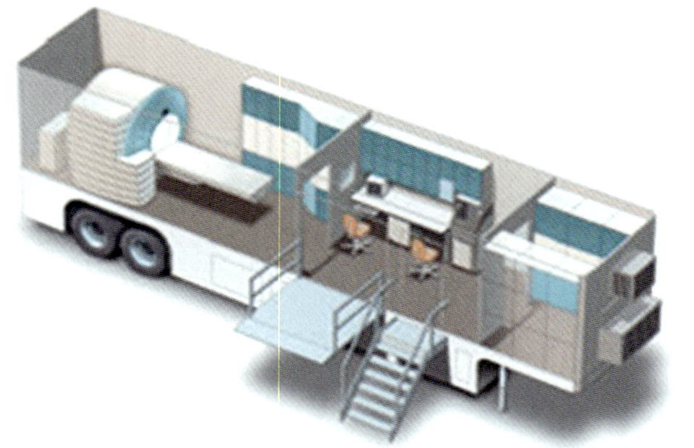

FIGURE 1.1 Suite design of a mobile breast MRI unit. *[From http://www.medical.siemens.com/webapp/wcs/stores/servlet/PSGenericDisplay~q_catalogId~e_-1~a_catTree~e_100001~a_langId~e_-1~a_pageId~e_76149~a_storeId~e_10001.htm.]*

certified MRI technologist, one day a week (Figure 1.1). This initial choice best minimized our risks, allowed us to incorporate the modality gradually, and allowed our staff to ease into MRI training while learning the technology firsthand. Within 2 years of initiation of our breast MRI practice, we needed more days to accommodate the patients, and this eventually grew to a full-time need. Because of this, we decided to build the addition to the building for the MRI suite that exists today.

Magnets and Breast Coils

Most sites use a magnet of at least 1.5 T in field strength to allow for the necessary speed and spatial resolution for breast MRI. It may be wise to consider that vendors are now making available 1.5 T magnets with larger bores, for accommodating larger patients.

A variety of coils are on the market and it may be beneficial to have more than one to accommodate different breast sizes. The coils should allow access to the breast for routine image positioning as well as for interventional procedures. For biopsies and localizations, it is essential to have a coil that will provide both lateral and medial access. However, it is just as important to look at the posterior access: how close to the chest wall can you get with a certain coil? The breast coil is an expensive purchase and is crucial in regards to image quality, so it is important to fully explore the options, features, and limitations of the products available. Listed below are some considerations when choosing breast coils:

- How comfortable is the coil? Have the vendor bring a sample coil for a demonstration to your facility. Have volunteers of different body habitus lie on it in the same position that would be used for the MRI. An uncomfortable patient will move and impair image quality.
- Is the breast coil easy to use? Are the moving parts easy to operate? Are they robust enough to hold up to daily use? Will they clean well after procedures?

Sixteen-channel coils have recently been introduced for optimizing signal-to-noise ratio. Some of these are designed with a closed cup construction, which surrounds the breast tissue, for best signal. This can make positioning a challenge, and a separate coil is used for biopsy. Others have coil elements built in to the compression paddles, which allows the elements to be customized to each patient. For biopsy with this construction, the paddle element is switched for a biopsy immobilization grid, thus turning the coil effectively into a seven-channel coil for the biopsy procedure.

Power Injector

Another piece of equipment that requires consideration is a power injector. When we first began breast MRI imaging, our nurse injected the contrast by hand. Our injection rate is 2 mL/second, with a 30 mL saline flush, also at 2 mL/second. Allowing true confidence in the consistency of the timing, a power injector will ensure that the injection is the same for every patient, every time. This is important for two reasons. First, the kinetic data gathered after the patient is injected is entirely dependent on timing. Second, many patients come for scanning on an annual basis and interpretation of a change on the MRI study from previous years is complicated when there is the possibility that variation may be due to differences in the injection rate. Using a power injector will remove this variable.

Our most noticeable change after we began using the power injector was that our patients moved less during injection, probably because the nurse no longer was injecting by hand. Minimizing patient movement led to better studies.

Implementing Breast Magnetic Resonance Imaging

Magnetic Resonance Imaging Staff

Patients that are referred to breast MRI have individualized concerns that need special considerations. Those being referred for an MRI to evaluate the extent of the disease are extremely anxious because of the recent diagnosis of breast cancer. Women who are at high risk of developing breast cancer or women with an inconclusive mammographic work-up will have increased anxiety as well, fearing the possibility of a finding that may be cancerous. Before the procedure, the physician should inform the patient of why the examination is being recommended as well as what might result from the procedure, such as follow-up MRI examinations or the need for an MRI biopsy.

Having dedicated scheduling staff is beneficial because they will be well versed in the specific needs of breast MRI patients. In our facility, two dedicated staff members assist patients with insurance preauthorization, scheduling, and patient check-in. Additionally, they inform patients about the examination—the length of time it will take and how to prepare—and inform them about the contrast injection. These trained staff members will discuss MRI contraindications, such as implantable devices and claustrophobia, and conduct a health-history survey that includes questions regarding prior contrast reaction, date of last menstrual cycle, and hormone use (Figure 1.2). This approach has helped minimize patient stress and, most important, gives the patient a contact person because many times this will be the first person the patient meets when arriving for the appointment. An information packet is sent through the mail before the appointment date; this includes much of the information covered over the phone by the MRI staff member (Figure 1.3).

Whether the MRI unit is dedicated to breast examinations or shared for other examinations, it is essential that the patient's needs and concerns be addressed. For example, a separate check-in line will minimize the anxiety of waiting in line with other patients. Our facility has a separate entrance to a private MRI suite (Figure 1.4) that facilitates individualized care with a quiet waiting room, away from the often busy main waiting room. All of this helps minimize the stress and anxiety that can accompany the breast MRI examination.

During selection of a technologist to staff a breast MRI program, the best-case scenario would be a technologist with background in all three involved disciplines: MRI, mammography, and breast biopsy. However, this is not always an option, especially when adding breast MRI to an existing MRI practice. Further, the ACR recommends that "technologists performing breast MRI hold the Current Basic Life Support certification, and be capable of using an automated external defibrillator."[7] Breast MRI patients require extra care, and their anxiety and questions will be best managed by a technologist with extensive breast imaging experience. In this respect, careful staffing can be a major time saver for the radiologist.

Magnetic Resonance Imaging Interventional Procedures

As mentioned, during selection of a breast coil, it is imperative that it allows access to both the medial and lateral aspects of the breast and also allows access to the posterior breast tissue. As with any imaging modality, it is crucial to have MRI biopsy and localization capabilities for areas of enhancement visualized only by MRI.

All supplies, needles, and any equipment needed for MRI interventional procedures must be MRI compatible.

It is very helpful to have a mammography technologist experienced with positioning the breast for needle localizations and core biopsies also assist with breast MRI interventional procedures.

Computer-aided detection (CAD) software is available that will facilitate biopsy targeting; thus it will be important to have a CAD monitor next to the scanner console, especially for a site that is new to performing biopsies.

Referring Physician Education and Communication

Referring physician education and communication is fundamental when implementing a new imaging modality such as breast MRI. Our facility began introducing breast MRI through newsletters, continuing medical education (CME) evenings, and presentations to referring doctors during the day. The newsletters and CME invitations went to all of our referring physicians, informing them that we were offering breast MRI examinations and inviting them to an educational MRI presentation at our facility, followed by a question-and-answer session. This introduced the community physicians to how breast MRI was being used at our facility through a discussion of ACR and local insurer guidelines and many case examples. This open communication

MAGNETIC RESONANCE (MR) PROCEDURE SCREENING FORM FOR PATIENTS

Name ______________________ Weight __________ Height __________

1. Do you have any pre-existing medical condition or concern? ______________ ☐No ☐Yes
2. Do you have a family history of breast cancer? ☐No ☐Yes
   If yes, what relation and at what age was it diagnosed? ______________
3. Have you had prior surgery or an operation (e.g. arthroscopy, endoscopy, etc.) of any kind? ☐No ☐Yes
   If yes, please indicate the date and type of surgery:
   Date ____ / ____ / ____ Type of surgery: ______________
   Date ____ / ____ / ____ Type of surgery: ______________
4. Have you had a prior diagnostic imaging study or examination (MRI, CT, ultrasound, x-ray, etc.)? ☐No ☐Yes
   If yes, please list: Body part Date Facility
   MRI ______________ ____ / ____ / ____ ______________
   CT/CAT Scan ______________ ____ / ____ / ____ ______________
   Nuclear Medicine/PET ______________ ____ / ____ / ____ ______________
5. Have you experienced any problem related to a previous MRI examination or MR procedure? ☐No ☐Yes
   If yes, please describe: ______________
6. Have you had an injury to the eye involving a metallic object or fragment (e.g., metallic slivers, shavings, foreign body, etc.)? ☐No ☐Yes
   If yes, please describe: ______________
7. Have you ever been injured by a metallic object or foreign body (e.g., BB, bullet, shrapnel, etc.)? ☐No ☐Yes
   If yes, please describe: ______________
8. Are you currently taking or have you recently taken any medication or drug? ☐No ☐Yes
   If yes, please list: ______________
9. Are you allergic to any medication? ☐No ☐Yes
   If yes, please list: ______________
10. Do you have a history of asthma, allergic reaction, respiratory disease, or reaction to a contrast medium or dye used for an MRI, CT, or x-ray examination? ☐No ☐Yes
11. Do you have anemia or any disease(s) that affects your blood, or seizures? ☐No ☐Yes
    If yes, please describe: ______________
12. Do you have diabetes? ☐No ☐Yes
13. Are you taking medication for diabetes? ☐No ☐Yes
    If yes, what are they? ______________
14. **Do you have hypertension?** ☐No ☐Yes
15. **Do you have kidney disease?** ☐No ☐Yes
16. Are you on dialysis? ☐No ☐Yes

For female patients:

17. Date of last menstrual period: ____ / ____ / ____ Post menopausal? ☐Yes
18. Are you pregnant or experiencing a late menstrual period? ☐No ☐Yes
19. Are you taking oral contraceptives or receiving hormonal treatment? ☐No ☐Yes
20. Are you taking any type of fertility medication or having fertility treatments? ☐No ☐Yes
    If yes, please describe: ______________
21. Are you currently breastfeeding? ☐No ☐Yes
22. Do you have implants? ☐No ☐Yes
    If yes, are they: ☐ saline or ☐ silicone?
    If known, what brand are the implants? ______________
23. Have you had a breast biopsy? ☐No ☐Yes
    If yes, on which breast? ☐ Right or ☐ Left
    Was a clip placed in your breast? ☐No ☐ Yes
    Where was it done? ______________
    When was it done? ____ / ____ / ____
    What was the outcome? ☐Benign ☐Malignant - Type, if known ______________
24. Have you recently or are you currently being treated with any of the following: ☐No ☐Yes

FIGURE 1.2 Example of an MRI procedure screening form and questionnaire for patients.

MRI Safety

Please review the following checklist prior to your exam:

- ☐ If you think you may be claustrophobic, ask your doctor to prescribe medication prior to the exam. If you do receive medication, bring someone with you to drive you home.
- ☐ You CANNOT have the exam if you have any of the following: cerebral aneurysm clips, certain heart valves, cochlear implants, metal filings in the eye, or pacemaker.
- ☐ If your occupational background includes metal work (welder, grinder, etc.) please be sure to tell the technologist prior to the exam.This may require you to have an orbital x-ray prior to your MRI appointment to ensure no foreign bodies are identified.
- ☐ You may eat, drink and take your usual medications before the exam.
- ☐ No metal is allowed in the MRI exam room. Safety pins, straight pins, metal hair pins and all jewelry must be removed before entering the room.
- ☐ We suggest bringing or wearing elastic waist pants which can be worn during the exam. You will be wearing a patient gown also.

Designated an ACR Breast Imaging Center of Excellence

ACR Gold Standard Accreditation in Breast MRI

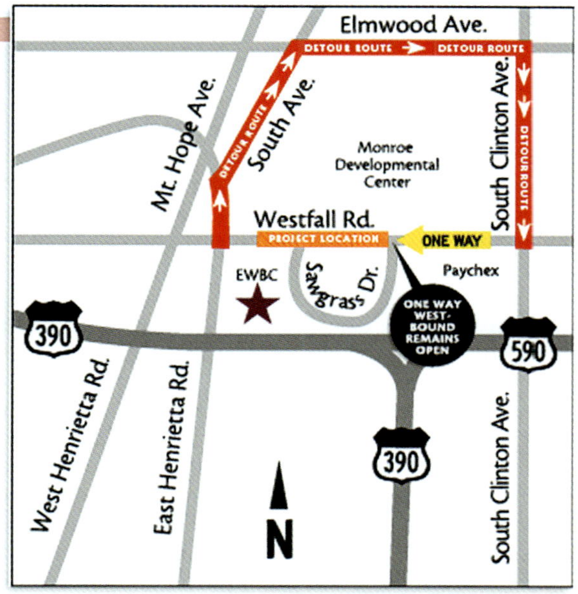

Directions to our Brighton office

(main office): 170 Sawgrass Drive | Rochester, NY 14620

PLEASE NOTE road construction on Westfall Road (between East Henrietta Rd and South Clinton Ave). Detour signs have been posted. Only one way traffic is allowed (westbound direction) to our office from South Clinton Avenue. Please allow an additional 15 - 20 minutes travel time if you are coming from East Henrietta Road due to the detour.

FROM THE NORTH/WEST

Travel 390 South to exit 16B (Rt. 15A - East Henrietta Rd.) ■ Turn left onto East Henrietta Rd.

FROM THE NORTH/EAST

Travel 590 South to 390 North. ■ Take 390 North to Exit 16 (Rt. 15A - East Henrietta Rd.)

FROM THE SOUTH/THRUWAY

Take the NYS Thruway to exit 46. ■ Travel 390 North toward the airport. ■ Get off at Exit 16 (Rt. 15A - East Henrietta Rd.) *Please note that there are two exits for East Henrietta Rd. on 390–be sure to take the second one, Exit 16.* ■ Turn right onto East Henrietta Rd.

Parking for MRI is on the far left side of the building. Enter up the handicap ramp through the side door, adjacent to MRI parking.

FIGURE 1.3 Example of a patient appointment information sheet.

allowed the attendees to see the benefits the technology could bring to the patients.

Patient Selection

It is important to recommend breast MRI for the appropriate patient populations because it is a time consuming, costly examination that requires intravenous contrast. MRI also has a lower specificity that may result in additional testing, ultimately increasing health care costs.[8]

A majority of patients referred will be for extent of disease or presurgical assessment. These patients have a recent diagnosis of breast cancer. At our facility, these patients are given the first available appointment. Bilateral contrast–enhanced breast MRI should be performed because this examination provides important diagnostic information for those considering lumpectomy and has been shown to detect occult contralateral carcinoma in up to 5% of patients.[9] This may generate a multitude of questions from the patient, allowing further discussion regarding the examination's potential. For example, clinicians should explain that based on the MRI findings, additional procedures such as targeted ultrasound and biopsy may be necessary.

Clinicians should also explain that breast MRI may allow diagnosis of multifocal or multicentric disease not visible with other studies, potentially altering surgical management. Breast MRI may allow better assessment of the extent of the disease than other imaging studies, such as mammography and ultrasonography, aiding in surgical planning. Additionally, studies have shown that MRI may allow for a more effective diagnosis of DCIS, with improved sensitivity at detecting multicentric disease compared with mammography.[10,11]

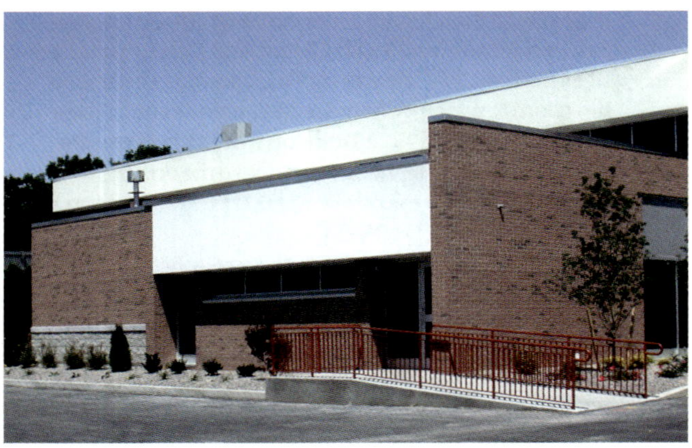

FIGURE 1.4 An MRI suite with a private entrance.

High Cancer–Risk Screening with Breast Magnetic Resonance Imaging

Breast MRI examinations for patients at high risk of developing cancer have increased over the last few years as patients and their primary care physicians are becoming more aware of their risk factors and the additional imaging procedures available to them. In 2008, 36% (370/1034) of all MRI examinations performed were for evaluating high-risk patients. Our use of high-risk screening with breast MRI has been increasing ever since as we identify patients at risk who will benefit from the examination, such as those with positive genetic testing, family history of breast cancer, or mantle radiation for Hodgkin disease. We experienced a 25 percentage point increase from initial incorporation in 2008 to 2011, with high-risk cases rising from 36% to 61%.

Identification of patients who have risk factors should be done by staff or referring physicians trained in the use of risk assessment models, as screening breast MRI may be recommended in women with more than a 20% lifetime risk of developing breast cancer. Because of this, facilities might consider using a health history form to flag those at increased risk. Our facility has a software application created by our programming consultant that allows the radiology information system (RIS) to flag patients with risk factors. The system will flag patients diagnosed with breast cancer at an age younger than 50 years, those diagnosed with cancer older than age 50 years and with a family member who has a prior diagnosis of breast or ovarian cancer, and those with two family members with either breast or ovarian cancer. Letters are generated for patients identified as having an increased risk for breast cancer stating that they may be a candidate for genetic counseling and/or additional screening tests (Figure 1.5). The referring physicians also receive a copy of this letter.

Dear,

Thank you for completing your Medical History Form. Based on the personal and family history information that you provided to us, risk factors have been identified (see below) that suggest you may benefit from further breast cancer risk assessment. Please keep in mind that this notification was generated by our preliminary screening process and is not based on a complete review of your medical history.

Many facilities in the area provide breast cancer risk assessment services. If you are interested in meeting with our genetic counselor to determine if you are a candidate for additional screening with breast MRI, genetic testing for hereditary breast cancer, or both, please contact our Genetic Counselor to schedule an appointment.

If you have already been evaluated for your eligibility for breast MRI and genetic testing for hereditary breast cancer, please feel free to disregard this letter. If you prefer not to be included in our high-risk screening process, please let a staff member know, and we will remove your name from further screening notifications.

Thank you for allowing us to participate in your health care.

Sincerely,

FIGURE 1.5 Letter sent to patients identified through the radiology information system as being at high risk of developing breast cancer.

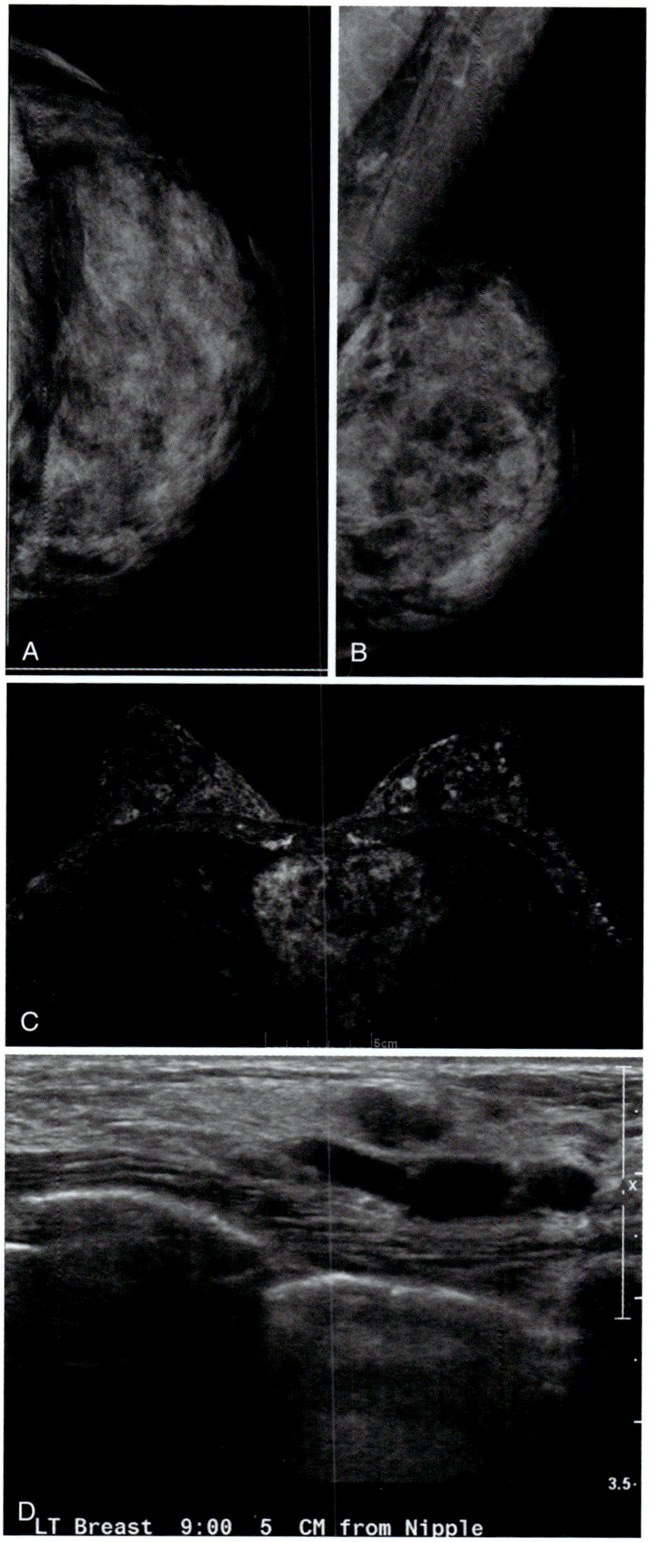

Implementing a genetic assessment program is beneficial in identifying which of those patients flagged as high risk fit the criteria to be screened with breast MRI. We implemented our own risk assessment program in 2009. Initially, a staff nurse or medical assistant fielded patient calls and set up genetic testing appointments. We found a high demand for the program and realized that we needed a dedicated genetic counselor on staff. In April of 2011, a certified genetic counselor was hired for 3 days a week, which quickly turned into 4 days because the patient response was much greater than expected. As stated previously, high-risk patients are identified through our RIS and flagged following National Comprehensive Cancer Network guidelines. Letters are sent to patients and their referring health care providers informing them that further risk assessment services are available, which include genetic counseling. The genetic counselor provides a risk assessment to identify possible high-risk, screening-MRI candidates. Staff and referring physician education are vital to the success of such a program. Staff need to be aware and knowledgeable to answer patient questions about risk and genetic counseling. Initially, referring physicians were apprehensive about the program we were offering to patients; however, once educated, they began referring patients.

In young women at high risk of developing cancer, such as those with *BRCA1* and *BRCA2* genetic mutations, breast MRI screening may be helpful because often these women have dense breasts in which mammography is limited (Figure 1.6, A-D). When high-risk patients are premenopausal, it is important to schedule the examinations on days 10 to 14 of their menstrual cycles. Published data from studies on the impact of breast MRI on breast cancer are limited in this population of patients; however, studies have reported a higher sensitivity for breast MRI compared with the sensitivity of mammography and/or ultrasound.[8]

Magnetic Resonance Imaging Patients and Imaging Protocols

As we have become more experienced in performing breast MRI, the indications for use have expanded. As mentioned previously, MRI for determining the extent of disease and for screening in women at high risk of developing breast cancer are the most common indications. As of 2011, in addition to performing MRI for patients

FIGURE 1.6 A 53-year-old patient's screening mammogram. A high-risk patient screening letter was generated because of her family history responses: breast cancer in her mother at age 67 years, maternal grandmother at age 68 years, and maternal aunt at age 80 years. The patient had personal risk assessment with a genetics counselor and was found to meet National Comprehensive Cancer Network guidelines for *BRCA* gene testing. The patient declined genetic testing because she did not have insurance coverage. The patient was referred for high-risk MRI at 6-month intervals between mammograms. **A** and **B**, Normal left mammogram of a high-risk 53-year-old patient. **C**, MRI at 6-month interval revealed a 7-mm mass in the patient who declined genetic testing. **D**. Targeted ultrasound finds a left 9 o'clock abnormality. Ultrasound-guided core biopsy was performed and revealed invasive ductal carcinoma.

before surgery and those with high-risk status, we also perform MRI for follow-up to previous abnormal MRI, to check implant integrity, and to search for an occult primary tumor (Figure 1.7). The choice of whom to image with breast MRI is influenced by guidelines set in place by radiologic societies such as the Society of Breast Imaging (SBI), ACR, and the American Cancer Society (ACS) in addition to local and national insurance carriers. The ACS does not recommend screening with MRI unless the patient has risk factors that meet its guidelines, at which point breast MRI is recommended as an adjunct to mammography (Figure 1.8).

Before initiating breast MRI services, we observed scanning protocols at Memorial Sloan-Kettering Cancer Center (New York, NY) and ultimately decided to adopt its imaging protocol. A routine dynamic protocol is used for almost all indications referred for MRI. The protocol consists of a localizer, followed by precontrast bilateral axial short tau inversion recovery (STIR) and axial T1 fat-suppressed images. A rapid bolus injection of a weight-based dose of gadolinium into the antecubital fossa is then administered using a power injector. Five imaging sequences are routinely performed after the injection: axial postcontrast T1 fat-suppressed, followed by a postcontrast sagittal T1 water excitation. All axial T1 fat-suppressed sequences are identical: one minute long, three-dimensional volumes with voxels that are approximately isotropic at 1 mm. The postcontrast sagittal T1 water excitation sequence consists of two three-dimensional volumes that yield high-resolution delayed images, approximately isotropic at 0 .8 mm. After the examination, the unenhanced images are subtracted from the enhanced images. A three-dimensional maximum intensity projection (MIP) reconstruction is also analyzed.

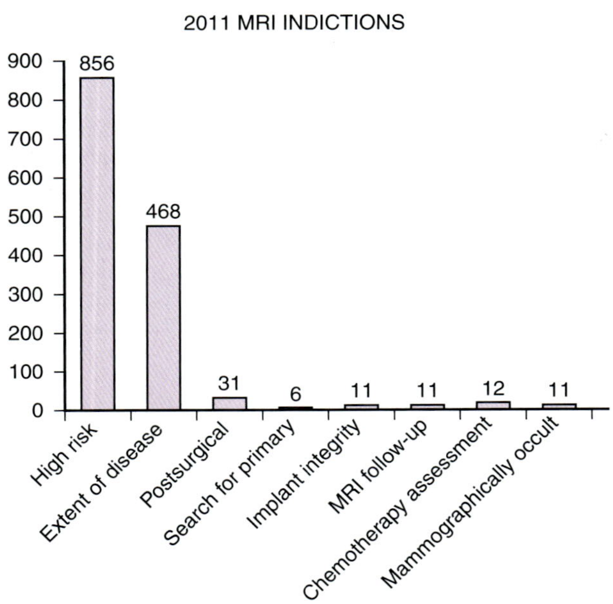

FIGURE 1.7 Indications for breast MRI examinations in 2011 at our facility (Elizabeth Wende Breast Care, LLC, Rochester, NY).

HIGH RISK MRI GUIDELINES (ACS)

- *BRCA* 1 or 2 mutation
- First degree relative with *BRCA* 1 or 2 and patient is untested
- Lifetime risk of breast cancer of 20–25% or more using standard risk assessment models
- Radiation treatment to the chest between ages 10 and 30
- Carry or have first-degree relative with genetic mutation in the *TP53* or *PTEN* genes (Li-Fraumeni, Cowden and Bannayan-Riley-Ruvalcaba syndromes)

FIGURE 1.8 American Cancer Society high cancer–risk MRI guidelines.

Breast Magnetic Resonance Imaging Interpretation, Imaging Correlation, and Comparison

It is imperative to have access to all earlier breast imaging studies (mammography, breast ultrasound, and MRI) for adequate correlation and comparison with the breast MRI examination. If a patient had any diagnostic imaging studies performed at other facilities, he or she should be asked to bring all reports and images for uploading or digitization into the Picture Archiving and Communication System (PACS) because this will allow easy access for the physician during MRI interpretation.

Early on, we read off film but found it a cumbersome process because there were many large films without reconstruction, color intensity, or MIP images for assistance. Soft-copy workstation review with breast MRI software/CAD is ideal for interpretation because there are about 2500 images to interpret per examination. Image manipulation, kinetic evaluation, and comparison with earlier MRI studies are all easily performed with this software. Some of these software packages have biopsy localization capabilities to ensure exact lesion location for MRI-guided interventional procedures.

In cases in which a patient is referred to MRI because of a recently diagnosed cancer (either before or after surgical evaluation), suspected recurrence, equivocal mammography/ultrasound, or follow-up of a previous abnormal MRI examination, it is beneficial for the initial radiologist to read the MRI examination for continuity because he or she is most familiar with the patient. However, this may not be practical or even possible, depending on the institution.

When relaying results to patients who need to return for additional procedures because of an abnormality found on a breast MRI examination, an effort is made for the radiologist who diagnosed the patient with cancer to call with the results. High-risk and follow-up patients receive result letters. When a patient is recalled because of a breast MRI abnormality, further imaging work-up should be performed before scheduling an MRI-guided biopsy. This may include additional views and targeted ultrasound. Studies have demonstrated the value of second look or targeted ultrasound in the evaluation of breast MRI abnormalities. A review of our institution's data showed that 70% (128/182) of breast lesions found on presurgical MRI examinations were visible at second look ultrasound and yielded 39 additional cancers.[12] LaTrenta and colleagues showed a 43% likelihood that MRI lesions associated with an ultrasound correlate represented carcinoma.[13]

Outcomes of Magnetic Resonance Imaging–Guided Breast Biopsy

As with any biopsy procedure, outcomes must be tracked for regulatory purposes. It is beneficial to track outcomes of MRI cores, for concordance and discordance to imaging. A process should be in place for review of all biopsies. At our institution, the radiologists review and sign all of their biopsy results and open surgical pathology reports. All information is entered into an outcomes program and is easily accessible for future reference, whether for patient care or yearly medical audits. If the core biopsy is discordant with imaging, the opportunity exists to re-biopsy at the earliest available time. For all benign MRI guided core biopsies, a facility should have a follow-up imaging protocol in place.

American College of Radiology Breast Magnetic Resonance Imaging Accreditation Requirements

Effective January 1, 2012, all MRI facilities that bill for advanced diagnostic services must be accredited to qualify for Medicare reimbursement. The process requires facilities to submit paperwork and images for any magnet used to perform breast MRI. Each unit must successfully pass for the facility to be accredited.

Besides the accreditation process, the ACR requires breast MRI facilities to perform mammographic correlation when reading breast MRI, to have the capacity to perform directed ultrasound of MRI abnormalities detected, and to have MRI-guided intervention capabilities or to refer patients to a site that does. Interpreting radiologists, MRI technologists, and medical physicists must meet specified qualifications as well as undergo continual experience and education.

The ACR does not require minimum field strength for the magnet, but the MRI must have a dedicated bilateral breast coil, simultaneous bilateral imaging capabilities, and meet state and federal performance requirements.

The facility's technologist must perform a prescribed weekly quality control process on the system, and physicist testing of the system is performed annually. As of this chapter writing, the ACR did not require phantom images to be submitted for accreditation, but clinical images must be submitted for approval.

The ACR is available for partnership and guidance, and can be a helpful resource in all aspects of setting up and maintaining the MRI program. Additional information regarding breast MRI accreditation can be found on the ACR website.[7]

Conclusion

Setting up a breast MRI practice can be a lengthy and involved process. Some helpful steps that worked for our breast MRI implementation were to designate key staff to help with identifying the equipment, the facility space, and the personnel needed for implementation and support. Many options are available; with diligent research you will find the equipment that will best suit your practice. For us, a gradual increase of breast MRI examinations helped build the workflow as well as staff confidence. The optimization process is ongoing; track your medical outcomes because this will help the learning process, and your breast MRI practice will continue to improve to best serve your patients. Adding breast MRI to our practice has allowed us to help our patients with surgical planning, high risk assessment, problem solving after inconclusive work-up, postsurgical evaluation, and treatment assessment during chemotherapy. The ability to provide this examination to our patients has made the addition of MRI invaluable to our practice.

References

1. Kaiser WA, Zeitler E: MR imaging of the breast: fast imaging sequences with and without Gd-DTPA, preliminary observations, *Radiology* 170:681–686, 1989.
2. Orel SG, Schnall MD, Newman RW, et al: MR Imaging-guided localization and biopsy of breast lesions: initial experience, *Radiology* 193:97–102, 1994.
3. Orel SG, Schnall MD, LiVolsi VA, Troupin RH: Suspicious breast lesions: MR imaging with radiologic-pathologic correlation, *Radiology* 190:485–493, 1994.
4. Liberman L, Morris EA, Lee MJ, et al: Breast lesions detected on MR imaging: features and positive predictive value, *AJR Am J Roentgenol* 179:171–178, 2002.
5. Zakhireh J, Gomez R, Esserman L: Converting evidence to practice: a guide for the clinical application of MRI for the screening and management of breast cancer, *Eur J Cancer* 44:2742–2752, 2008.
6. American College of Radiology: *ACR Guidance Document for Safe MR Practices*, 2007, http://www.acr.org/~/media/ACR/Documents/PDF/QualitySafety/Radiation%20Safety/Guidance%20Document%20on%20MR%20Safe%20Practices.pdf. Accessed May 25, 2012.
7. American College of Radiology: *Breast MRI Accreditation Program Requirements*, http://www.acr.org/~/media/ACR/Documents/Accreditation/BreastMRI/Requirements.pdf. Accessed May 25, 2012.
8. Elmore JG, Armstrong K, Lehman CD, Fletcher SW: Screening for breast cancer, *JAMA* 293(10):1245–1256, 2005.
9. Lehman CD, Gatsonis C, Kuhl CK, et al: ACRIN 6667 group MRI evaluation of the contralateral breast in women with recently diagnosed breast cancer, *N Engl J Med* 356(13):1295–1303, 2007.
10. Kuhl CK, Schrading S, Bieling HB, et al: MRI for diagnosis of pure ductal carcinoma in situ: a prospective observational study, *Lancet* 370:485–492, 2007.
11. Santamaria G, Velasco M, Farrus B, et al: Preoperative MRI of pure intraductal breast carcinoma—A valuable adjunct to mammography in assessing cancer extent, *Breast* 17(2):186–194, 2008.
12. Destounis S, Arieno A, Somerville PA, et al: Community-based practice experience of unsuspected breast magnetic resonance imaging abnormalities evaluated with second-look sonography, *J Ultrasound Med* 28:1337–1346, 2009.
13. LaTrenta LR, Menell JH, Morris EA, et al: Breast lesions detected with MR imaging: utility and histopathologic importance of identification with US, *Radiology* 227:856–861, 2003.

CHAPTER 2

Optimizing the Breast MRI Protocol

Robert A. Pooley

Optimizing the breast magnetic resonance imaging (MRI) protocol requires many decisions to be made about image acquisition techniques, types of pulse sequences, and sequence parameters used to control image quality and acquisition speed. Fundamental trade-offs exist among spatial resolution, acquisition speed, and signal-to-noise ratio, and these trade-offs must be understood in order to optimize quality and speed consistent with diagnostic goals. Image contrast is controlled by the pulse sequence and its acquisition parameters through manipulation of the magnetic resonance (MR) signal from hydrogen protons in tissue. To understand how acquisition techniques, pulse sequences, and pulse sequence parameters can be used to optimize the breast MRI protocol, it is important to first understand the fundamentals of MRI. This chapter will begin with a review of these fundamentals, followed by information on pulse sequences and acquisition techniques. These elements will be summarized with recommendations for optimizing the overall breast MRI protocol.

Fundamentals of Magnetic Resonance Imaging

Protons and the Main Magnetic Field

The strong magnetic field associated with the MR scanner is typically called the main magnetic field or the B_0 ("B zero") field. This B_0 field typically points in a direction called the longitudinal direction or *z* direction (Figure 2.1). The plane perpendicular to this direction is defined by the *x* and *y* directions, and is called the transverse plane (see Figure 2.1). The *z* direction is horizontal for high field strength cylindrical bore scanners.

Protons act like tiny bar magnets and align with or against the longitudinal direction when brought in the vicinity of the strong magnetic field of the MR scanner. Because some protons are aligned with B_0 and some are aligned in the opposite direction, the small magnetic fields associated with many of these protons will cancel out. A proportion of protons remains, aligned in the longitudinal direction and resulting in a net magnetization. This net magnetization is manipulated by the pulse sequence and becomes the MR signal that is measured by the MR coils, producing the tissue contrast in the acquired images.

Protons also precess when in the vicinity of a strong magnetic field. This precession (like the precession of a child's spinning top) occurs at a certain frequency, ω_0, determined by the Larmor equation, $\omega_0 = B_0 \times \gamma$ (gamma is a constant called the gyromagnetic ratio).

Radiofrequency Pulse

Radiofrequency (RF) energy is transmitted by the RF coil (located in the bore of the scanner). This transmitted RF energy can be turned on and off and is called an RF pulse. If the frequency of this RF pulse matches the precessional frequency of the protons, ω_0, resonance occurs and the protons will absorb some of this energy. Recall that the net magnetization is aligned in the longitudinal direction. This net magnetization is also called longitudinal magnetization.

As energy is absorbed, the net magnetization rotates away from the longitudinal direction. How far the net magnetization rotates depends on the strength and duration of the RF pulse. If an RF pulse is provided that rotates the net magnetization to the transverse plane, then a 90° RF pulse was used (Figure 2.2). If the net magnetization rotates to the -*z* direction, then a 180° RF pulse was used.

After the RF pulse turns off, the protons begin to release energy in a process called relaxation. There are two types of relaxation, called T1 relaxation and T2 relaxation.

T1 Relaxation and Contrast

Let's assume a 90° RF pulse is used to rotate the net magnetization to the transverse plane. The net magnetization is no longer pointing in the longitudinal direction, but slowly the protons will begin to realign in this direction of the main magnetic field. After a "long" time (several seconds), most of the magnetization will have realigned in the longitudinal direction. The realignment in this direction is called T1 relaxation or longitudinal relaxation. The amount of magnetization that has realigned in this direction can be shown on a graph (Figure 2.3). The realignment occurs at a rate that is characterized by a time constant, T1, called the T1 relaxation time.

A key point is that the protons or magnetization associated with different tissues will realign with the longitudinal direction at different rates (Figure 2.4) and thus will have different T1 relaxation times. This is the source of contrast in T1-weighted images, in which tissues with shorter T1 relaxation times will be brighter than tissues with longer T1 relaxation times. The T1 relaxation time of fluid is longer than that for fibroglandular tissue. Thus cysts are darker than fibroglandular tissue on T1-weighted images. The T1 relaxation time of a tissue depends on the strength of the magnetic field surrounding that tissue. T1 relaxation times for various breast tissues at 1.5 tesla (T) and 3.0 T magnetic field strengths are listed in Table 2.1.

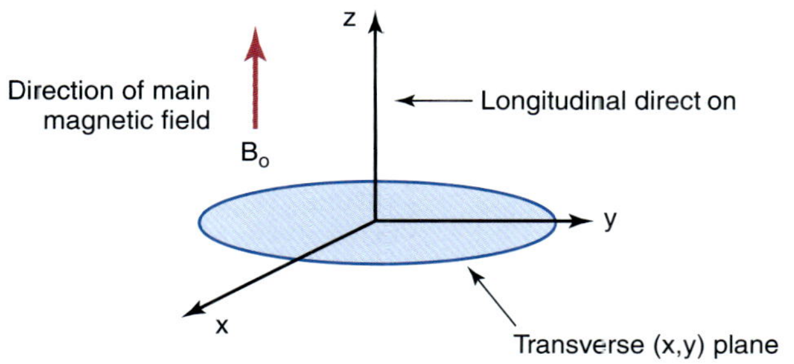

FIGURE 2.1 In a coordinate system, for a typical 1.5 Tesla cylindrical bore imaging unit, the *z* axis (longitudinal direction) is often aligned with the main magnetic field; the plane perpendicular to this is called the transverse plane.

T2 Relaxation and Contrast

Let's assume again that a 90° RF pulse has just been applied. As before, the net magnetization rotates from the longitudinal direction to the transverse plane. This magnetization in the transverse plane is called transverse magnetization. T2 relaxation is a simultaneous and independent process involving the magnetization just rotated to the transverse plane. Recall that this magnetization is made up of many different protons. The protons are all precessing, but because of several factors (mentioned below) these protons are not all precessing at the same frequency. The slightly different frequencies of the protons cause the transverse magnetization to dephase (Figure 2.5). The transverse magnetization ultimately provides the actual MR signal that is measured by the receive RF coils. Just after the 90° RF pulse, when the protons are all in-phase, the MR signal is strong. As the transverse magnetization begins to dephase, the MR signal decreases as shown in Figure 2.5.

Several factors make the protons precess at slightly different frequencies. These factors (which will not be discussed in detail here) include spin-spin interactions, magnetic field inhomogeneities, chemical shift, and magnetic susceptibility. The dephasing due to each of these can be reversed—except

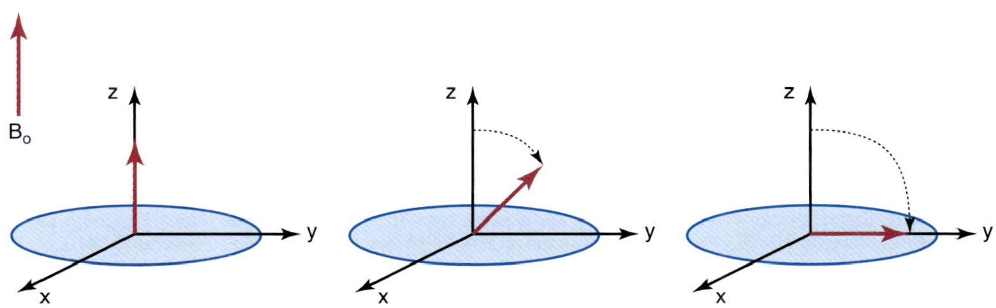

FIGURE 2.2 As the net magnetization (*red arrows*) absorbs RF energy, it rotates away from the longitudinal direction. A 90° RF pulse will rotate the net magnetization to the transverse plane.

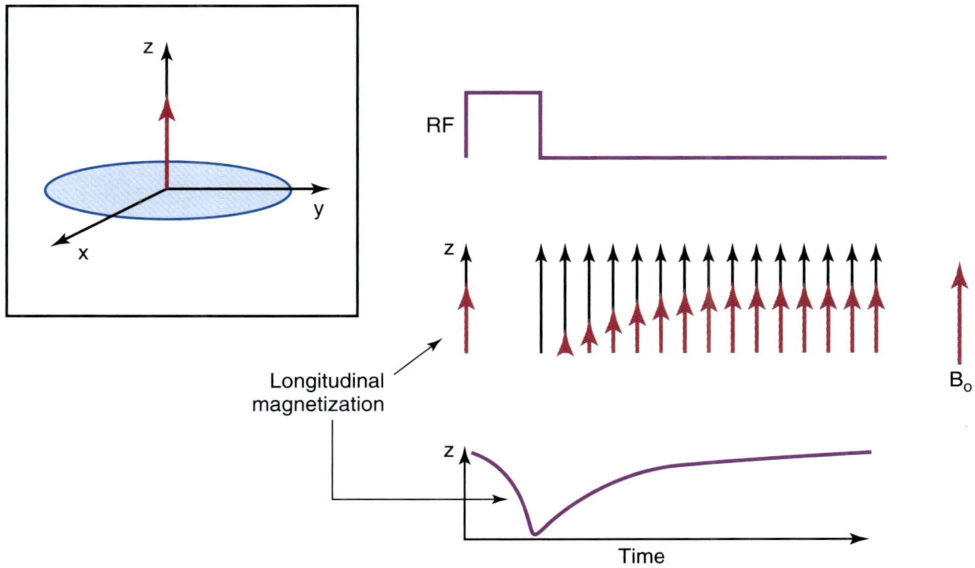

FIGURE 2.3 Application of a 90° RF pulse causes longitudinal magnetization to become zero. Over time, the longitudinal magnetization will grow back in a direction parallel to the main magnetic field. This is called longitudinal (T1) relaxation.

for spin-spin interactions—using an SE technique as discussed below. The dephasing due to spin-spin interactions cannot be reversed. The decrease in signal due only to spin-spin interactions occurs at a rate that is characterized by a time constant, T2, called the T2 relaxation time. The rate of decrease in signal due to all factors is characterized by the T2* relaxation time.

A key point is that different tissues will have different T2 relaxation times, as shown in Figure 2.6. This is the source of contrast in T2-weighted images, in which tissues with longer T2 relaxation times will be brighter than tissues with shorter T2 relaxation times. Thus cysts are brighter than fibroglandular tissue on T2-weighted images. The T2 relaxation time of a tissue is a characteristic of that tissue. T2

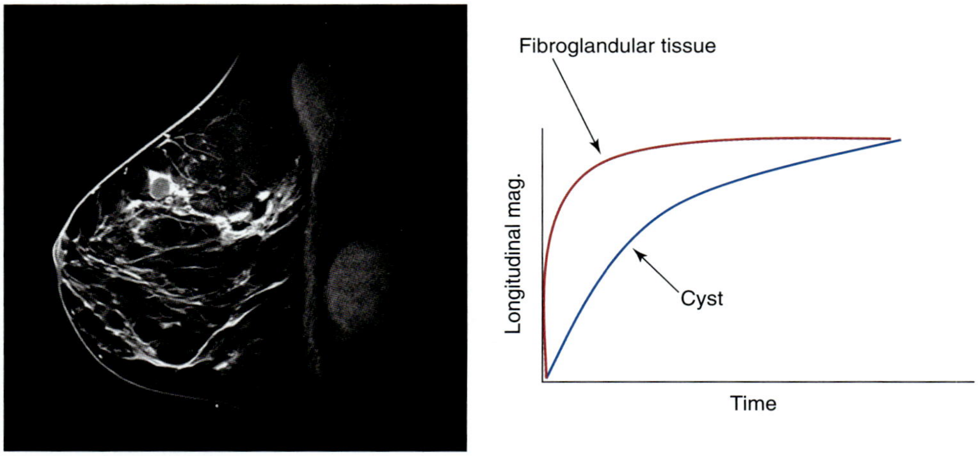

FIGURE 2.4 Different tissues have different rates of T1 relaxation. An image obtained at a time when the relaxation curves are widely separated will have maximum T1-weighted contrast.

Table 2.1 T1 and T2 Relaxation Times for Breast Tissues at 1.5 and 3.0 Tesla Magnetic Field Strengths

Tissue	1.5 T		3.0 T	
	T1	*T2*	*T1*	*T2*
Fat	250 ms	60-80 ms	423 ms	154 ms
Normal fibroglandular tissue	700 ms	60-80 ms	1680 ms	71 ms
Cyst	3000 ms	300 ms	—	—
Lesion	800-1000 ms	80-100 ms	—	—
Enhanced lesion	200-400 ms	—	—	—

Hendrick RE: *Breast MRI: fundamentals and technical aspects,* New York, 2010, Springer; Edden RA, Smith SA, Barker PB: Longitudinal and multi-echo transverse relaxation times of normal breast tissue at 3 Tesla. *J Magn Reson Imaging* 32:982-987, 2010.

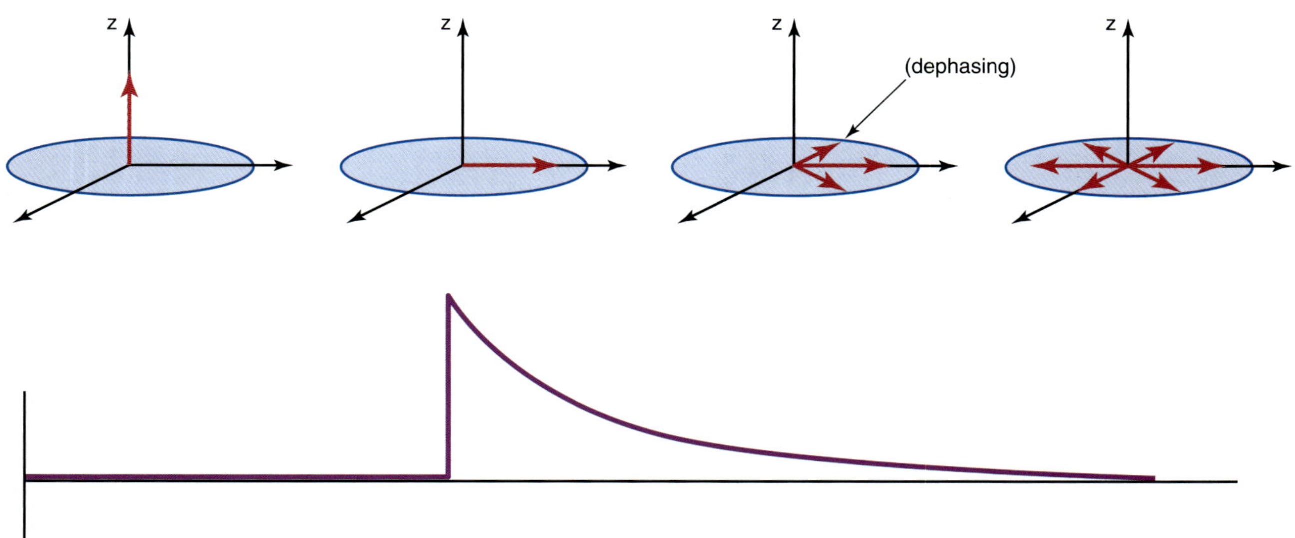

FIGURE 2.5 In transverse (T2*) relaxation, immediately after application of a 90° RF pulse, transverse magnetization is maximized and then begins to dephase. The signals from these dephasing protons begin to cancel out, and the MR signal decreases.

relaxation times for various breast tissues are listed in Table 2.1. Knowledge of T1 and T2 relaxation times is important for understanding how to optimize contrast in breast MR images.

Understanding Pulse Sequences

Pulse sequences take advantage of the different relaxation times (T1 and T2) of various tissues and manipulate the net magnetization in a way that produces desired image contrast. Several different types of pulse sequences exist, including spin echo, fast spin echo (or turbo spin echo), and gradient echo. Each pulse sequence has several parameters that can be adjusted to control contrast, spatial resolution, scan time, signal-to-noise ratio, and so on.

An aid to understanding the various types of pulse sequences is found in the use of diagrams that display the main features of the pulse sequence. Basic diagrams will be shown with each type of pulse sequence below. The features of a pulse sequence will be described using the spin echo pulse sequence as an example. Figure 2.7 shows the pulse sequence diagram for the spin echo pulse sequence. Time moves across horizontally. The top line shows the placement in time of RF pulses. A 90° and a 180° RF pulse are shown. The second line displays the transverse magnetization or MR signal that can be measured by the receive RF coil. The 90° RF pulse produces transverse magnetization that dephases because of the processes mentioned above, and the 180° pulse is used to reverse transverse magnetization, which reverses the effects of everything except spin-spin interactions, and produces the "spin echo" as shown.

Lines 3 to 5 of Figure 2.7 show gradient magnetic field operation, which is used to divide the MR signal into image slices and pixels (or voxels). Three gradients are responsible for splitting the signal into three orthogonal directions. These gradients are called the slice select gradient,

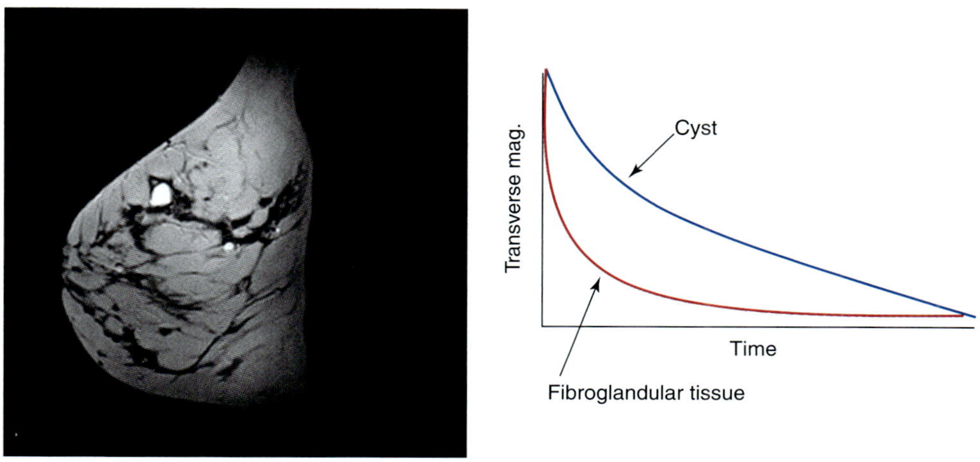

FIGURE 2.6 Different tissues have different rates of T2 relaxation. An image obtained at a time when the relaxation curves are widely separated will have maximum T2-weighted contrast.

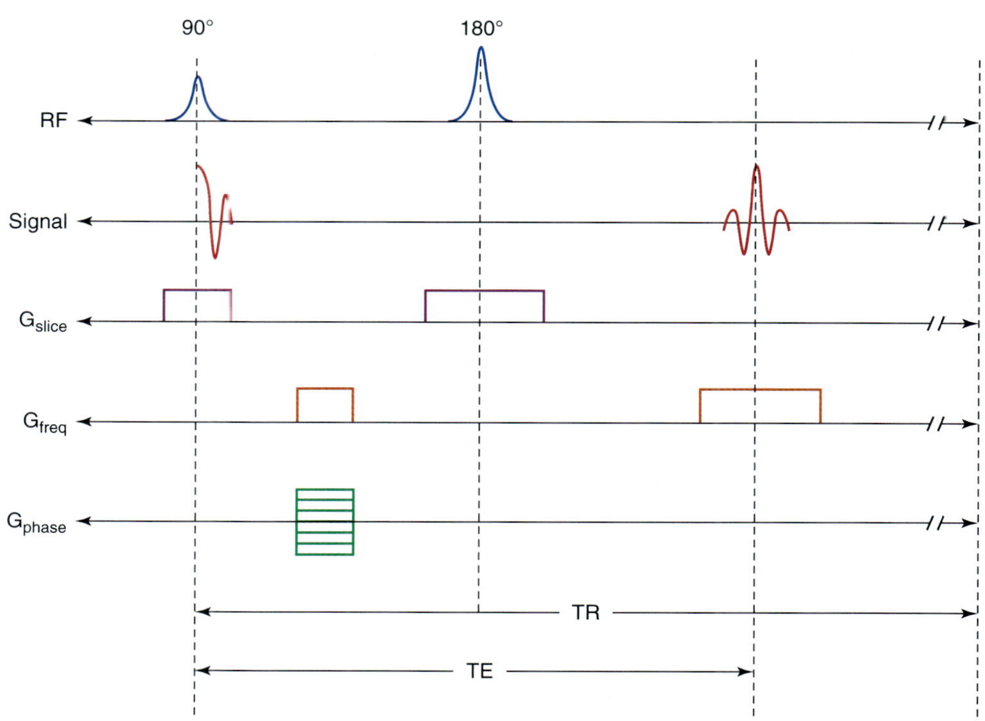

FIGURE 2.7 A spin echo pulse sequence diagram shows the relative timing of events during MR acquisition. The timing of RF pulses, the signal formed from these pulses, and application of gradient magnetic fields are shown. Application of 90° and 180° RF pulses result in a spin echo at time TE. The TR is the length of time it takes to go through the pulse sequence one time.

frequency-encoding gradient, and phase-encoding gradient. The slice select gradient is turned on during the 90° and 180° RF pulses (in two-dimensional [2-D] acquisition mode) and is responsible for exciting the protons in the slice of interest so that signal comes only from these protons.

The frequency-encoding gradient is turned on during signal acquisition of the SE and is responsible for dividing up the signal along the frequency-encoding direction. The echo is sampled at this time, and these data are entered into one line of "k-space," which stores the raw data for reconstruction into images. The pulse sequence must be repeated a number of times to collect all the information needed to produce an image. For a 256 by 256 image this pulse sequence would be repeated 256 times.

The phase-encoding gradient is adjusted each time the pulse sequence is repeated and is responsible for placing data in each line of k-space. The time from the 90° RF pulse to the center of the SE is the echo time or TE (see Figure 2.7). The time that it takes to run the pulse sequence one time is the repetition time or TR. TE and TR are user-selectable parameters of a pulse sequence that are used to determine image contrast.

Contrast Formation

To illustrate the importance of TE and TR we turn back to graphs showing T1 and T2 relaxation (Figure 2.8), which occur simultaneously and independently. The height of these curves is related to the tissue signal (image brightness) measured during the pulse sequence; the vertical separation is related to the contrast between tissues. TR is used to select the amount of T1 weighting on the curves labeled T1 Relaxation, and TE is used to select the amount of T2 weighting on the curves labeled T2 Relaxation.

Placing TR at position *A* in Figure 2.8 maximizes T1-related contrast by taking advantage of the large separation in T1 relaxation for these tissues. Placing TR at position *B* minimizes T1 contrast by imaging when the difference in relaxation for these tissues is minimal.

Placing TE at position C minimizes T2 contrast by imaging when T2 relaxation for these tissues is not very different. Placing TE at position D maximizes T2-related contrast by taking advantage of the large separation in the T2 relaxation for these tissues.

Thus, to obtain T1-weighted contrast, TE and TR would be placed as shown in Figure 2.9 to maximize T1 effects and minimize T2 effects. To obtain T2-weighted contrast, TE and TR would be placed as shown in Figure 2.10 to maximize T2 effects and minimize T1 effects. Positioning TE and TR to minimize both T1 and T2 relaxation effects (Figure 2.11) results in spin density contrast, in which image brightness is related to the density of hydrogen protons in the tissue. An important part of optimizing the breast MRI protocol includes optimizing the pulse sequence to obtain the maximum contrast possible. This is done primarily through optimizing the values of TE and TR.

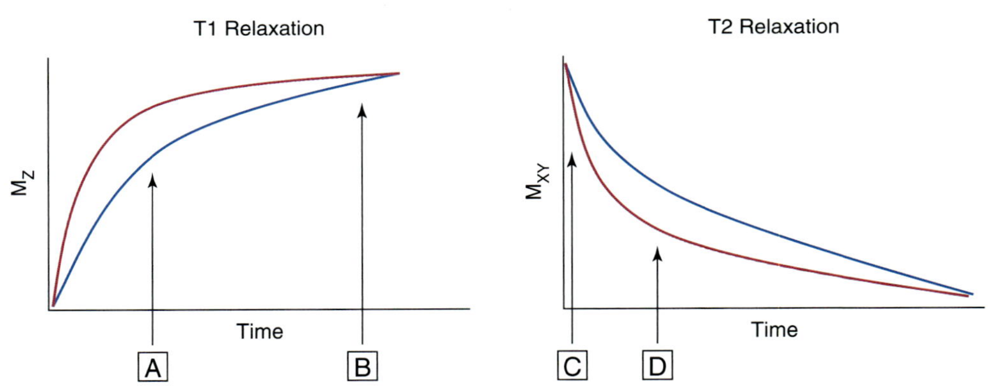

FIGURE 2.8 These diagrams show T1 and T2 relaxation curves. T1-weighted contrast is obtained by maximizing contrast due to T1 relaxation (*position A*) and minimizing contrast due to T2 relaxation (*position C*). T2-weighted contrast is obtained by maximizing contrast due to T2 relaxation (*position D*) and minimizing contrast due to T1 relaxation (*position B*). Spin density contrast is obtained by minimizing contrast due to both T1 and T2 relaxation effects (*positions B and C*). M_Z and M_{XY} refer to the longitudinal and transverse magnetizations, respectively.

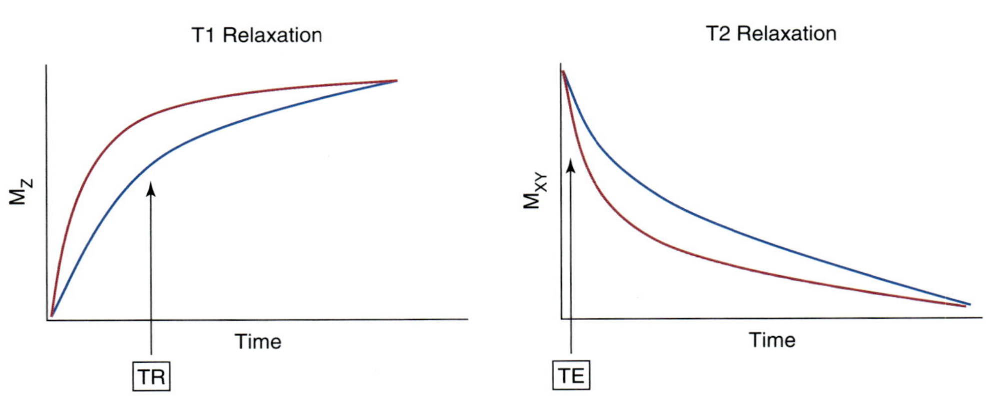

FIGURE 2.9 T1-weighted image contrast is obtained by using short TE (to minimize T2 effects) and short TR (to maximize T1 effects). M_Z and M_{XY} refer to the longitudinal and transverse magnetizations, respectively.

MR contrast agents using gadolinium can be used to increase the image brightness of tissue and lesions that take up the contrast material. Gadolinium has seven unpaired electrons that affect the magnetic field near the gadolinium atoms and shorten the T1 and T2 relaxation times of nearby tissue. Because a tissue with a shorter T1 will be brighter than adjacent tissue with longer T1, a lesion that has taken up gadolinium will be brighter than surrounding tissue. Because the change in the rate of T1 relaxation is more significant than the change in the rate of T2 relaxation, contrast injected imaging is primarily done with T1-weighted imaging.[1] Additional information regarding the fundamental physics of MR can be found in the suggested readings.[2-4]

Fundamental Trade-offs

Fundamental trade-offs exist among image resolution, scan time, and signal-to-noise ratio. Managing these trade-offs is critical when optimizing the breast MRI protocol. Given a minimum adequate level of signal, high resolution imaging is typically achieved at the expense of longer scan time. On the other hand, if reduced scan time is a priority, this is often accomplished at the expense of resolution.

Resolution

The spatial resolution of an imaging study is controlled by several acquisition parameters in the pulse sequence. Spatial resolution is directly related to pixel size and slice thickness, which together make up the size (volume) of an image voxel. Spatial resolution improves as voxel volume decreases, that is, as pixel size and/or slice thickness decrease. Smaller pixel size (area) provides better in-plane resolution. Pixel size in one direction is equal to the field of view (FOV) in that direction divided by the number of pixels in that direction. The pixel size in the "x" direction, $Px = FOVx / Nx$. As shown in Figure 2.12, increasing the number of pixels while keeping FOV the same (A) or decreasing the FOV while keeping the number of pixels the same (B) will decrease pixel size and improve spatial resolution.

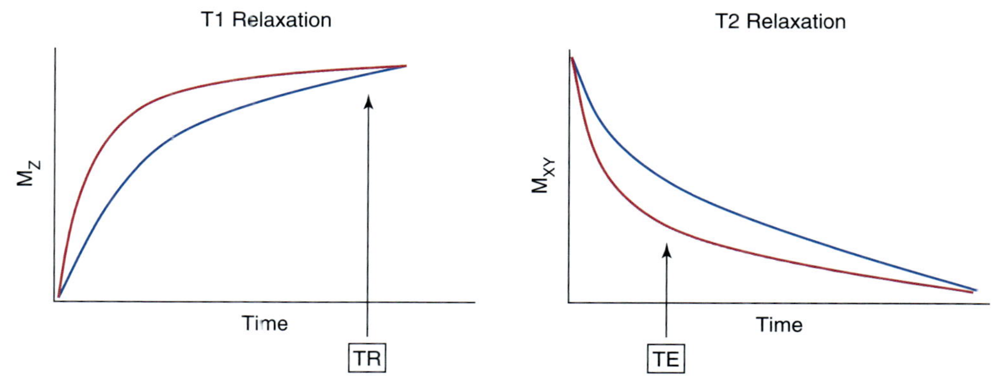

FIGURE 2.10 T2-weighted image contrast is obtained by using long TE (to maximize T2 effects) and long TR (to minimize T1 effects). M_Z and M_{XY} refer to the longitudinal and transverse magnetizations, respectively.

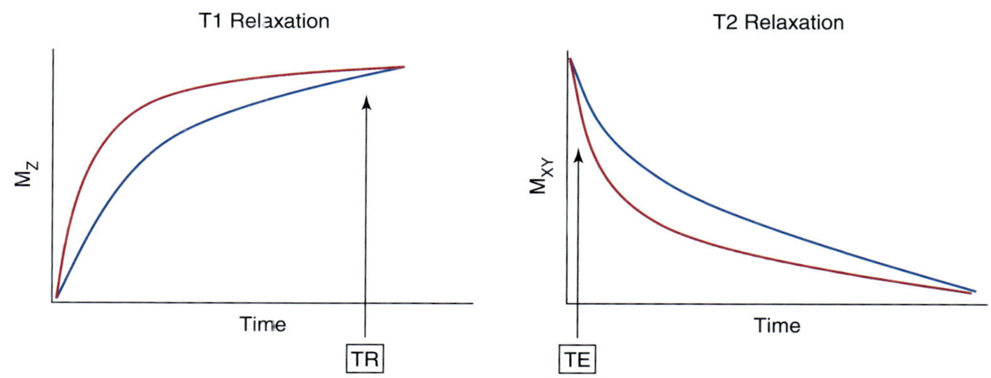

FIGURE 2.11 Spin density–weighted image contrast is obtained by using short TE and long TR to minimize both T1 and T2 effects. M_Z and M_{XY} refer to the longitudinal and transverse magnetizations, respectively.

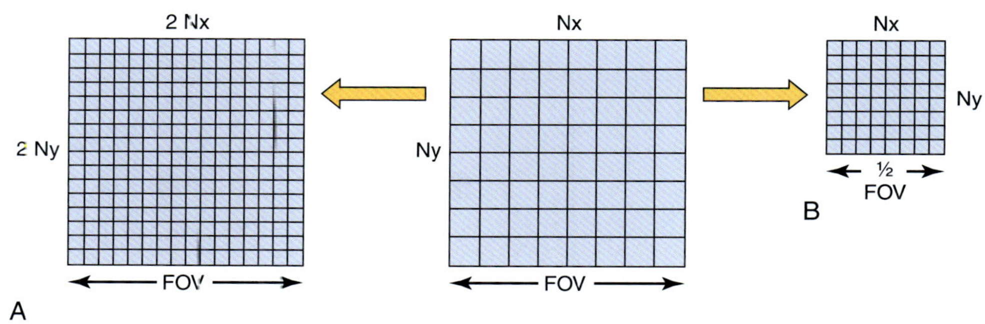

FIGURE 2.12 The effect on resolution of FOV and the number of pixels shows that increasing the number of pixels with the same FOV (**A**) or decreasing the FOV with the same number of pixels (**B**) will decrease pixel size and increase in-plane spatial resolution.

Thinner slice thickness decreases partial volume effect and allows small objects to be seen more clearly and edges to appear sharper (Figure 2.13). Partial volume effect occurs when an object is smaller than the thickness of one slice. The signal in the voxel that contains the object also has contributions from other material in the same voxel, decreasing its visibility in the image, especially in the presence of noise. A protocol with thinner slice thickness will cover less anatomy in the slice direction. If the same anatomical coverage is required, additional slices must be added and this may increase scan time.

Scan Time

It is always important in MRI to keep protocol scan time (acquisition duration) as short as possible to improve patient comfort and decrease motion artifacts. Dynamic breast MRI protocols add additional constraints to scan time. The goal in dynamic imaging is to acquire image volumes fast enough to properly characterize contrast wash-in and wash-out effects. MR image-acquisition parameters related to scan time include repetition time (TR), the number of phase-encoding steps, number of signal averages (NSA), and echo train length (ETL).

TR is determined primarily by the type of pulse sequence and the desired image contrast. TR may be reduced to shorten scan time if desired contrast weighting is maintained. For a basic pulse sequence, the number of phase-encoding steps equals the number of pixels in the phase-encoding direction. Thus a direct relationship exists between scan time and spatial resolution in this direction. If the number of pixels in the phase-encoding direction is increased, then the number of phase-encoding steps (Np) must also be increased, which increases the number of times the pulse sequence is repeated. This adds significant time to acquire all data. If the NSA is increased from 1 to 2, this means the pulse sequence is repeated at each phase-encoding step and the data are averaged in to the same line of k-space. This significantly reduces image noise but directly increases scan time. Thus, for fast dynamic imaging, the number of signal averages is typically not greater than 1. Finally, for turbo SE pulse sequences (discussed below), multiple echoes may be acquired during one time through the pulse sequence. This allows multiple lines of k-space to be filled, reducing scan time. If the number of echoes (ETL) is equal to 8, this will reduce scan time by a factor of 8. Thus for 2-D acquisitions, in which the slice-encoding gradient is used to select anatomical sections, scan time = TR × NSA × Np / ETL.

In summary, scan time will increase as TR and NSA increase and as the number of pixels in the phase-encoding direction increases because of the additional phase-encoding steps. Further, if slice thickness is decreased, which decreases partial volume effect and increases edge sharpness, anatomical coverage will decrease. Additional slices may be needed, which may increase scan time, depending on the type of pulse sequence used.

Signal-to-Noise Ratio

Many factors have an effect on image signal, noise, and the signal-to-noise ratio (SNR). These include the type of pulse sequence, TE, TR, voxel volume (resolution), NSA, type of RF coil, magnetic field strength, and so on. Only the relationships between resolution, scan time, and SNR will be discussed here. SNR is directly proportional to voxel volume. Any parameter that is changed that affects the size of the voxel will have an effect on SNR. If the pixel size is decreased by half in both directions, for example by doubling the number of pixels in both directions, resolution will increase, SNR will decrease by a factor of 4, and scan time will double with the increased number of phase encodes. If slice thickness is doubled, resolution

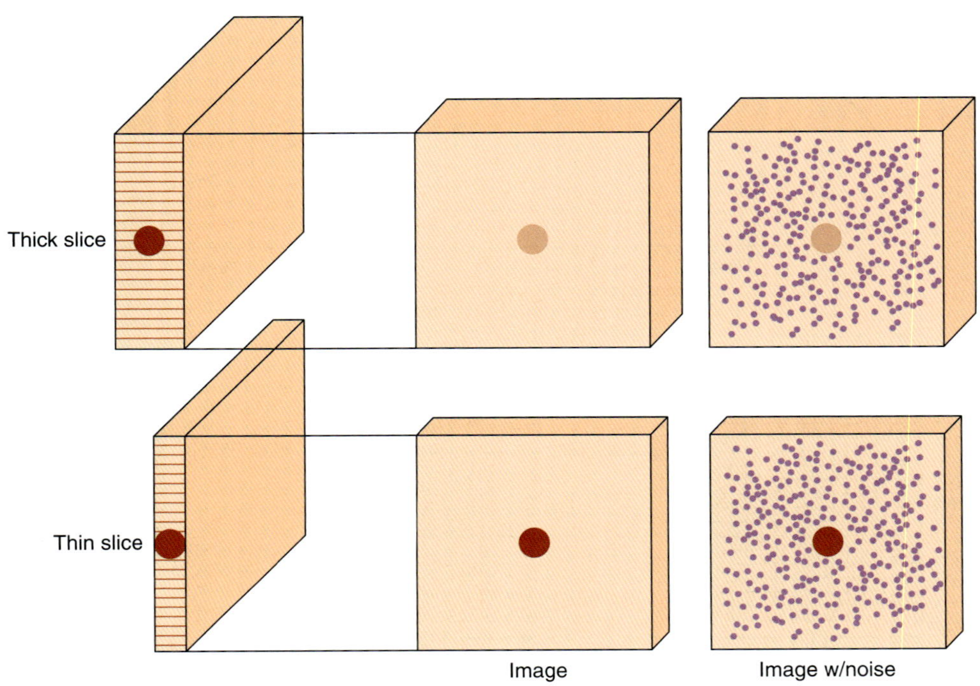

FIGURE 2.13 Partial volume effect occurs when an object is smaller than the thickness of one slice, decreasing its visibility in the image, especially in the presence of noise. Thinner slice thickness decreases partial volume effect and allows small objects to be seen more clearly and edges to appear sharper.

Table 2.2 Effect of Pulse Sequence–acquisition Parameter Changes on Resolution, Signal-to-noise Ratio, and Scan Time

Pulse Sequence Parameter	Parameter Change	Resulting Change		
		Resolution	*SNR*	*Scan Time*
FOV*x*	↓	↑	↓	—
FOV*y*	↓	↑	↓	—
N*x*	↑	↑	↓	—
N*y**	↑	↑	↓	↑
Slice thickness	↓	↑	↓	(↑)**
TE	↑	—	↓	—
TR	↓	—	↓	↓
NSA	↓	—	↓	↓
ETL	↑	(↓)	—	↓

*Assuming *y* is the phase-encoding direction.
**( ) denotes indirect effect.
ETL, Echo train length; FOV*x*, field-of-view in *x* direction; FOV*y*, field-of-view in *y* direction; NSA, number of signal averages; N*x*, number of pixels in *x* direction; N*y*, number of pixels in *y* direction; SNR, signal-to-noise ratio; TE, echo time; TR, relaxation time.

will decrease (partial volume effect will be worse), SNR will double, and it might be possible to decrease scan time because fewer slices are needed to cover the anatomy. A summary of parameter changes and the effect on resolution, SNR, and scan time is shown in Table 2.2. Knowing these relationships is useful when optimizing protocols for high resolution and low scan time. We may wish to improve resolution, but this should be done only if adequate SNR remains and scan time is as low as desired.

Pulse Sequences

Spin Echo

The main features of the SE pulse sequence (see Figure 2.7) were described above and include an initial 90° RF pulse and a 180° RF pulse, which produce an SE at time TE. The 180° pulse occurs at a time TE/2. The signal from the SE is measured by a receive RF coil, and these data are placed in one line of raw data called k-space. This pulse sequence must be repeated a number of times in order to fill all of k-space.

The SE sequence can produce T1 or T2-weighted images, depending on the selection of TE and TR. T1 weighting is used to demonstrate the structure of fat and glandular tissue in non–fat-suppressed acquisitions. T2-weighted SE scans show fluid as bright, which is useful in identifying cysts. An advantage of the SE sequence is that dephasing due to magnetic field inhomogeneities, magnetic susceptibility, and chemical shift can be rephased by the 180° RF pulse, which results in increased signal and decreased artifacts and contrast more directly related to tissue characteristics (spin-spin interactions) than to system factors.[4] A disadvantage of the SE sequence is that scan times are longer than scan times of the other sequences described below. Acquisition of precontrast, non–fat-suppressed, T1-weighted scans will improve visualization of fat in benign lymph nodes, fat necrosis, and areas near metallic clips used to mark biopsy sites.[5,6,7] T2-weighted scans without contrast injection are useful in identifying benign, high T2 signal lesions such as cysts and fibroadenomas.[7,8,9] Cysts appear bright on T2-weighted sequences because of their high water content, which results in increased T2 relaxation time compared with T2 relaxation time in other tissue.[1]

Optimizing pulse sequence acquisition parameters includes adjusting TE and TR for optimum contrast, while achieving the best trade-offs of signal, noise, resolution, and scan time. In SE imaging, to achieve T1-weighted contrast, TE and TR would be selected to maximize T1 effects and minimize T2 effects. This is accomplished by selecting a TE as short as allowed by the pulse sequence (typically a few milliseconds [ms]) and a relatively short TR (300 to 600 ms).[4] T2-weighted contrast is obtained by selecting TE and TR to minimize T1 effects and maximize T2 effects. This is done by selecting a relatively long TE (80 to 120 ms) and a very long TR (2 to 3 seconds).[4] Minimizing both T1 and T2 effects by selecting a very short TE and very long TR results in spin density contrast.

Inversion Recovery

An inversion recovery (IR) pulse sequence is shown in Figure 2.14. This sequence is characterized by an initial 180° RF pulse that inverts the longitudinal magnetization from the +*z* direction to the -*z* direction (Figure 2.15). There is some flexibility in the rest of the pulse sequence because the inversion pulse could be followed by a spin echo sequence (see Figure 2.14) or another type of sequence. The primary purpose of the IR pulse sequence is to null the signal from some tissue, most often fat in breast imaging. This is done by waiting a certain amount of time (called the inversion time [TI]) after the initial inversion pulse and then continuing with a 90° RF pulse, rotating the magnetization to the transverse plane.

To null the signal from fat, for example, TI is set to a time when the signal from fat is crossing through zero, about 180 ms at 1.5 T. The 90° RF pulse then rotates all non-zero magnetization into the transverse plane. Because no fat signal is rotated into the transverse plane, no fat signal is generated in the image. System limitations prevent perfectly homogeneous fat suppression, but this method is fairly robust and is less affected by magnetic field inhomogeneities compared with effects of inhomogeneities of other methods. Fat suppression techniques will be further discussed below.

Turbo Spin Echo

The turbo spin echo (also known as fast spin echo) pulse sequence allows more lines of raw data to be filled in k-space

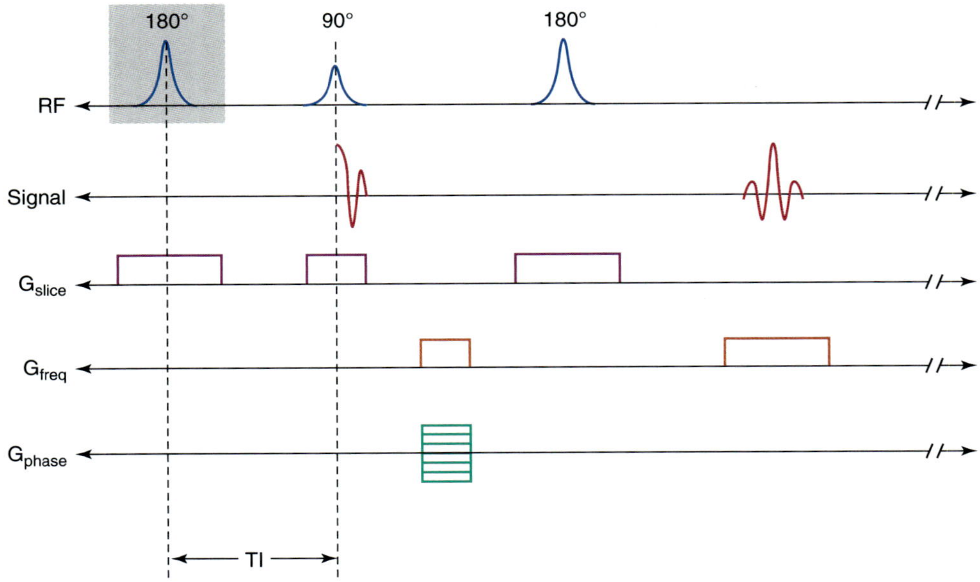

FIGURE 2.14 Inversion recovery pulse sequence is characterized by an initial RF inversion pulse and is used to null unwanted signals (e.g., from fat, fluid).

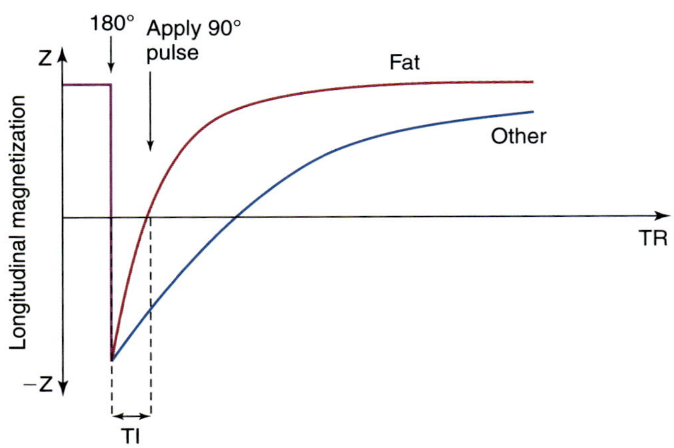

FIGURE 2.15 Inversion of longitudinal magnetization shows that after initial inversion of the longitudinal magnetization, T1 relaxation occurs and the signals from different tissues cross the zero axis at different times. When the signal to be suppressed crosses the zero axis, a 90° RF pulse will rotate all other signals into the transverse plane for image formation.

per TR period compared with the number of such data lines with the SE pulse sequence. This is accomplished by using multiple 180° RF refocusing pulses, generating multiple spin echo signals, measuring each with a receive RF coil, and placing the data into different lines of k-space (Figure 2.16). Now, instead of one line of k-space being filled for each TR period of the pulse sequence, multiple lines of k-space can be filled for each TR period. If we have eight 180° RF refocusing pulses, generating eight echoes and filling eight lines of k-space, we have an ETL of eight, and the scan can be performed eight times faster than the equivalent spin echo pulse sequence.

This sequence can produce both T1- and T2-weighted contrast like the spin echo sequence, and it is used to acquire image data more rapidly than the spin echo sequence. The continued rephasing of signal with each 180° RF pulse helps to reduce artifacts (e.g., metal artifact) compared with artifacts produced by the gradient echo sequences described below. However, some additional blurring of the image is seen because multiple lines of k-space are filled.

Gradient Echo

A gradient echo sequence is characterized by having an initial RF pulse less than 90° and by not having a 180° refocusing pulse, as shown in Figure 2.17. The RF pulse is less than 90° and moves some of the longitudinal magnetization to the transverse plane, but it also leaves a significant component of the magnetization in the longitudinal direction. Instead of using a 180° refocusing pulse to generate an echo, the gradients are used to dephase and rephase the signal, generating a gradient echo that is measured by an RF receive coil. These two features allow this pulse sequence to generate signal very quickly, allowing short TR periods and rapid scan times. The lack of a 180° RF pulse means that the dephasing caused by spin-spin interactions and the other factors listed above is not rephased in the echo, making this sequence sensitive to magnetic field inhomogeneities, chemical shift, and susceptibility artifacts. This sequence generates T1- or T2*-weighted contrast.

The short TR of gradient echo imaging not only allows large volumes to be imaged in significantly less time than spin echo but also results in increased T1 contrast and increased sensitivity to T1 shortening effects from gadolinium compared with these effects in spin echo.[6,9] Thus gradient echo sequences are primarily used for T1-weighted acquisition of contrast enhanced volumes. The short TR can be used to acquire very high-resolution volumes or very rapid acquisitions in the case of dynamic imaging, in which the same tissue volume is repeatedly scanned, capturing the time course of changing levels of enhancement of tissue and lesion. All contrast-enhanced imaging is done with types of gradient echo sequences.[10]

Image contrast depends on selection of TE and TR and also on the choice of flip angle. For T1-weighted imaging, TE should typically be minimized to decrease T2* effects; however, for non–fat-suppressed imaging, TE should be

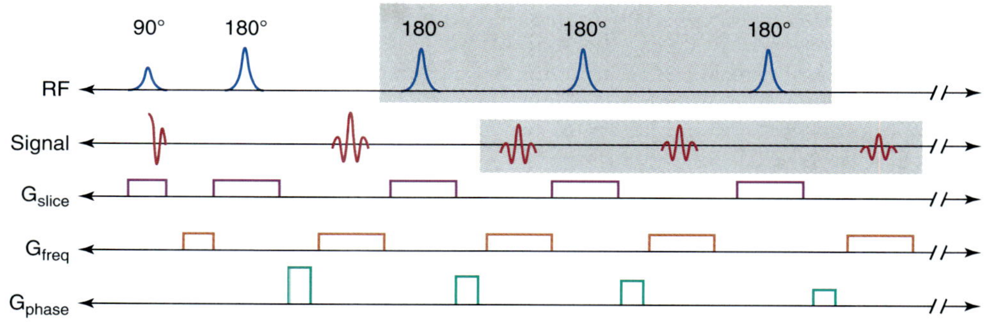

FIGURE 2.16 Turbo spin echo pulse sequence uses a 90° RF pulse with multiple 180° RF pulses. Multiple echoes are formed, and these data are used to create a single data set. Multiple rows of raw data are filled during one TR period; this feature allows the pulse sequence to be run fewer times, saving imaging time.

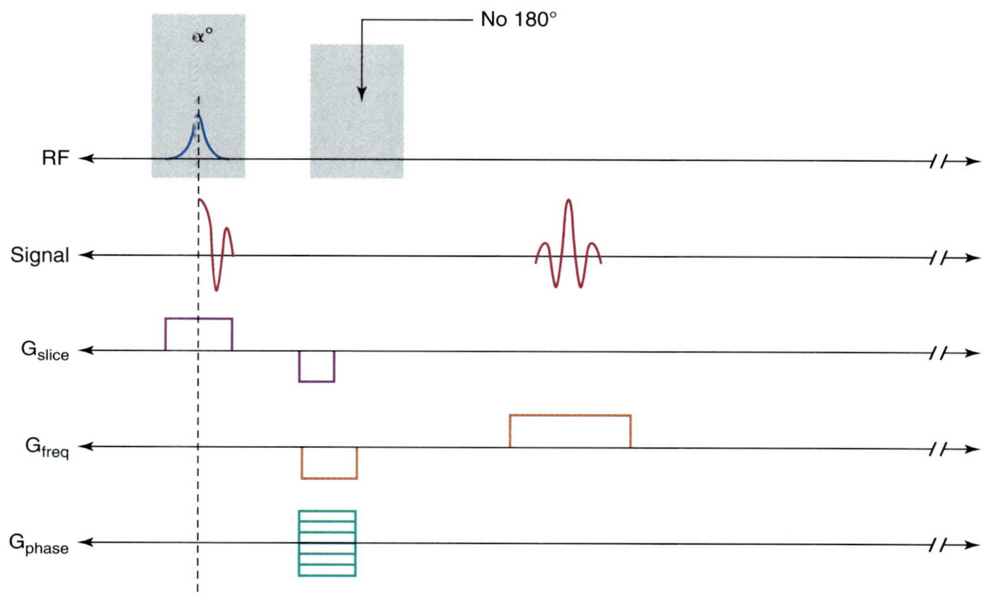

FIGURE 2.17 Gradient echo pulse sequence is characterized by an initial pulse of less than 90° and the absence of a 180° RF refocusing pulse. Signal dephasing and rephasing by means of gradient pulses results in formation of a gradient echo, which is used to produce T1- or T2*- weighted images.

set to 4.6 ms to image fat and water in phase at 1.5T.[10] If fat and water spins are not in phase, resulting artifactual decreased signal will be seen in pixels containing both fat and water. TR and flip angle must be chosen together to maximize T1 contrast. If minimizing acquisition speed is a priority, the shortest TR possible is selected and then the appropriate flip angle based on this TR is selected to maximize T1 contrast.[4]

A primary purpose of gradient echo sequences is to acquire image data rapidly. When TR is so short, signal may remain in the transverse plane at the end of the TR period, before the sequence is repeated to fill additional lines of k-space. This signal can be removed through a process called "spoiling," which can be accomplished with gradients or another RF pulse. The purpose of spoiling is to completely dephase any remaining signal in the transverse plane. Spoiled gradient echo sequences can produce more heavily T1-weighted contrast. An alternative to spoiling the remaining signal in the transverse plane is to use this signal in a controlled way during the next TR period in "steady state" gradient echo imaging. TE, TR, and flip angle can be chosen to result in image contrast related to T2/T1. Steady state gradient echo imaging has not found widespread use in breast MRI. Clinicians' desire for heavily T1-weighted contrast enhanced acquisitions has led to the use of spoiled gradient echo imaging in breast MRI.

Acquisition Techniques

Optimizing breast MR images requires choices to be made between many acquisition technique options. These options are described below along with discussion of advantages and disadvantages.

Bilateral Versus Unilateral Imaging

Choosing between bilateral and unilateral imaging involves both technical and clinical considerations. Bilateral acquisition allows the simultaneous imaging of both breasts. This requires a much larger FOV (and must include all signal-producing tissue to avoid signal wrap), resulting in decreased in-plane resolution compared with unilateral acquisition with a smaller FOV. The use of parallel imaging and fast sequences with bilateral acquisition can be used to compensate for this; using this technique over the past several years has resulted in images with increased resolution.[5,11] Unilateral imaging allows a smaller FOV and thus allows higher in-plane resolution. The magnetic field of the smaller FOV is more homogeneous and allows more uniform fat suppression. Bilateral axial image data can be reconstructed into sagittal views, but the acquired slice thickness (typically >1 mm) results in poor sagittal in-plane resolution. Unilateral sagittal images can be acquired with high in-plane resolution and submillimeter pixel size.

An advantage of bilateral imaging is that the contrast agent has had the same amount of time to be taken up in each breast, allowing direct comparison of degree of enhancement in left and right breasts. This is a more efficient use of contrast.[10] For unilateral contrast enhanced imaging, one breast will have more time to take up contrast, compared with contrast uptake in the other, making direct comparison of enhancement more challenging. Bilateral imaging also facilitates interpretation of breast symmetry (e.g., enhancement patterns related to hormone levels in premenopausal women) and may allow detection of cancer in the contralateral breast that otherwise may have been missed with unilateral imaging.[1,5,6,10,11] However, using bilateral imaging with large FOV and decreased resolution may decrease diagnostic accuracy. Unilateral imaging may be used when following up specific findings in a single breast.[11] American College of Radiology and European Society of Breast Imaging guidelines recommend bilateral imaging except in the case of mastectomy or for evaluation of a specific finding in a single breast.[12,13]

Acquisition Plane

The choice of acquisition plane is closely related to the choice of bilateral or unilateral acquisition. Acquisition of submillimeter isotropic voxels can result in low SNR; thus clinicians at many facilities choose to have section thicknesses of 2 to 3 mm. Therefore the acquisition plane will have highest in-plane resolution, and careful consideration must be made as to which plane view is preferred.[7] Sagittal or axial acquisition allows correlation with mammography views and provides good visualization of ducts and glandular tissue.[1,7,9] Sagittal acquisition is a natural viewing orientation and requires smaller FOV, resulting in higher in-plane resolution. The smaller FOV allows a more homogeneous magnetic field across the image and should result in more uniform fat suppression.[6,7,10] Bilateral sagittal acquisition requires more slices and longer scan time, so sagittal acquisitions may be limited to a single breast.[7,10,13] Bilateral imaging can be done in axial or coronal planes. Although imaging in the coronal plane can reduce artifacts caused by cardiac motion, this plane is more susceptible to respiratory motion and is less easily correlated with mammography.[9,10,13] Thus bilateral imaging is most often accomplished in the axial plane, and unilateral imaging is often accomplished in the sagittal plane.

Two-Dimensional Versus Three-Dimensional Views

MRI allows data to be collected in two-dimensional (2-D) or three-dimensional (3-D) acquisition modes. Two-dimension acquisition mode uses RF pulses (e.g. 90° and 180° in the SE pulse sequence) applied at the same time as the slice-encoding gradient (see Figure 2.7). This excites a thin section of frequency- and phase-encoded protons, resulting in the viewed image corresponding to that section. The acquired signal comes only from that section. Three-dimension acquisition mode uses RF pulses to excite a large volume of protons. This volume is then divided into voxels in three dimensions using a frequency-encoding gradient and two phase-encoding gradients. In this case, acquired signal comes from the entire volume. The scan time for a 3-D acquisition must also include the additional number of phase encodes in the slice direction, Nslice, resulting in scan time = TR × NSA × Nslice × Np / ETL.

Because signal is collected from the entire volume, 3-D acquisition has the advantage of higher SNR compared with SNR in 2-D imaging.[1,10] Using the additional phase-encoding gradient results in the volume being split into sections with a rectangular profile, an advantage over 2-D imaging, in which the slice profile is not rectangular, resulting in additional blurring in the slice direction. This also allows 3-D acquisition to be capable of thinner slices with no gap (no spacing between slices).[7] The short TRs of gradient echo imaging has allowed 3-D acquisition of large volumes to become possible. The short TRs also allow 3-D acquisitions to have stronger T1 weighting and contrast.[7,10,13] However, 2-D acquisitions result in fewer artifacts related to motion and pulsation.[13] Because 3-D acquisitions can accommodate large FOV, magnetic field homogeneity may be decreased compared with magnetic field homogeneity in smaller-FOV imaging, resulting in poorer fat suppression. Further, with 3-D imaging and the additional phase encoding in the slice direction, it is now possible to have wrap-around artifact in the slice direction. This is mitigated by slice oversampling and limited excitation of protons outside the dedicated breast coils.

Fat Suppression

Fat suppression is a required component of breast MRI because enhancing lesions may have the same brightness as fat.[1,10] Several types of fat suppression exist, each with advantages and disadvantages, including fat saturation, water excitation, inversion recovery, and subtraction. Generally, a very homogeneous magnetic field is required to produce uniform fat suppression; however, some suppression techniques are less sensitive to inhomogeneities than others. A large FOV has a less homogeneous magnetic field than a small FOV; therefore uniform fat suppression is more challenging in bilateral imaging than in unilateral imaging.[10]

Fat Saturation

Fat and water resonate at slightly different frequencies (about 220 Hz apart at 1.5 T). Fat saturation takes advantage of this difference by using an RF pulse at the beginning of the pulse sequence to excite only the protons associated with fat. The magnetization associated with fat is subsequently spoiled (destroyed) so that fat provides no signal as the pulse sequence continues. Fat saturation is compatible with many types of pulse sequences but requires a very homogeneous magnetic field to provide uniform fat suppression.[14,15] The fat-saturation RF pulse also adds significant time to the pulse sequence, which results in an increase in the minimum TR.[14]

Water Excitation

The water-excitation technique uses the different resonant frequencies of fat and water and selects only the water protons for excitation and subsequent signal acquisition. This does not require preliminary pulses prior to the normal pulse sequence but substitutes special RF pulses designed to select only water protons.[14] Water excitation adds less time to the pulse sequence compared with the time needed for fat saturation; as a result, this technique works well with 3-D fast gradient echo and bilateral imaging.

Inversion Recovery

A common type of inversion recovery sequence for fat suppression is STIR (short TI inversion recovery), which takes advantage of the different T1 relaxation times of fat and other tissues in the breast. As previously described, a 180° RF inversion pulse is used to invert the longitudinal magnetization of all tissue (see Figures 2.14 and 2.15). The magnetization of fat and other tissue begins to realign to the direction of the main magnetic field because of T1 relaxation. At a certain time, the magnetization from fat will cross zero. At this time, called TI, a 90° pulse is applied, tipping magnetization from all other tissue except fat into the transverse plane, and the rest of the pulse sequence is continued. Thus all tissue except fat contributes to signal in the image. This technique is not sensitive to magnetic field inhomogeneities, but the additional inversion pulse and delay due to inversion time increase TR and decrease the maximum number of slices that can be acquired.[14] Also, because the magnetization from all tissues is inverted, the resulting image contrast shows inverted T1 contrast.

Because of the added time, this technique was limited to 2-D acquisition; however, new implementations allow inversion recovery with 3-D acquisitions. Additionally, gadolinium cannot be used because signal from tissue with shorter T1 from gadolinium may be suppressed along with fat. Another type of inversion recovery sequence uses a special RF inversion pulse that selects only fat magnetization for inversion, allowing magnetization from other tissue to remain positive. After the TI delay, the pulse sequence continues, resulting in the measurement of signal from tissues other than fat. This technique is also insensitive to magnetic field inhomogeneities and has the added benefit of producing normal T1-weighted contrast because the magnetization from tissues other than fat are not inverted.

Subtraction

Image subtraction may be used to subtract the precontrast data set from the enhanced postcontrast data set. Subtraction does not add time to the acquisition, which allows this technique to work well with bilateral fast gradient echo imaging. The technique is also not sensitive to magnetic field inhomogeneities but is very sensitive to patient motion.[6,9,10] The other fat suppression techniques mentioned previously are less sensitive to patient motion. Pre- and postcontrast dynamic series may be acquired with or without other fat suppression techniques before subtraction. Subtraction is then used to visualize enhancing tissue. Clinicians at some facilities prefer to subtract data without other fat suppression to save time and reduce fat suppression artifacts.[7] It is important to acquire the pre- and postcontrast data with exactly matching acquisition parameters, including receiver settings.[10]

Parallel Imaging

Parallel imaging can be used to decrease acquisition time. Recall that the MR signal from a section is divided into pixels using frequency and phase encoding, and a different phase-encoding step is required to place data in each line of k-space (raw data). The pulse sequence must be repeated with different phase-encoding steps until all data have been collected. Parallel imaging takes advantage of multiple receiver coils to provide additional spatial localization that is used to acquire data with fewer phase-encoding steps. This reduction directly reduces scan time, typically by a factor of two to three.[6,7] The decreased scan time can reduce patient motion but also results in decreased SNR.[7,11] Further, when this technique is used to reduce scan time by a large factor, increased parallel imaging artifacts may result.[6,7]

1.5 Tesla Versus 3.0 Tesla

Performing breast MRI exams at 3 T holds the promise of increased SNR, increased resolution, and decreased scan time,[7] but several other factors should be considered before moving a breast MRI practice from 1.5 T to 3.0 T. The increased magnetic field strength of 3-T scanners inherently provides an increase in SNR of approximately a factor of two, and this increased SNR can be used to decrease acquisition time, increase resolution, or see subtle lesions requiring higher SNR.[1,6,7,16] Additionally, the separation in resonant frequencies of fat and water is doubled compared with those frequencies at 1.5 T, and this can be used to improve the homogeneity of fat suppression.[6,7]

On the other hand, 3-T scanners have increased nonuniformity in the RF pulses (dielectric effect) used to excite protons, which can lead to nonuniform signal intensity across the image.[6,16] Work continues to improve inhomogeneity from this effect. Other effects which can cause artifacts and nonuniformity such as chemical shift and susceptibility are greater at 3 T as well.[6,16] Special attention must be paid to acquisition protocols to minimize artifacts from these effects.

Tissue heating is higher at 3 T, which can limit the number and strength of RF pulses.[6] Higher-field–strength magnets also necessitate additional limitations on medical devices, potentially limiting the number of patients who can be scanned at 3 T. Although T2 relaxation times of tissue are similar at 1.5 and 3.0 T, tissue T1 relaxation times are increased. This also must be accounted for in acquisition protocols at 3 T,[6,16] in which TR can be extended or flip angle decreased for gradient echo imaging. At 3 T, the T1 of fat in breast increases about 24% and the T1 of fibroglandular tissue increases about 14%. However, the T1 of gadolinium does not change as much as breast tissue does, so improvement in contrast could be realized at 3 T.[17] Although several articles have described experiences at 3 T, with reports of improvement in image quality and increased diagnostic confidence, additional work must be done to fully optimize protocols at 3 T.[6,7,16]

Contrast Injection

Injection of contrast agent is used to increase the visibility of lesions that take up the agent and also to aid in the differentiation of benign and malignant lesions. Because the contrast agent shortens the T1 relaxation time, these lesions will become brighter than surrounding tissue. Some lesions take up contrast rapidly, becoming bright very quickly, and other lesions take up contrast more slowly. The contrast may then wash out quickly or slowly. Enhancing lesions allows two basic types of analysis: morphologic (evaluation of structure) and kinetic (evaluation of enhancement pattern over time). Typically a combination of morphologic and kinetic analysis is used because this has been shown to increase specificity.[18] When morphologic analysis is performed, high spatial resolution images are desired and enhancement allows improved visualization of lesion detail. Contrast between lesion and background is best early after contrast administration, before background tissue has had time to enhance.

The time course of enhancement (rate of contrast wash-in and wash-out) can be measured with MRI, and this information can add specificity to determination of malignant versus benign lesions. There is correlation between shape of contrast enhancement curve and lesion suspicion, in which lesions with fast uptake and wash-out are more likely to be malignant and lesions with slow uptake are more likely to be benign lesions. There is some overlap of curve shape for benign and malignant lesions, and analysis of morphology can be used to increase diagnostic confidence and specificity. To measure time-course shape with MR, a series of pre- and postcontrast studies are acquired. If the acquisition duration is too long, the shape of the enhancement curves may not be properly determined, leading to misinterpretation. This can make a rapid uptake and wash-out curve appear more like slow uptake and wash-out. An adequately short scan time must be used to properly determine shape of the wash-in and wash-out time course curves. To capture the peak of contrast enhancement, it is recommended that scanning should begin within 1 to 2 minutes after contrast injection, and scan duration should be less than 2 minutes. This should adequately capture peak enhancement for lesions with relatively fast uptake, which may occur within 90 to 180 seconds after injection.[1,7,10]

Protocol Optimization

The previous sections provided information fundamental to understanding the many aspects involved in optimizing the breast MRI protocol. Investigators generally agree regarding implementation of many of these aspects, which will be discussed later.[1,4,6,7,13,18] Discussion continues regarding other aspects of the breast MRI protocol, primarily those related to exact degree of trade-off to be made between temporal and spatial resolution in the contrast enhanced series.

In general there is agreement regarding the importance of implementing the following features in every breast MRI protocol. A high field strength magnet (≥1.5 T) with very uniform magnetic field should be used. The high field strength allows higher SNR compared with SNR of lower field strength magnets, and this SNR can be used to increase spatial and temporal resolution while maintaining adequate SNR. The use of 3-T magnets will require careful adjustment of protocol parameters to optimize image quality. A uniform magnetic field is required for uniform fat suppression.

Another feature that should be employed is the use of a dedicated multi-channel bilateral breast coil for imaging patients in the prone position. These coils promote high SNR (which can be used to increase spatial and temporal resolution) and allow comfort to the patient with stabilization of breasts (through mild compression) to decrease potential patient motion. Multiple coil elements are also needed for the use of parallel imaging. Modern scanners allow parallel imaging that can be used to increase the temporal resolution of sequences, usually by two or three times (the acceleration factor). Higher acceleration factors result in lower SNR and increased artifacts.[7]

Choice of phase-encoding direction should not be in the anterior-posterior direction for axial and sagittal acquisition planes to minimize cardiac motion artifacts. Thus the phase-encoding direction would be left to right for axial imaging and head to foot for sagittal imaging. For coronal imaging, phase-encoding direction could be head to foot or left to right; however, a rectangular field of view may be used with coronal imaging, which maintains pixel size (resolution) while reducing scan time when the phase-encoding direction is head to foot.

Finally, there is general agreement regarding the use and purpose of several different pulse sequences in the overall protocol. There should be a set of precontrast images that are used not only to define the architecture of the breast tissue, including fat, but also to identify cysts and characterize high T2-signal solid masses such as fibroadenomas and lymph nodes. A precontrast non–fat-suppressed T1-weighted image can be used to define fat, and a precontrast fat-suppressed T2-weighted image can be used to separate cysts from solid mass. Further, there should be a dynamic series of pre- and postcontrast T1-weighted 3-D spoiled gradient echo acquisitions to identify enhancing lesions. Bilateral acquisitions allow simultaneous evaluation of both breasts for asymmetries in contrast enhancement. And subtraction of pre- from postcontrast allows an increase in brightness of enhancing lesions compared with brightness of the background. These features of the breast MRI protocol may be implemented with little trade-off or compromise.

Other aspects of the breast MRI protocol still require some degree of trade-off to be made. These aspects primarily relate to temporal and spatial resolution of the contrast enhanced set of acquisitions. Technology continues to improve so that we can scan at higher spatial resolution at faster speeds than in the past. Although the trade-off between spatial and temporal resolution is less now than it has been, discussion of this trade-off continues as we push to obtain even higher spatial resolution images in a short time. Kuhl[18] reported in 2005 that diagnostic confidence and accuracy increased when in-plane pixel size (mm) was decreased from 1.25 × 1.25 to 0.8 × 0.6 with a loss in temporal resolution from 69 seconds to 116 seconds (slice thickness remained 3 mm in both cases). This enabled identification of subtle morphologic features of enhancing lesions not observed on lower spatial resolution images, although temporal resolution remained adequate to capture time course characteristics. The decreased temporal resolution reduced the ability to capture enhancement rates, but this was considered less valuable clinically because of an overlap of benign and malignant lesions.

This set a standard subsequently reported by several authors[1,6,7] against which future protocols could be compared. These recommendations for the pre- and postcontrast enhanced set of acquisitions include the following: In-plane pixel size should be less than 1mm with slice thickness of less than 3 mm. Acquisition time should be 1 to 2 minutes, and postcontrast acquisitions should extend out to 6 to 7 minutes. Still, a trade-off is made in the final protocol between spatial and temporal resolution. As scanner technology continues to improve, these diverging goals will come closer together. Protocol optimization involves using the best technology available and making decisions that involve trade-offs that are consistent with the goals of diagnostic interpretation.

References

1. Rausch DR, Hendrick RE: How to optimize clinical breast MR imaging practices and techniques on your 1.5-T system, *Radiographics* 26(5):1469–1484, Sep-Oct 2006.
2. Jacobs MA, Ibrahim TS, Ouwerkerk R: AAPM/RSNA physics tutorials for residents: MR imaging: brief overview and emerging applications, *Radiographics* 27(4):1213–1229, Jul-Aug 2007.
3. Pooley RA: AAPM/RSNA physics tutorial for residents: fundamental physics of MR imaging, *Radiographics* 25(4):1087–1099, Jul-Aug 2005.
4. Hendrick RE: *Breast MRI: fundamentals and technical aspects*, New York, NY, 2010, Springer.
5. Harvey JA, Hendrick RE, Coll JM, Nicholson BT, Burkholder BT, Cohen MA: Breast MR imaging artifacts: how to recognize and fix them, *Radiographics* 27(Suppl. 1):S131–S145, Oct 2007.
6. Chatterji M, Mercado CL, Moy L: Optimizing 1.5-Tesla and 3-Tesla dynamic contrast-enhanced magnetic resonance imaging of the breasts, *Magn Reson Imaging Clin North Am* 18(2):207–224, May 2010. viii.
7. Weinstein S, Rosen M: Breast MR imaging: current indications and advanced imaging techniques, *Radiol Clin North Am* 48(5): 1013–1042, Sep 2010.
8. Kuhl CK, Klaschik S, Mielcarek P, Gieseke J, Wardelmann E, Schild HH: Do T2-weighted pulse sequences help with the differential diagnosis of enhancing lesions in dynamic breast MRI? *J Magn Reson Imaging* 9(2):187–196, Feb 1999.
9. Orel SG, Schnall MD: MR imaging of the breast for the detection, diagnosis, and staging of breast cancer, *Radiology* 220(1):13–30, Jul 2001.
10. Kuhl C: The current status of breast MR imaging. Part I. Choice of technique, image interpretation, diagnostic accuracy, and transfer to clinical practice, *Radiology* 244(2):356–378, Aug 2007.
11. Friedman PD, Swaminathan SV, Herman K, Kalisher L, Breast MRI: the importance of bilateral imaging, *AJR Am J Roentgenol* 187(2):345–349, Aug 2006.
12. American College of Radiology. ACR Practice Guideline for the Performance of Contrast-enhanced Magnetic Resonance Imaging (MRI) of the Breast. Res. 25–2008. Available at: http://www.acr.org/guidelines.
13. Mann RM, Kuhl CK, Kinkel K, Boetes C, Breast MRI: guidelines from the European Society of Breast Imaging, *Eur Radiol* 18(7):1307–1318, Jul 2008.
14. Hauger O, Dumont E, Chateil JF, Moinard M, Diard F: Water excitation as an alternative to fat saturation in MR imaging: preliminary results in musculoskeletal imaging, *Radiology* 224(3): 657–663, Sep 2002.
15. Hylton NM, Kinkel K: Technical aspects of breast magnetic resonance imaging, *Top Magn Reson Imaging* 9(1):3–16, Feb 1998.
16. Kuhl CK, Jost P, Morakkabati N, Zivanovic O, Schild HH, Gieseke J: Contrast-enhanced MR imaging of the breast at 3.0 and 1.5 T in the same patients: initial experience, *Radiology* 239(3):666–676, Jun 2006.
17. Rakow-Penner R, Daniel B, Yu H, Sawyer-Glover A, Glover GH: Relaxation times of breast tissue at 1.5T and 3T measured using IDEAL, *J Magn Reson Imaging* 23(1):87–91, Jan 2006.
18. Kuhl CK, Schild HH, Morakkabati N: Dynamic bilateral contrast-enhanced MR imaging of the breast: trade-off between spatial and temporal resolution, *Radiology* 236(3):789–800, Sep 2005.

CHAPTER 3

Computer-Aided Detection for Breast MRI

Christopher E. Comstock
Janice S. Sung

Optimal breast magnetic resonance imaging (MRI) interpretation depends on the image reader's ability to both detect and accurately characterize contrast enhanced breast lesions. Detecting areas of enhancement involves the tedious process of comparing the precontrast and postcontrast sequences. This process can be facilitated with subtraction images; however, even a small amount of patient motion can degrade subtraction images, limiting their utility.

Once an abnormality is detected, lesion characterization on breast MRI, similar to mammography and ultrasound, relies heavily on morphologic analysis (lesion shape, margins and internal pattern). Because of the considerable overlap in the morphologic features of benign and malignant lesions, reliance on morphology alone has its limitations. Besides using morphology, incorporating a lesion's enhancement kinetics (enhancement time curve) improves specificity.[1] Although kinetic analysis can be performed subjectively by visually assessing the change of a lesion's signal intensity between the early to late postcontrast sequences, visual estimation of enhancement kinetics is inaccurate, especially because many breast lesions contain a mixture of kinetic patterns. Therefore quantitative methods to objectively characterize and analyze a lesion's enhancement kinetics are necessary.

Unfortunately, quantitative kinetic analysis is not possible on most generic picture archiving and communication system (PACS) workstations. Computer-aided detection (CAD) systems have been developed to both improve detection of areas of enhancement and facilitate the extraction and analysis of kinetic information. This chapter will discuss the use of CAD methods to improve breast MRI interpretation.

Principles of Breast Magnetic Resonance Imaging Interpretation

The sensitivity of breast MRI for detecting breast cancer is high, within the range of 93% to 100%. The primary limitation of dynamic contrast enhanced MRI is a relatively low specificity, reported to be between 37% and 97%.[2-4] Almost all malignant lesions will enhance after gadolinium administration, and comparing the precontrast and postcontrast sequences to detect areas of enhancement is essential in detecting malignancies. In subtraction images, the precontrast images are subtracted from the postcontrast images, making areas of enhancement more apparent. However, because both benign and malignant breast lesions can enhance, identification of enhancement alone is not sufficient.

Breast MRI specificity relies on analysis of a lesion's morphological features to distinguish a benign from malignant lesion. Benign lesions tend to be oval with smooth margins and homogeneous internal enhancement, whereas malignant lesions tend to have a round or irregular shape with irregular margins and heterogeneous internal enhancement.

Besides using morphology, breast MRI specificity may be further improved by analyzing lesion kinetics. Some malignant lesions produce angiogenic factors, such as vascular endothelial growth factor (VEGF), that induce the growth of existing capillaries and the formation of vessels to allow the tumor to grow and invade the tissue.[5,6] The vessels formed by tumor angiogenesis are abnormal and are more porous or leaky than native vessels. Increased enhancement of some cancers relative to the normal, surrounding parenchyma may result from both an increased supply of gadolinium through this proliferative network of vessels and their increased permeability. Increased vascular permeability also results in earlier wash-out of contrast from malignant lesions than from normal breast parenchyma. Therefore lesions on MRI that demonstrate rapid early enhancement followed by a wash-out pattern raise suspicion for associated angiogenesis. For detecting enhancing lesions and assessing their enhancement patterns over time, dynamic contrast-enhanced MRI (DCE-MRI) requires a precontrast and multiple postcontrast sequences (usually three to five).

Computer-Aided Detection for Registration Correction

Many radiologists prefer to interpret subtracted images (postcontrast minus precontrast) because only areas of enhancement in the breast are displayed, reducing distractions and facilitating detection of enhancing lesions (Figure 3.1). However, the quality of subtracted images is significantly affected by patient motion. Most MRI CAD

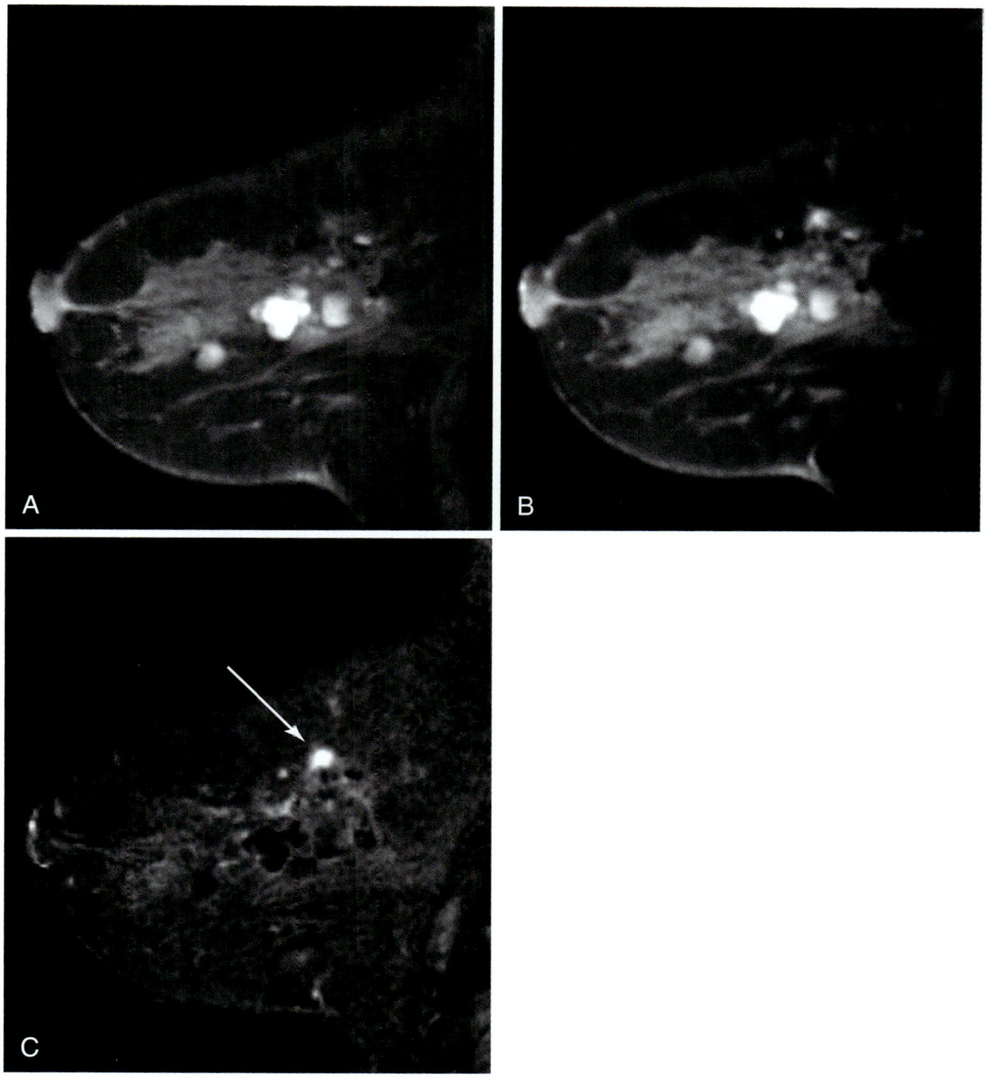

FIGURE 3.1 Image subtraction is shown in this precontrast (**A**) and postcontrast (**B**) fat-saturated T1-weighted image, which demonstrates a subtle 5 mm enhancing focus that is difficult to distinguish from other nonenhancing areas of high T1 signal intensity representing proteinaceous/hemorrhagic cysts. The focus (*arrow*) is easily appreciated on the subtraction image (**C**), in which only areas of enhancement appear as areas of high signal. Evaluation for enhancing lesions using subtracted images is less distracting and less tedious than back-and-forth comparison of the precontrast and postcontrast images. However, once an area of enhancement is identified, assessment of morphology is best done on the original unsubtracted images.

systems, which were developed to allow automated kinetic analysis, provide image registration correction to improve alignment of sequences affected by slight patient motion and reduce subtraction artifact (Figure 3.2). MRI CAD systems usually can correct only for two-dimensional patient motion (the patient rolling left-right or in-out of the coil), not for three-dimensional patient motion (the patient sliding up or down in the magnet). Registration correction is particularly important for breast MRI studies in which fat suppression is not performed and subtraction images are heavily relied upon. Additionally, image registration correction allows for improved three-dimensional image reformation and maximal intensity projection (MIP) generation. However, significant patient motion can lead to erroneous findings on the subtraction images that cannot be overcome by MRI CAD registration correction algorithms. In those instances, interpretation should be based on the source images rather than the subtracted images. Generally, subtraction images should be used only to help detect enhancing lesions. Once detected, the unsubtracted (source) images should be used for analysis of lesion morphology.

Enhancement Curves

Breast tumors tend to demonstrate early enhancement, whereas normal breast parenchyma enhances slowly. Therefore neoplasms are most discernible in the early postcontrast phase, about 60 to120 seconds after contrast injection. If the MR acquisition time is longer than 2 minutes, the first postcontrast images may be acquired too late to depict the true time-signal intensity curve of a lesion (low temporal resolution), leading to inaccurate kinetic results.

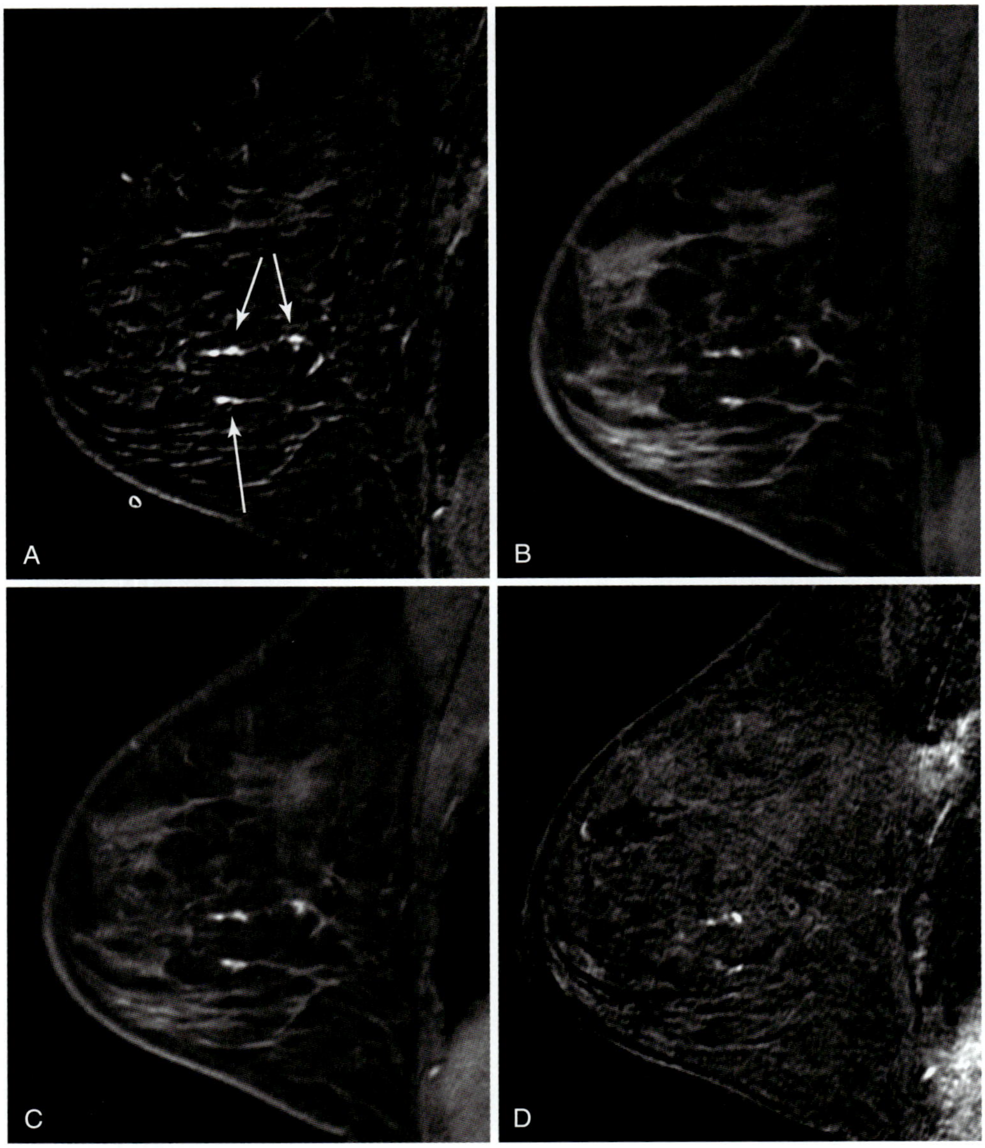

FIGURE 3.2 Registration can be corrected for motion artifact. Subtraction image (**A**) demonstrates an area of apparent non-mass enhancement in a ductal configuration (*arrows*), suspicious for ductal carcinoma in situ (DCIS). However, this area has high signal intensity on both the precontrast (**B**) and postcontrast (**C**) fat-saturated T1-weighted images, consistent with proteinaceous/hemorrhagic debris within retroareolar ducts. This is an example of patient motion causing artifactual areas of high signal–simulating enhancement on the subtraction images. Registration-correction algorithms that improve alignment of sequences can reduce this subtraction artifact (**D**).

In DCE-MRI, enhancement curves are divided into two phases of enhancement: early phase, between contrast injection and the second postcontrast minute; and late phase, after the second postcontrast minute (Figure 3.3). The American College of Radiology Breast Imaging Reporting and Data System (BI-RADS) lexicon characterizes kinetic curves obtained during the initial early phase of enhancement as slow, medium, or rapid. Typically, malignant lesions exhibit a higher rate of initial enhancement than benign lesions do. The time course of enhancement during the late phases can also be analyzed using time-intensity curves, which are classified into three types:

- Progressive (type I): Enhancement continues throughout the dynamic series.
- Plateau (type II): Enhancement reaches a steady state after the early phase. Peak enhancement is reached immediately after the early phase, with little signal variation during the late phases.
- Washout (type III): Enhancement decreases after reaching early-phase peak enhancement.

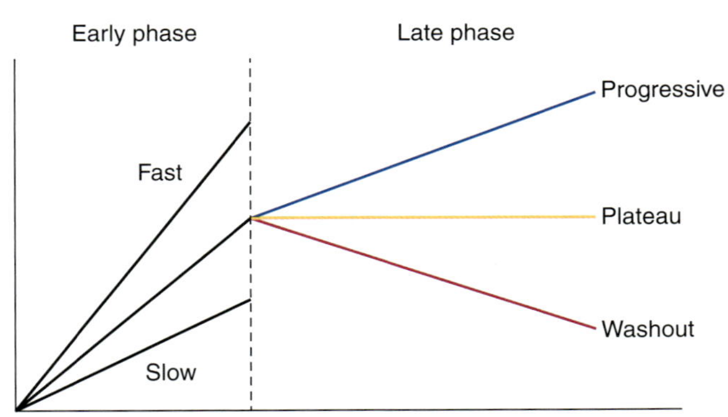

FIGURE 3.3 The signal time course of a dynamic series is divided into early and late phases of enhancement. Lesion enhancement during the early phase is described as having slow, intermediate, or fast wash-in rates. The enhancement pattern in the late phase is categorized as progressive when enhancement continues over the entire dynamic series, plateau when enhancement reaches a steady state after the initial phase, or wash-out when the enhancement decreases after the initial phase.

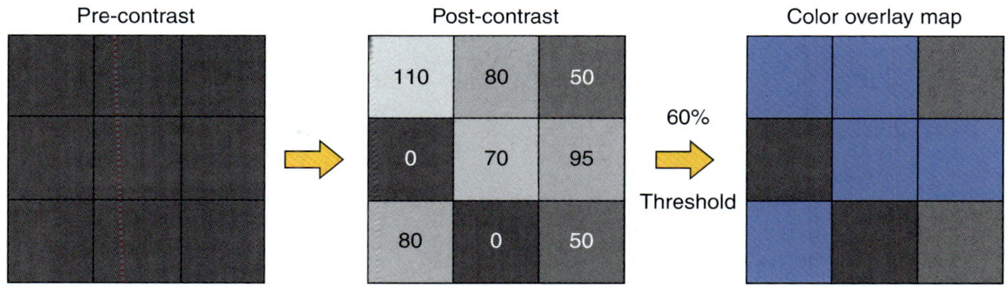

FIGURE 3.4 MRI CAD systems allow selection of a threshold for which pixels are color coded. In this example, the threshold is set at 60%, so that only pixels that increase above this threshold in intensity from the precontrast to the first postcontrast series will be color coded.

Because lesions on MRI often contain multiple kinetic patterns, the most suspicious pattern within a lesion is usually described.

Computer-Aided Detection for Quantitative Kinetic Analysis

At least three time points— precontrast, early postcontrast, and a more delayed postcontrast— are needed to analyze lesion kinetics. Although kinetic analysis is improved when more than three time points are obtained, there is a trade-off between higher temporal resolution and lower spatial resolution. Visual estimates of a lesion's kinetic pattern on a gray-scale workstation are inaccurate.[7] If used to accurately influence breast MRI interpretation, lesion kinetics should be obtained through quantitative methods. This can be done using analysis utilities on the MRI-scanner workstation to place regions of interest on the lesions being evaluated. However, this process is time consuming and not practical to incorporate into the daily workflow. Several third-party vendors have developed standalone software packages that allow automated breast MRI kinetic analysis, which has been termed *MRI CAD*. Unlike CAD used in mammography, the majority of these systems do not perform neural network–type analysis based on lesion morphology to detect cancer, but rather help readers to visualize kinetic information with color mapping and to analyze the information with graphical and quantitative representations.

The basic function of MRI CAD systems is to analyze image pixel intensity throughout the precontrast and postcontrast sequences. An arbitrary threshold, generally between 50% and 100%, is set to select which pixels are coded (Figures 3.4 and 3.5). Only pixels that increase in intensity above the threshold from the precontrast to the first postcontrast sequences will be color coded. However, the optimal enhancement threshold has not been established.[1,8] Several studies have reported improved specificity in discriminating benign from malignant lesions using CAD to exclude lesions with low threshold enhancement.[1,8,9] Increasing the threshold improves specificity (rate of true negative results) but reduces sensitivity (rate of true positive results).

The color assigned to each color-coded pixel depends on the late-phase enhancement pattern of that pixel once the threshold has been reached. A common color scheme is blue or green for progressive enhancement, yellow for a plateau pattern, and red for a wash-out pattern. Wash-out is usually defined as a decrease in intensity of more than 10% relative to the maximal enhancement at the 60 to 120 second time point. Besides color mapping and curve plotting, most MRI CAD systems can perform lesion segmentation to quantify lesion volume and percentage composition of the various enhancement patterns.

Interpretation Using Kinetics

Although lesion morphology is the main determinant of specificity on breast MRI, reliance on morphology alone is limited by the considerable overlap of morphologic features between benign and malignant lesions. Specificity is improved by incorporating a lesion's enhancement kinetics together with its morphological features. However, as with morphology, the kinetic patterns of benign and malignant lesions overlap considerably, with some malignant lesions displaying a benign kinetic pattern and some benign lesions displaying a wash-out kinetic pattern (Figure 3.6). As many as 9% to 45% of cancers demonstrate a benign persistent enhancement pattern.[10,11] This is particularly true for invasive lobular carcinoma and ductal carcinoma in situ (DCIS), which commonly exhibit weak and persistent benign kinetic enhancement patterns.[12-15] Conversely, benign entities including fibroadenomas, papillomas, intramammary lymph nodes, radial scars, and fat necrosis may demonstrate suspicious wash-out kinetics. Consequently, the kinetic pattern of a lesion cannot be used as an absolute, and lesions deemed suspicious based on morphology should be biopsied regardless of their enhancement kinetics.

Generally, the kinetic pattern should be incorporated into lesion analysis after first evaluating its morphology and composition (fat or fluid content on T1- and T2-weighted sequences).[10] Kinetic information may be most useful in determining management of lesions characterized as probably benign based on their morphology. For example, suspicious wash-out kinetics in a lesion with probably benign morphological features may prompt biopsy, whereas a short-term follow-up may be considered if that same low-suspicion lesion demonstrates a benign progressive enhancement pattern.

Pitfalls of Computer-Aided Detection

Patient motion during image acquisition results in blurred images and may lead to errors in kinetic analysis, particularly for very small lesions. It is important to assess for patient motion before relying on subtracted images and the CAD kinetic results. Motion should be suspected when

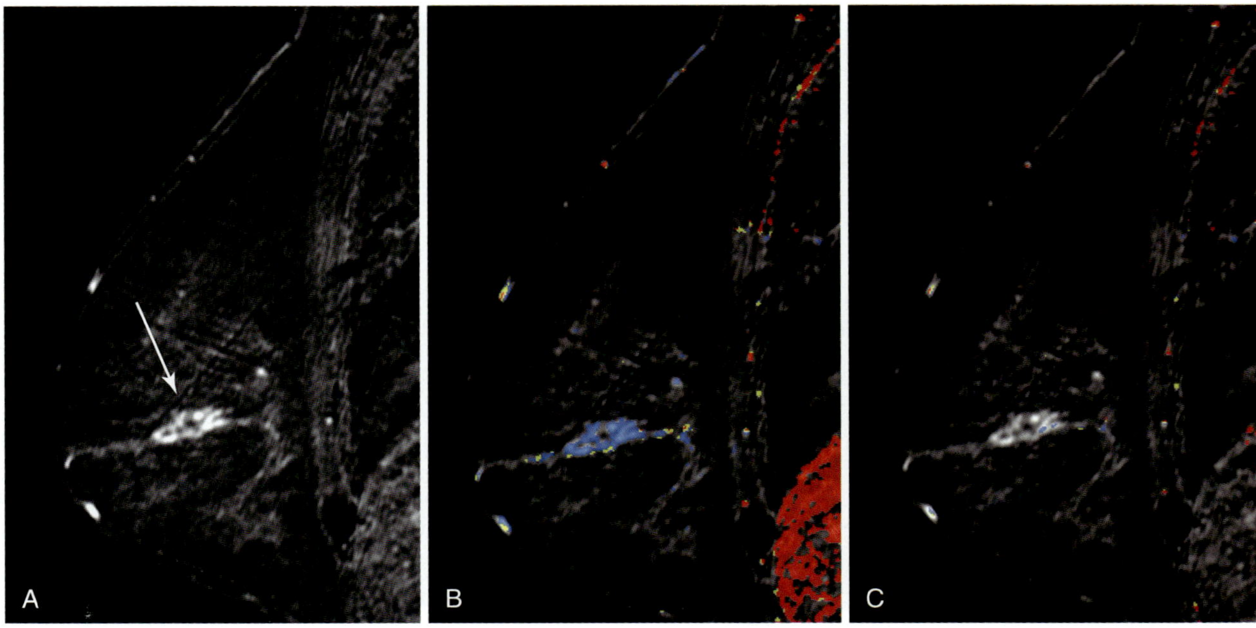

FIGURE 3.5 A threshold case shows a subtraction image demonstrating an area of focal nonmass enhancement (*arrow*) in the patient's central right breast (**A**). At a 50% threshold, the area of nonmass enhancement is color coded blue (**B**). But at a 100% threshold, the lesion's increase in signal intensity does not meet the threshold and is not assigned a color (**C**).

color coding or a trilaminar (red-yellow-blue) kinetic color overlay is seen extending along the edge of a lesion. This trilaminar appearance occurs when a patient moves during the later postcontrast sequences, causing an enhancing lesion to shift in its pixel location. The CAD system is unable to attribute this change to patient motion and misrepresents the decrease in intensity of the vacated pixels as wash-out (Figure 3.7). In such cases, visual inspection of the enhancement pattern, location of the color overlay map, and degree of motion usually confirm the erroneous kinetic results. Additionally, using motion-correction software algorithms may reduce this error Figure 3.8.

Various artifacts, including phase noise and uneven signal or fat suppression, also can affect breast MRI CAD results. Selection of phase-encoding direction is important because phase noise may be color coded and misinterpreted as an area of suspicious enhancement. To prevent cardiac phase noise overlying the breast image, phase encoding should be directed left to right when scanning in the axial plane and superior to inferior with a sagittal acquisition. Occasionally, uneven signal or inconsistent fat suppression from sequence to sequence may lead to erroneous color coding. It is important to check for evidence of a true lesion in the areas of color coding on all of the sequences when artifact is suspected.

Conclusion

Using breast MRI for cancer detection and staging continues to increase. Besides the morphologic analysis of lesions, incorporation of kinetic analysis can improve the accuracy of breast MRI interpretation.[16] CAD-based analysis has been reported to improve specificity compared with the specificity of manual analysis.[8] Additionally, MRI CAD systems facilitate quantitative kinetic analysis at the workstation and provide image registration–correction methods for improved image subtraction. An understanding of MRI CAD methods will help to avoid pitfalls caused by improper system settings, artifacts, and patient motion. New and future systems continue to evolve, incorporating kinetic, morphologic, and neural-network based information that only improve not only detection but also diagnosis.

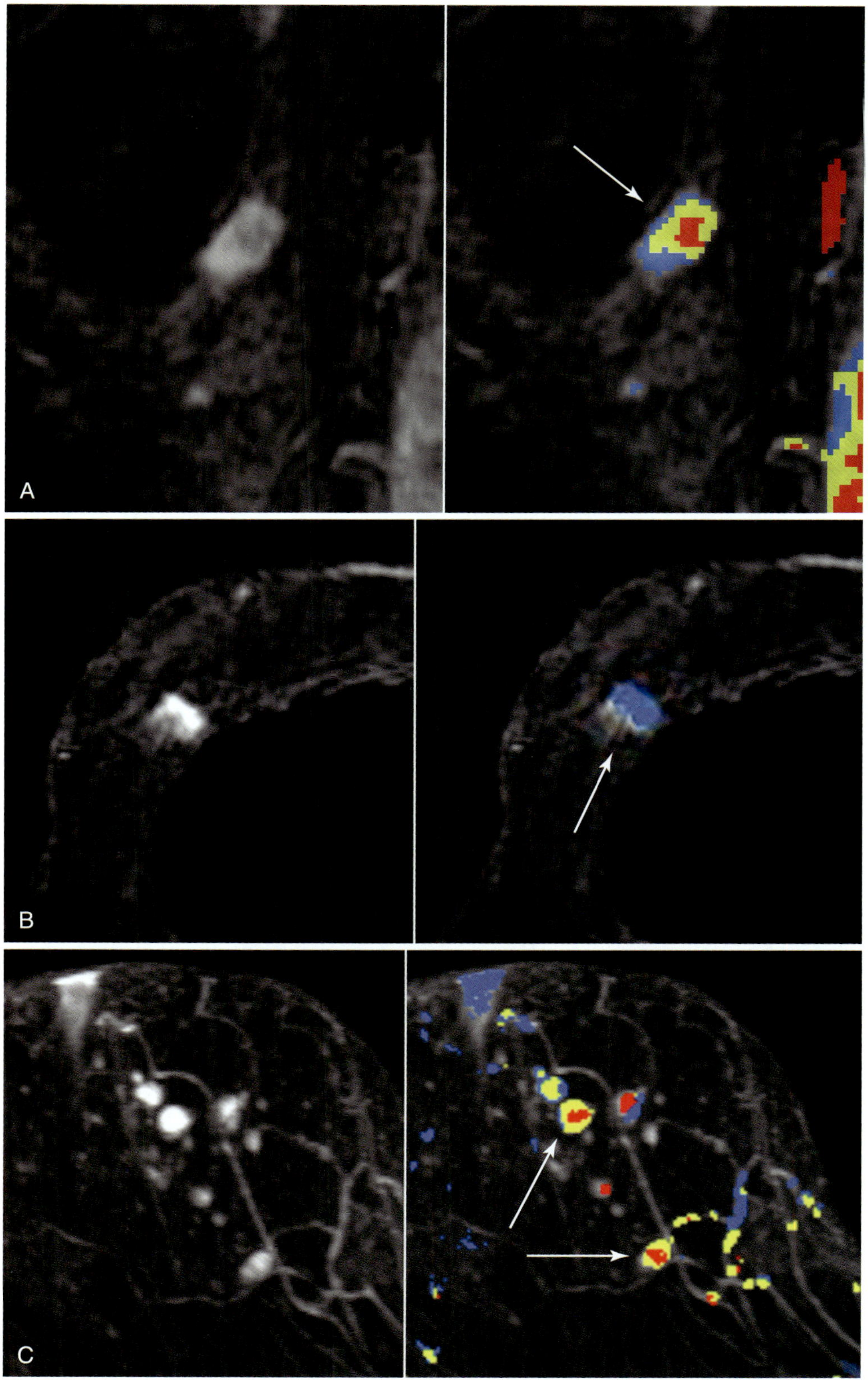

FIGURE 3.6 **A,** Invasive ductal carcinoma appearing as an irregular rimmed, enhancing mass with an area of central contrast wash-out depicted as red on the color overlay (*arrow*). **B,** Invasive ductal carcinoma appearing as an irregular mass with progressive enhancement kinetics depicted as blue on the color overlay (*arrow*). Some cancers may have a benign kinetic pattern, and therefore the decision to biopsy should be based on lesion morphology. **C,** Two benign papillomas appearing as circumscribed enhancing masses with central wash-out kinetics (*arrows*). This case demonstrates that benign lesions may also occasionally display suspicious kinetics.

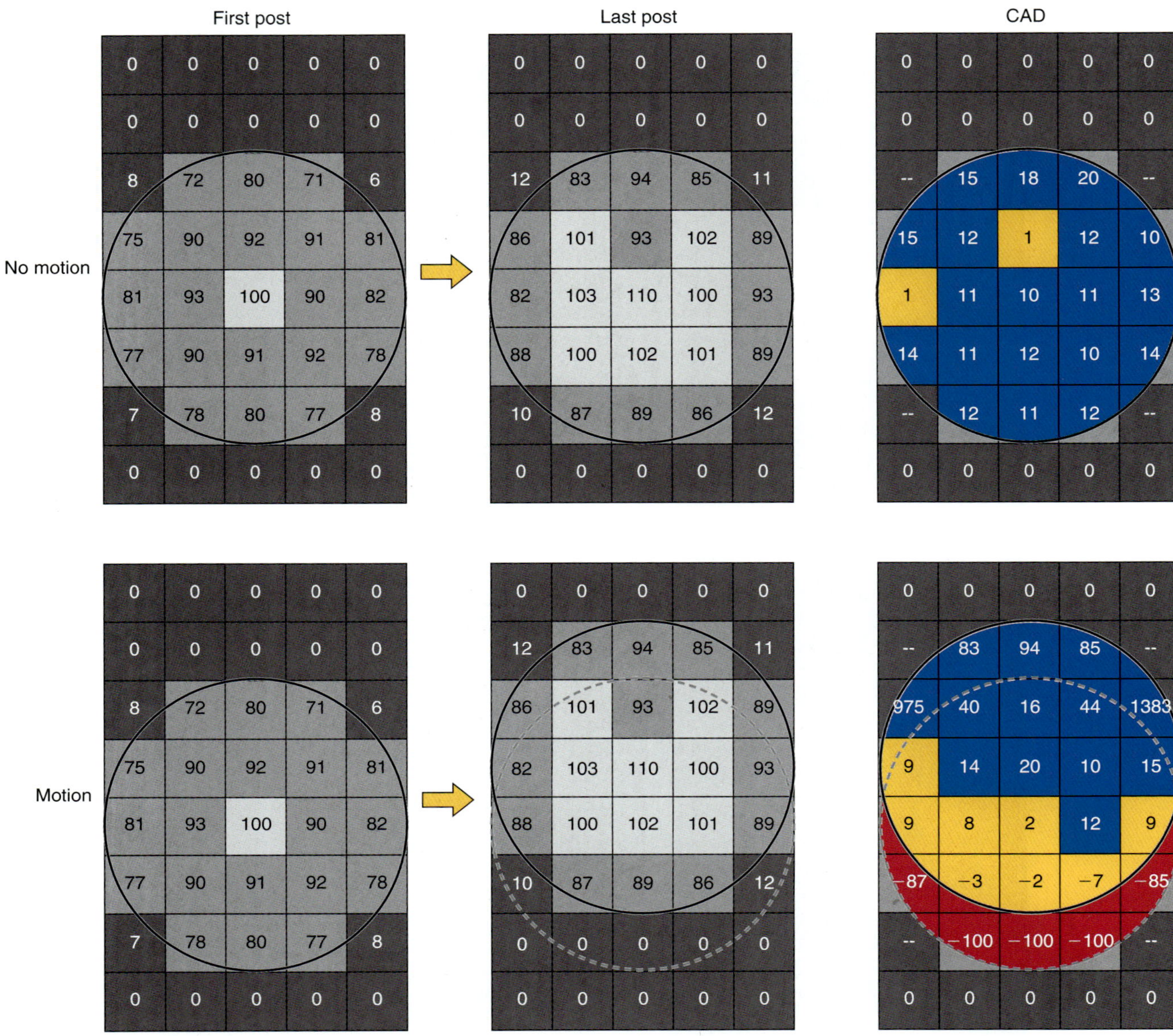

FIGURE 3.7 Motion artifact shows as trilaminar area. Top row (no motion) demonstrates pixel intensity of a lesion (*circle*) on the first and delayed postcontrast images. Only pixels that reach an arbitrary threshold are assigned a color. The numeric values on the CAD image demonstrates the percentage change in pixel intensity, which determines the color assigned: blue for progressive enhancement kinetics if the pixel intensity increases by more than10%, yellow for persistent kinetics if the pixel intensity increases or decreases by less than 10%, or red for wash-out kinetics if the pixel intensity decreases by more than 10%. Bottom row (motion) shows the patient moving superiorly between the first and delayed postcontrast images, resulting in a trilaminar appearance. This artifactual color overlay occurs because the CAD system tracks each individual pixel in the image separately and assigns the color pattern without being able to take into consideration lesion motion.

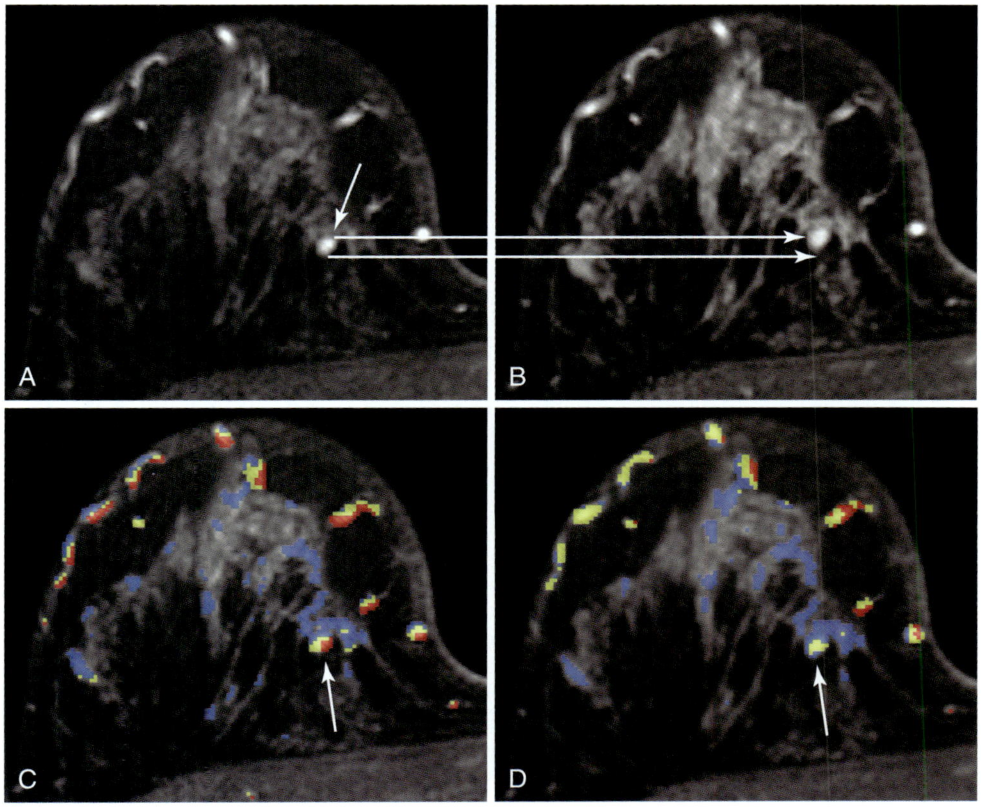

FIGURE 3.8 Images corrected for patient motion are shown. Early (**A**) and late (**B**) postcontrast fat-saturated T1-weighted images demonstrate a 5 mm enhancing mass (*arrow*). However, the patient has moved slightly anteriorly between the two sequences (*white lines*). Initial color overlay on the mass demonstrates a trilaminar appearance (**C**, *arrow*), where portions of the lesion demonstrate progressive, plateau, and washout kinetics, suggesting motion artifact. Following application of registration correction algorithms to correct for patient motion, the mass now demonstrates plateau kinetics depicted as yellow on the color overlay (**D**, *arrow*).

References

1. Williams TC, DeMartini WB, Partridge SC, Peacock S, Lehman CD: Breast MR imaging: computer-aided evaluation program for discriminating benign from malignant lesions, *Radiology* 244:94–103, 2007.
2. Bluemke DA, Gatsonis CA, Chen MH, et al: Magnetic resonance imaging of the breast prior to biopsy, *JAMA* 292:2735–2742, 2004
3. Kuhl CK, Schrading S, Leutner CC, et al: Mammography, breast ultrasound, and magnetic resonance imaging for surveillance of women at high familial risk for breast cancer, *J Clin Oncol* 23:8469–8476, 2005.
4. Newell D, Nie K, Chen JH, et al: Selection of diagnostic features on breast MRI to differentiate between malignant and benign lesions using computer-aided diagnosis: differences in lesions presenting as mass and non-mass-like enhancement, *Eur Radiol* 20:771–781, 2010.
5. Schneider BP, Miller KD: Angiogenesis of breast cancer, *J Clin Oncol* 23:1782–1790, 2005.
6. Weidner N, Semple JP, Welch WR, Folkman J: Tumor angiogenesis and metastasis–correlation in invasive breast carcinoma, *N Engl J Med* 324:1–8, 1991.
7. Comstock CE, Middleton MS, Lundell A: Accuracy of visual estimates of lesion kinetics during interpretation of dynamic breast MR images on a workstation: RSNA, 2005.
8. Meeuwis C, van de Ven SM, Stapper G, et al: Computer-aided detection (CAD) for breast MRI: evaluation of efficacy at 3.0 T, *Eur Radiol* 20:522–528, 2010.
9. Deurloo EE, Muller SH, Peterse JL, Besnard AP, Gilhuijs KG: Clinically and mammographically occult breast lesions on MR images: potential effect of computerized assessment on clinical reading, *Radiology* 234:693–701, 2005.
10. Schnall MD, Blume J, Bluemke DA, et al: Diagnostic architectural and dynamic features at breast MR imaging: multicenter study, *Radiology* 238:42–53, 2006.
11. Kuhl CK, Mielcareck P, Klaschik S, et al: Dynamic breast MR imaging: are signal intensity time course data useful for differential diagnosis of enhancing lesions? *Radiology* 211:101–110, 1999.
12. Kinkel K, Hylton NM: Challenges to interpretation of breast MRI, *J Magn Reson Imaging* 13:821–829, 2001.
13. Kuhl C: The current status of breast MR imaging. Part I. Choice of technique, image interpretation, diagnostic accuracy, and transfer to clinical practice, *Radiology* 244:356–378, 2007.
14. Qayyum A, Birdwell RL, Daniel BL, et al: MR imaging features of infiltrating lobular carcinoma of the breast: histopathologic correlation, *AJR Am J Roentgenol* 178:1227–1232, 2002.
15. Raza S, Vallejo M, Chikarmane SA, Birdwell RL: Pure ductal carcinoma in situ: a range of MRI features, *AJR Am J Roentgenol* 191:689–699, 2008.
16. Lehman CD, Peacock S, DeMartini WB, Chen X: A new automated software system to evaluate breast MR examinations: improved specificity without decreased sensitivity, *AJR Am J Roentgenol* 187:51–56, 2006.

CHAPTER 4

Screening for Breast Cancer with MRI

Samantha L. Heller
Linda Moy

Breast cancer remains the second leading cause of cancer death in women. Mammography is the single large-scale method currently employed in screening for breast cancer in asymptomatic women. Although the effect of mammography in decreasing mortality is debated, multiple studies have shown its efficacy,[1-3] particularly in patients aged 50 to 69 years.[4] But mammographic imaging has limitations, including patient exposure to ionizing radiation and low sensitivity, especially in women with dense breasts.[5,6] Between 10% and 15% of cancers may not be detected on mammography because of density of the breast tissue. Additionally, diffuse cancers and lobular carcinomas are often difficult to differentiate from normal glandular tissue on mammography.[1] For this reason, contrast-enhanced magnetic resonance imaging (MRI), which is more sensitive than mammography, has been increasingly employed for screening purposes, in particular in populations with a relatively high lifetime risk of malignancy.[7,8]

However, MRI is more logistically complex than mammography: screening MRI demands the use of intravenous contrast agent and requires exclusion of patients with magnetic resonance (MR)-incompatible hardware in their bodies. Additionally, for optimal imaging, scans should be timed for days 7 to 14 of the patient's menstrual cycle to decrease confounding background parenchymal enhancement.[9] Most crucially, MRI is more costly than mammography and may also lead to larger numbers of false-positive determinations and unnecessary biopsies.[10]

In this chapter, we discuss the available literature evaluating MRI breast screening, review current guidelines for MRI breast screening, and consider controversies regarding which populations are considered appropriate candidates for screening.

Search Criteria

In evaluating the literature, we performed a search of the PubMed database using the Medical Subject Heading (MeSH) terms "early detection of cancer," and/or "breast neoplasms/diagnosis," and/or "breast," and/or "magnetic resonance imaging," and "sensitivity and specificity"; this resulted in 1564 results. After we removed duplicate entries, unrelated articles, case studies, and articles not published in English, a total of 132 articles remained.

High-Risk Groups

At present, the 2007 American Cancer Society (ACS) guidelines recommend annual MRI breast cancer screening for those with a *BRCA1* or *BRCA2* mutation or those with a first-degree relative with a *BRCA* mutation. MRI screening is also recommended for people who have a clinical history of radiation to the chest between 10 and 30 years of age and those with specific genetic mutations known to increase the risk of breast cancer such as Li-Fraumeni syndrome (*TP53* gene mutations) and Cowden and Bannayan-Riley-Ruvalcaba syndromes (*PTEN* gene mutations), or their first-degree relatives (Table 4.1).

Although these known genetic mutations are associated with a lifetime risk of cancer estimated at 50% to 80%, the majority of women with a family history of breast cancer do not have an identified genetic mutation.[11] The ACS recommends annual screening for those with a 20% to 25% or greater lifetime risk of breast cancer,[7] a risk usually assessed by applying models that evaluate family history. Commonly used risk-prediction models include the Gail model, Claus model, and Tyrer-Cuzick model. However, a recent meta-analysis of breast cancer risk-prediction models of 18 prediction models and 7 validating studies found only consistently poor to fair discriminatory accuracy in internal and external validation.[12] Although those models are imperfect, they remain the standard means of assessing risk for the majority of the high-risk population.

The bulk of the large prospective studies evaluating MRI sensitivity and specificity in the literature have been performed on this high-risk population (Table 4.2). Table 4.3 shows that in these studies, MRI specificity (81.0% to 97.2% across studies) is consistently lower than for mammography (93.0% to 99.8%). However, MRI sensitivity (77% to 91% across studies) has consistently been shown to be greater than that of mammography (32.6% to 50.0%). As Table 4.4 shows, the yield for cancer detected on MRI alone in the compared studies ranges from 1.2% to 3.6%.

BRCA1 and *BRCA2* Mutation Carriers

Molecular genetic testing is available to determine mutations in germline *BRCA1* and *BRCA2* in women with a family history of or relatives with known *BRCA* mutations, although it is important to realize that not all identified mutations have the same clinical presentation.[3] BRCA1 tumors are frequently estrogen receptor (ER) and progesterone receptor (PR) negative as well as HER2/neu receptor negative and are often high grade. Cancers in this group have been shown to grow rapidly and to be larger at diagnosis in an annual screening setting than tumors in other high-risk cases (Figure 4.1).[14] BRCA2 tumors are more likely to be ER and PR positive and to be similar to sporadic cancers (Figure 4.2).[15,16] If the patient desires treatment rather than surveillance, prophylactic mastectomy, and/or oophorectomy may be pursued. Chemopreventive treatment with tamoxifen has been shown to reduce the risk of receptor-positive tumors for women who are known *BRCA1* or *BRCA2* mutation carriers.[17]

Of the seven studies we compare in Table 4.2, five were performed on *BRCA1* and *BRCA2* mutation carriers in women with a high-risk family history and two were on *BRCA1* and *BRCA2* mutation carriers alone.[45,46] The number of mutation carriers in the studies ranges from 43/529 (8%) to 100% of the total. Some screening trials have shown that when these *BRCA1* and/or *BRCA2* mutation carriers are analyzed as a subset distinct from other women at high risk of developing cancer, there may be an even greater relative increase in sensitivity of MRI compared with the sensitivity of mammography. For example, Kuhl and colleagues showed that sensitivity for cancer detection was 91% in all women with MRI versus 33% with mammography, but in the cohort of women who were mutation carriers, 100% sensitivity was noted with MRI versus 25% sensitivity with mammography.[36] Of note, however, there were only 8 patients in this subgroup. Kriege and colleagues, who divided their cohort into mutation carriers (50% to 85% lifetime risk), women at high risk of developing breast cancer (20% to 29% lifetime risk), and women at moderate risk (15% to 20% lifetime risk) found the highest cancer detection rate (26.5/1000) to be in women with known genetic mutations (*BRCA1*, *BRCA2*, *PTEN*, and *TP53*) as opposed to women in the non–mutation-carrier high-risk group (5.4/1000) or moderate-risk group (15% to 20% risk; 7.8/1000).[44] Leach and colleagues found that contrast-enhanced MRI was particularly sensitive for BRCA1 cancers relative to mammography (77% for MRI vs. 40% for mammography for all patients and 92% vs. 23% for BRCA1 carriers (13 cancers),[18] probably because of the lower sensitivity of mammography for BRCA1 cancers, as described previously.

Table 4.1 American Cancer Society 2007 Guidelines for MRI Breast Cancer Screening

Risk	Recommendation
High risk ≥20%-25% lifetime risk of developing breast cancer *BRCA1*, *BRCA2* or untested first-degree relatives of *BRCA* mutation carriers Lifetime risk of 20%-25% or more using a breast cancer risk model History of radiation to chest between age 10 and 30 years Presence of genes known to cause Li-Fraumeni, Cowden, Bannayan-Riley-Ruvalcaba, or first-degree relatives of such carriers	Annual MRI breast cancer screening
Moderate risk 15%-20% lifetime risk of developing breast cancer	Insufficient evidence for or against annual MRI
Low risk <15% lifetime risk of developing breast cancer	No screening

Saslow D, Boetes C, Burke W, et al.: American Cancer Society guidelines for breast screening with MRI as an adjunct to mammography. *CA Cancer J Clin* 57:75-89, 2007.

Table 4.2 Prospective Studies Evaluating MRI Breast Screening: Patient Demographics

Study	Year	Number of Patients	Risk	Mutation Carriers	Number of Patients with a Personal History of Cancer	Modalities
Sardanelli et al.[24]	2011	501	≥25%	330	218 breast and/or ovary	Annual MRI, mammography, ultrasound, CBE x at least 2 rounds*
Hagen et al.[46]	2007	491	*BRCA*	All	None	Annual mammography, MRI
Lehman et al.[8]	2007	195	*BRCA* or ≥20% chance of carrying *BRCA* mutation	80	47	Annual mammography, MRI, ultrasound
Kuhl et al.[36]	2005	529	*BRCA* or suspected *BRCA*	43	139	Annual mammography, MRI, 6-month CBE, ultrasound
Leach et al.[18]	2005	649	≥25%	120	None	Annual mammography, MRI
Kriege et al.[44]	2004	1909	≥15%	358	None	Annual mammography, MRI, 6-month CBE
Warner et al.[45]	2004	236	*BRCA1* and *BRCA2*	All	Breast 70 Ovary 22	Annual mammography, MRI, ultrasound, 6-month CBE

CBE, Clinical breast examination.
*Clinical breast examination for at least two rounds of screening.

Chest Irradiation

Fewer studies have been dedicated to evaluating MRI sensitivity in the subset of women with a history of chest irradiation. Sung and colleagues performed a retrospective review of 247 screening examinations in 91 women who had a history of chest irradiation. Ten cancers were identified in the study period, four on MRI alone (invasive carcinomas) and three with mammography alone (ductal carcinoma in situ [DCIS] and DCIS with microinvasion). The sensitivity of MRI and mammography was identical (66.7%), and the authors conclude that MR imaging is a useful adjunct to mammography (Figure 4.3).[19]

Estimated Size of High-risk Population

How many women fit the aforementioned high-risk criteria for MRI screening in the United States? Using data from the 2000 and 2005 National Health Interview Survey and the National Cancer Institute Breast Cancer Risk Assessment Tool (Gail model 2), Graubard and colleagues calculated that 1.09% of women aged 30 to 84 years have a lifetime absolute breast cancer risk of 20% or more, which at the time of the study entailed 880,063 U.S. women eligible for MRI screening.[20]

Moderate-Risk Groups

It is worth evaluating the data on screening in the moderate-risk group, women with a risk of between 15% and 20% for whom the ACS has found insufficient evidence to recommend either for or against MRI screening. This group includes patients with a personal history of invasive or in situ breast cancer; those with a history of atypical

Table 4.3 Prospective Studies Evaluating Sensitivity, Specificity, and Positive Predictive Value of Breast Cancer Screening Modes

Study	Year	MRI: Sensitivity Specificity PPV (%)	Mammography: Sensitivity Specificity PPV (%)	Clinical Breast Exam: Sensitivity Specificity PPV (%)	Ultrasound: Sensitivity Specificity PPV (%)
Sardanelli et al.[24]	2011	91.0 96.7 56.0	50.0 99.0 71.4	17.6 99.3 56.3	52.0 99.0 71.4
Hagen et al.[46]	2007	86.0 NR NR	50.0 NR NR	—	—
Kuhl et al.[36]	2005	91.0 97.2 50.0	32.6 96.8 23.7	—	39.5 90.5 11.3
Leach et al.[18]	2005	77.0 81.0 NR	40.0 93.0 NR	—	—
Kriege et al.[44]	2004	79.5 89.8 60.0*	33.3 95.0 100*	17.9 98.1 50.0*	—
Warner et al.[45]	2004	77.0 95.4 42.0†	36.0 99.8 83.0†	9.1 99.3 NR	33.0 96.0 23.0†

NR, not reported; PPV, positive predictive value.
*PPV was analyzed per American College of Radiology Breast Imaging Reporting and Data System (BI-RADS) categories or level of suspicion. Numbers are taken from the BI-RADS 5 or suspicious clinical breast examination category.
†PPV was analyzed per screening year. Percentages are given for year 1.

Table 4.4 Magnetic Resonance Imaging Cancer Detection and Cancer Yield

		Cancers			Cancers Found		
Study	**Year**	*Total*	*Invasive Breast*	**Interval Cancers**	*With MRI*	*With Mammography*	**Cancer Yield for MRI Alone (%)**
Sardanelli et al.[24]	2011	52	44	3	48	25*	16/501 (3.2)
Hagen et al.[46]	2007	25	21	5	18	10	8/491 (1.6)
Lehman et al.[8]	2007	6	6	NA (No FUP)	6	2	4/171 (2.3)
Kuhl et al.[36]	2005	43	34	1	39	14†	19/529 (3.6)
Leach et al.[18]	2005	35	29	2	19	6	19/649 (2.9)
Kriege et al.[44]	2004	51‡	44	4	32	18	22/1909 (1.2)
Warner et al.[45]	2004	22	16	1	17	8	7/236 (3.0)

FUP, follow-up; N/A, not applicable.
*Seventeen cancers were found with film screen mammography and eight with digital mammography.
†Fourteen cancers were identified by mammography alone, and an additional 21 were identified with combined mammography and ultrasound.
‡One of the 51 cancers detected was non-Hodgkin lymphoma. Five cancers were excluded from analysis of the modalities.

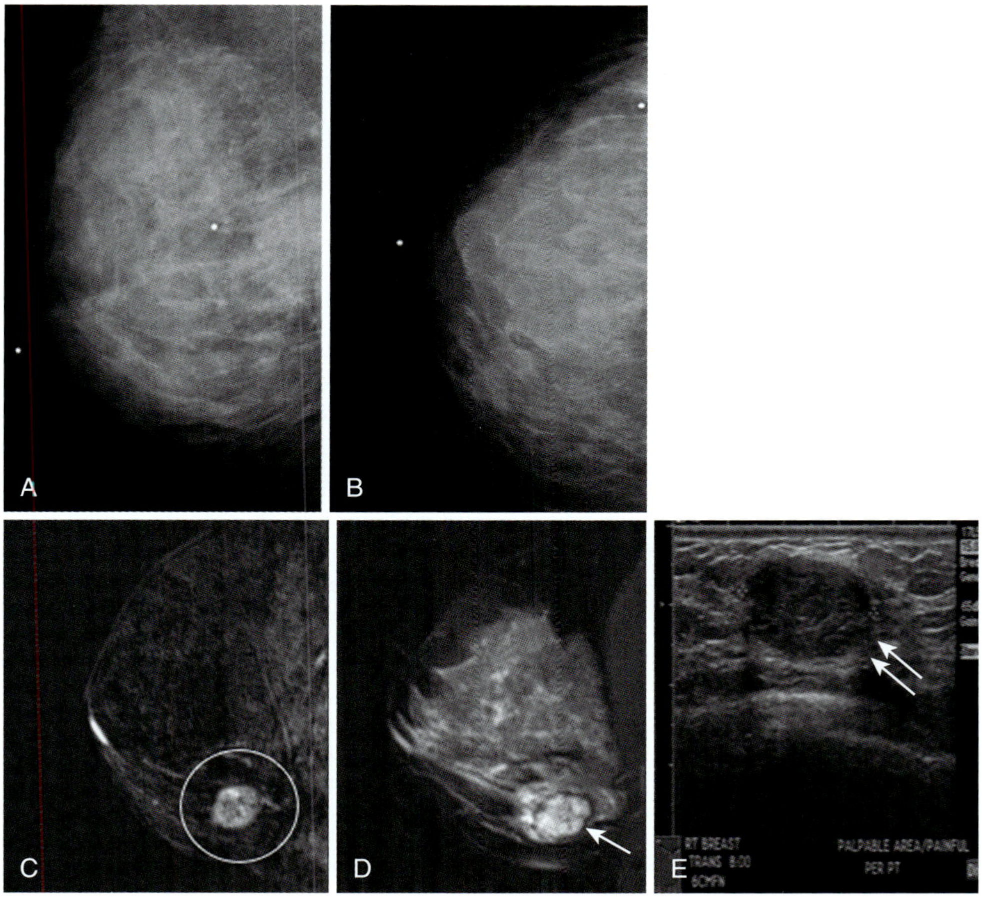

FIGURE 4.1 This 26-year-old *BRCA1* carrier presented with a palpable mass. The parenchyma is extremely dense, and the lesion is occult on mediolateral oblique (*A*) and craniocaudal (*B*) mammographic images. **C,** Post-contrast T1-weighted subtraction image demonstrates an oval enhancing mass (*circle*). **D,** The mass is hyperintense on the T2-weighted image (*arrow*). **E,** Targeted ultrasound shows an oval hypoechoic mass with circumscribed margins and posterior acoustic enhancement (*double arrows*). Final pathology was triple negative invasive ductal carcinoma.

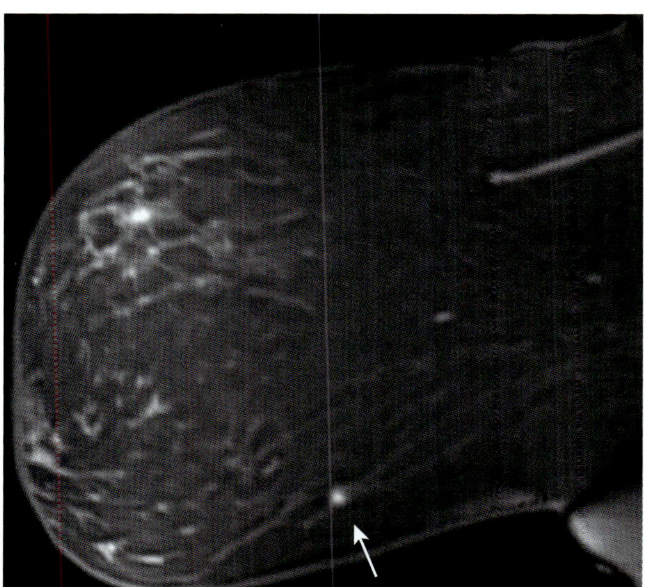

FIGURE 4.2 This 61-year-old *BRCA2* mutation carrier presented on screening MRI with a new 6 mm mass seen in the left breast at 5 o'clock (*arrow*) on this T1-weighted postcontrast sagittal image. The mass demonstrated a type II (plateau) kinetic curve. MR-guided biopsy was performed, indicating invasive ductal carcinoma.

ductal hyperplasia (ADH) or lobular carcinoma in situ (LCIS) or atypical lobular hyperplasia (ALH), and women with heterogeneously dense or extremely dense breasts on mammography. Of note, the American College of Radiology (ACR)/Society for Breast Imaging (SBI) 2010 guidelines say that screening MRI "may be considered in women with between 15% and 20% lifetime risk for breast cancer," specifically in women with either a personal history of breast cancer (invasive and DCIS), ovarian cancer, ADH, LCIS, or biopsy-proven ALH, and that at present, individual facilities in conjunction with referring clinicians may be in the best position to decide whether to screen these patients.[21]

Personal History

Several recent studies have suggested value in screening women with a personal history of breast cancer (Figure 4.4). Brennan and colleagues[22] performed a retrospective review of 144 women with a personal history of breast cancer and no family history who had received screening MRIs. Eighteen cancers were identified in 17 women (12% of women) with a positive predictive value (PPV) of MRI screening of 39%. Ten cancers were detected solely on MRI and were more likely to be DCIS (4/10) or minimal breast cancers (7/10), defined as DCIS or node-negative invasive cancer less than 1 cm in size. DeMartini and colleagues[23] performed a retrospective review of initial screening breast MRI examinations of 1026 women from January 2004 to June 2009. Of the women, 327 had a genetic or family history of breast cancer and 646 had a personal history of treated breast cancer. The cancer yield in the women with a personal history of breast cancer (3.1%) was double that of the women with a genetic or family history (1.5%). The PPV of biopsy was also higher in the personal history group, with 35.7% of biopsies yielding cancer, compared with only 12.2% in the other group.

Additional value in MRI screening may be possible for women with a personal history of breast cancer as well as a *BRCA* mutation. Sardanelli and colleagues,[24] for example, showed that women at high risk of developing cancer who had previous personal breast cancer had a cancer incidence of 4.3%, borderline significantly higher than that in women without such a history of previous breast cancer (2.5%).

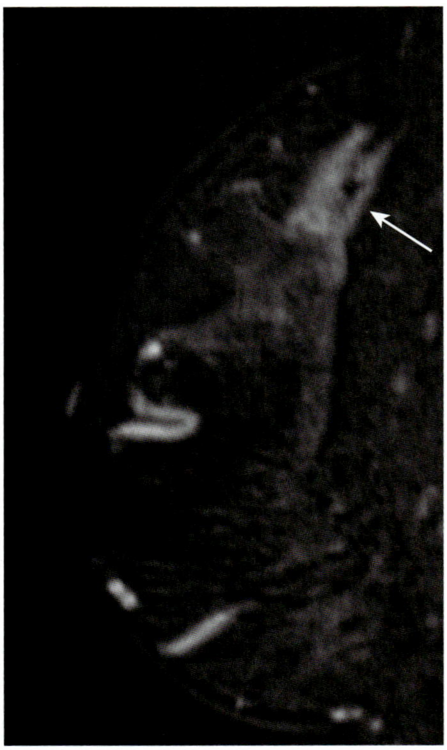

FIGURE 4.3 This 40-year-old woman had a history of Hodgkin lymphoma and chest irradiation. Postcontrast T1-weighted subtraction MRI scan demonstrates newly diagnosed right 12 o'clock enhancing mass (*arrow*) with susceptibility artifact from biopsy clip. Pathology was invasive ductal carcinoma.

Lobular Carcinoma in Situ, Atypical Lobular Hyperplasia, and Atypical Ductal Hyperplasia

Two recent, relatively large retrospective studies addressed patients with a history of LCIS. Friedlander and colleagues performed a retrospective review of 445 examinations in 198 patients. Cancer was detected in 1.6% (5/307) screening studies and in 3.8% (5/133) patients with a PPV for screening studies for which biopsy was recommended of 18.5%.[25] Sung and colleagues[26] retrospectively evaluated 670 screening studies in 220 women with a history of LCIS and found 17 cancers in the study period, 12 of which were identified only by MRI (9 invasive; 3 DCIS) and 5 of which were identified only by mammography (2 invasive; 3 DCIS). Both authors conclude that MRI appears useful as an adjunct screening method for women with a history of LCIS, similar to high-risk populations (Figure 4.5). However, we are aware of no existent prospective studies that have assessed this population.

Scant data exist on screening MRI in patients with a history of ADH. Yet, evidence shows that multiple centers are performing screening MRI on women with a history of high-risk lesions regardless of the ACS recommendations.[27] Current recommendations by the ACS arise in large part from a 2007 paper by Port and colleagues.[28] The authors retrospectively analyzed patients with a history of LCIS who had received screening MRIs and compared results of this group with the results of mammographically screened patients with a history of ADH. They concluded that there was only a slight benefit in using MRI to screen for LCIS over mammography and none for using MRI versus mammography to screen patients with ALH or ADH.[28] Of note, this study was retrospective and also categorized women with a history of either ALH or ADH in the same group without differentiating between them; there is, perhaps, room for future studies to tease out the differences between these two entities and the potential role of screening MRI.

Dense Breasts

Increased mammographic density is known to be an independent risk factor for breast cancer[29,30]; however, at this

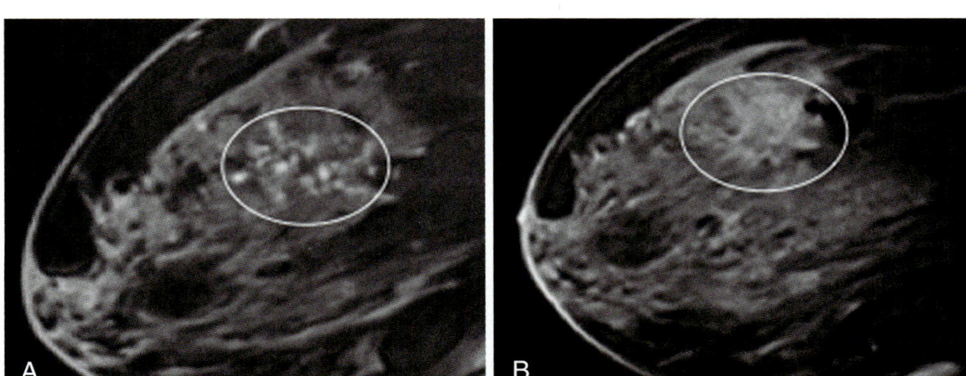

FIGURE 4.4 This 71-year-old woman had a personal history of right breast cancer. **A,** Screening MRI postcontrast T1-weighted fat-suppressed image demonstrates clumped nonmass enhancement (*circle*), which proved to be DCIS after surgical excision. **B,** Image taken after MRI-guided biopsy shows postbiopsy changes in same location (*circle*). The cancer was mammographically occult.

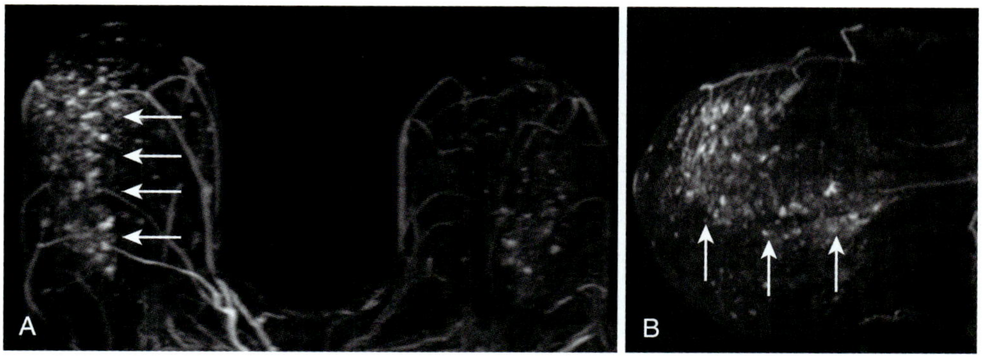

FIGURE 4.5 This 45-year-old woman had a history of LCIS in the right breast. Maximum-intensity projection image (**A**) and postcontrast T1-weighted subtraction image (**B**) from MRI screening study performed 5 years later show asymmetric stippled enhancement in the right breast (*arrows*); this proved to be DCIS on MRI-guided biopsy. The patient underwent bilateral mastectomy, and extensive DCIS was found in the right breast. No cancer was identified in the left breast

time, there are no large or prospective studies directly evaluating the value of MRI in a screening population with a risk factor of mammographic density alone. Sardanelli and colleagues evaluated the effectiveness of MRI versus mammography in a group of women with known cancer and planned mastectomy and found that MRI was more sensitive than mammography in dense breasts (81% for MRI vs. 60% for mammography); no significant difference in sensitivity was found between the two in fatty breasts (80% for MRI vs. 75% for mammography; $P < .001$ for both).[31]

Wright and colleagues performed a small retrospective study evaluating MRI cancer detection in premenopausal versus postmenopausal women. They found a significant number of cancers were detected on MRI and not mammography in the premenopausal group (35%) versus the postmenopausal group (6%; $P = .002$)[32] and implied that this was due to the increased breast density of the premenopausal population. However, the authors did not specifically correlate premenopausal status with mammographic density.

Berg and colleagues evaluated the additive value of annual ultrasound or a single screening MRI in asymptomatic women with heterogeneously dense or extremely dense breast tissue and at least one other high or intermediate risk factor. Of the original 2662 women who had undergone mammogram and ultrasound screenings, a subset of 612 women who agreed to a contrast-enhanced MRI examination were included in the MRI screening analysis. Out of 111 cancers found in the entire study, 33/111 (30%) were detected on mammography only, 32 (29%) by ultrasound, and 9/111 (8%) by MRI; 11/111 (10%) were detected clinically. Adding MRI resulted in 14.7 additional cancers/1000 screening examinations, and adding ultrasound resulted in 4.3/1000 screens with each screening round. However, MRI resulted in higher false positives, a recall rate of 20%, and biopsy rate of 7% (43/612); the mammogram biopsy rate was 2%. Of this group, 8/43 (19%) had cancer. It is important to note, however, that MRI was performed after three consecutive screening rounds of mammography and ultrasound and was performed only on women whose studies had been negative by these modalities. Ultrasound, on the other hand, resulted in a 7% recall rate of which 242/4814 (5%) needed biopsy; of this group, cancer was found in 18/242 (7%).[10] Specificity decreased with the addition of both MRI and ultrasound.[10]

Low-Risk Groups

At present there are no data to support using MRI to screen women with a less than 15% lifetime risk of breast cancer and such screening is not recommended by either the ACS or ACR/SBI.[7,21]

Mortality

To date, no study has definitively demonstrated decreased mortality with MRI screening.[33,34] Multiple studies have shown that MRI is more sensitive than mammography, able to detect cancers that mammography cannot (see Table 4.4),[10] including smaller cancers,[35] and node-negative disease[36]; however, it remains unclear what ultimate benefit this will have.[37] Warner and colleagues began to address this question in their 2011 prospective study examining breast cancer incidence in women with *BRCA1* or *BRCA2* mutations.[35] The authors assessed 1275 women over a mean of 3.2 years, of whom 445 were screened annually with MRI and 830 were not screened with MRI. Their hypothesis was that advanced-stage breast cancer incidence should be decreased in the women undergoing MRI screening. They found that the cumulative incidence of DCIS was 13.8% and that of stage II to stage IV breast cancer was 1.9% in the MRI group and DCIS was 7.2% and stage II to stage IV breast cancer was 6.6% in the comparison group. Additionally, a statistically significant decrease (70%) was seen in the incidence of large or node-positive invasive disease in the 6-year period after screening was initiated with an adjusted hazard ratio of 0.3 (95% confidence interval, 0.12 to 0.72; $P = .008$) for stage II to stage IV breast cancer associated with MRI screening. Although these are promising data, as the authors themselves acknowledge, more studies are needed before a mortality benefit can be proved.

Other Considerations

When To Screen and Screening Intervals

The large prospective studies employ annual mammography and annual MRI (see Table 4.2). Some authors recommend yearly simultaneous screening with MRI and mammography because the two modalities can be easily cross-referenced. On the other hand, alternating 6-month MRI and mammography regimens have also been advocated because this allows more frequent surveillance.[38] However, as Lowry and colleagues point out, it is very difficult to perform a randomized controlled study to address the optimal screening frequency and regimen. To this end, the authors performed a comparative effectiveness analysis using computer modeling to determine the optimal multimodality strategy for screening. They analyzed film mammography (FM), digital mammography (DM), FM and MRI, or DM and MRI in contemporaneous and alternating regimens, initiated at 25, 30, 35, or 40 years of age, as well as annual MRI with delayed/alternating DM/FM versus clinical follow-up. When radiation risk was factored in, they found that annual MRI starting at age 25 and delayed/alternating DM at age 30 was the most effective screening strategy in *BRCA* mutation carriers.[39]

Cost-Effectiveness

Several studies have investigated the cost-effectiveness of MRI for screening, with the majority of studies focused on women with a high lifetime risk of developing breast cancer, in particular *BRCA1* and *BRCA2* mutation carrier populations. The UK MARIBS study found the most cost-effective screening regimen was targeted toward BRCA1 and BRCA2 subgroups compared to other high-risk groups.[40] Plevritis and colleagues found in a study published in 2006 that the cost of annual mammography and MRI versus mammography alone for women aged 35 to 54 years in cost per quality-adjusted life year (QALY) terms was $55,420 for *BRCA1* carriers and $130,695 for *BRCA2* carriers. If women with dense breasts are considered, the cost decreased to $41,183 for *BRCA1* carriers and $98,454 for *BRCA2* carriers.[41] The difference in BRCA1 and BRCA2 findings is attributed to the fact that *BRCA1* mutations tend to result in cancers with a more benign mammographic appearance. Lee and colleagues compared three screening strategies for 25-year-old *BRCA1* mutation carriers and looked at QALY and lifetime costs for FM, MR imaging, and combined MR imaging and FM. They found that annual combined screening using MR and mammography was the most effective (44.62 QALYs vs. 44.50 QALYs for MRI alone and 44.46 QALYs for mammography alone), but was also more expensive ($110,973 combined vs. $108,641 for MRI and $100,336 for mammography alone).[42]

It is very difficult to determine the true cost-effectiveness for the group of women at moderate lifetime risk of developing breast cancer, given the difficulty in truly determining risk in this group.[43]

Conclusion

At present, data exist to support the greater sensitivity of MRI compared with the sensitivity of mammography in the high-risk populations as described above, particularly in *BRCA1* and *BRCA2* mutation carriers. More prospective and randomized controlled studies are needed to demonstrate both the value of screening MRI in the moderate-risk population and the overall benefit of screening MRI in terms of mortality.

References

1. Heywang-Kobrunner SH, Hacker A, Sedlacek S: Advantages and Disadvantages of Mammography Screening, *Breast Care (Basel)* 6:199–207, 2011.
2. Hendrick RE, Smith RA, Rutledge JH 3rd, Smart CR: Benefit of screening mammography in women aged 40-49: a new meta-analysis of randomized controlled trials, *J Natl Cancer Inst Monogr* 22:87–92, 1997.
3. Hackshaw A: EUSOMA review of mammography screening, *Ann Oncol* 14:1193–1195, 2003.
4. Warner E: Clinical practice. Breast-cancer screening, *N Engl J Med* 365:1025–1032, 2011.
5. Samei E, Saunders RSJ, Baker JA, Delong DM: Digital mammography: effects of reduced radiation dose on diagnostic performance, *Radiology* 243:396–404, 2007.
6. Fenton JJ, Taplin SH, Carney PA, et al: Influence of computer-aided detection on performance of screening mammography, *N Engl J Med* 356:1399–1409, 2007.
7. Saslow D, Boetes C, Burke W, et al: American Cancer Society guidelines for breast screening with MRI as an adjunct to mammography, *CA Cancer J Clin* 57:75–89, 2007.
8. Lehman CD, Gatsonis C, Kuhl CK, et al: MRI evaluation of the contralateral breast in women with recently diagnosed breast cancer, *N Engl J Med* 356:1295–1303, 2007.
9. Liberman L: Breast cancer screening with MRI—what are the data for patients at high risk? *N Engl J Med* 351:497–500, 2004.
10. Berg WA, Zhang Z, Lehrer D, et al: Detection of breast cancer with addition of annual screening ultrasound or a single screening MRI to mammography in women with elevated breast cancer risk, *JAMA* 307:1394–1404, 2012.
11. Klijn JG: Early diagnosis of hereditary breast cancer by magnetic resonance imaging: what is realistic? *J Clin Oncol* 28:1441–1445, 2010.
12. Anothaisintawee T, Teerawattananon Y, Wiratkapun C, et al: Risk prediction models of breast cancer: a systematic review of model performances, *Breast Cancer Res Treat* 133:1–10, 2012.
13. Petrucelli N, Daly MB, Feldman GL: BRCA1 and BRCA2 hereditary breast and ovarian cancer. In Pagon RA, Bird TD, Dolan CR, et al: *GeneReviews™ [Internet]*, Seattle (WA), 1993-1998 Sep 04, University of Washington, Seattle. [updated 2011 Jan 20].
14. Tilanus-Linthorst MM, Obdeijn IM, Hop WC, et al: BRCA1 mutation and young age predict fast breast cancer growth in the Dutch, United Kingdom, and Canadian magnetic resonance imaging screening trials, *Clin Cancer Res* 13:7357–7362, 2007.
15. Lakhani SR, Jacquemier J, Sloane JP, et al: Multifactorial analysis of differences between sporadic breast cancers and cancers involving BRCA1 and BRCA2 mutations, *J Natl Cancer Inst* 90:1138–1145, 1998.
16. Gilbert FJ, Warren RM, Kwan-Lim G, et al: Cancers in BRCA1 and BRCA2 carriers and in women at high risk for breast cancer: MR imaging and mammographic features, *Radiology* 252:358–368, 2009.
17. Boetes C: Update on screening breast MRI in high-risk women, *Obstet Gynecol Clin North Am* 38:149–158, 2011. viii-ix.
18. Leach MO, Boggis CR, Dixon AK, et al: Screening with magnetic resonance imaging and mammography of a UK population at high familial risk of breast cancer: a prospective multicentre cohort study (MARIBS), *Lancet* 365:1769–1778, 2005.
19. Sung JS, Lee CH, Morris EA, et al: Screening breast MR imaging in women with a history of chest irradiation, *Radiology* 259:65–71, 2011.
20. Graubard BI, Freedman AN, Gail MH: Five-year and lifetime risk of breast cancer among U.S. subpopulations: implications for magnetic resonance imaging screening, *Cancer Epidemiol Biomarkers Prev* 19:2430–2436, 2010.
21. Lee CH, Dershaw DD, Kopans D, et al: Breast cancer screening with imaging: recommendations from the Society of Breast Imaging and the ACR on the use of mammography, breast MRI, breast ultrasound, and other technologies for the detection of clinically occult breast cancer, *J Am Coll Radiol* 7:18–27, 2010.
22. Brennan S, Liberman L, Dershaw DD, Morris E: Breast MRI screening of women with a personal history of breast cancer, *AJR Am J Roentgenol* 195:510–516, 2010.
23. Kalish G, DeMartini WB, Peacock S, et al: *Screening MRI for high risk women: should patients with a treated personal history of breast cancer be screened?*. Presented at the Radiological Society of North America (RSNA) 96th Scientific Assembly and Annual Meeting, November 28-December 3, 2010, Chicago, Il. Abstract SSAO1–01.

24. Sardanelli F, Podo F, Santoro F, et al: Multicenter surveillance of women at high genetic breast cancer risk using mammography, ultrasonography, and contrast-enhanced magnetic resonance imaging (the high breast cancer risk Italian 1 study): final results, *Invest Radiol* 46: 94–105, 2011.
25. Friedlander LC, Roth SO, Gavenonis SC: Results of MR imaging screening for breast cancer in high-risk patients with lobular carcinoma in situ, *Radiology* 261:421–427, 2011.
26. Sung JS, Malak SF, Bajaj P, et al: Screening breast MR imaging in women with a history of lobular carcinoma in situ, *Radiology* 261:414–420, 2011.
27. Bassett LW, Dhaliwal SG, Eradat J, et al: National trends and practices in breast MRI, *AJR Am J Roentgenol* 191:332–339, 2008.
28. Port ER, Park A, Borgen PI, et al: Results of MRI screening for breast cancer in high-risk patients with LCIS and atypical hyperplasia, *Ann Surg Oncol* 14:1051–1057, 2007.
29. Boyd NF, Martin LJ, Yaffe MJ, Minkin S: Mammographic density and breast cancer risk: current understanding and future prospects, *Breast Cancer Res* 13:223, 2011.
30. McCormack VA, dos Santos Silva I: Breast density and parenchymal patterns as markers of breast cancer risk: a meta-analysis, *Cancer Epidemiol Biomarkers Prev* 15:1159–1169, 2006.
31. Sardanelli F, Giuseppetti GM, Panizza P, et al: Sensitivity of MRI versus mammography for detecting foci of multifocal, multicentric breast cancer in fatty and dense breasts using the whole-breast pathologic examination as a gold standard, *AJR Am J Roentgenol* 183:1149–1157, 2004.
32. Wright H, Listinsky J, Rim A, et al: Magnetic resonance imaging as a diagnostic tool for breast cancer in premenopausal women, *Am J Surg* 190:572–575, 2005.
33. Lord SJ, Lei W, Craft P, et al: A systematic review of the effectiveness of magnetic resonance imaging (MRI) as an addition to mammography and ultrasound in screening young women at high risk of breast cancer, *Eur J Cancer* 43:1905–1917, 2007.
34. Narod SA: Screening of women at high risk for breast cancer, *Prev Med* 53:127–130, 2011.
35. Warner E, Hill K, Causer P, et al: Prospective study of breast cancer incidence in women with a *BRCA1* or *BRCA2* mutation under surveillance with and without magnetic resonance imaging, *J Clin Oncol* 29:1664–1669, 2011.
36. Kuhl CK, Schrading S, Leutner CC, et al: Mammography, breast ultrasound, and magnetic resonance imaging for surveillance of women at high familial risk for breast cancer, *J Clin Oncol* 23:8469–8476, 2005.
37. Morrow M, Waters J, Morris E: MRI for breast cancer screening, diagnosis, and treatment, *Lancet* 378:1804–1811, 2011.
38. Warner E: The role of magnetic resonance imaging in screening women at high risk of breast cancer, *Top Magn Reson Imaging* 19:163–169, 2008.
39. Lowry KP, Lee JM, Kong CY, et al: Annual screening strategies in *BRCA1* and *BRCA2* gene mutation carriers: a comparative effectiveness analysis, *Cancer* 118:2021–2030, 2012.
40. Griebsch I, Brown J, Boggis C, et al: Cost-effectiveness of screening with contrast enhanced magnetic resonance imaging vs X-ray mammography of women at a high familial risk of breast cancer, *Br J Cancer* 95:801–810, 2006.
41. Plevritis SK, Kurian AW, Sigal BM, et al: Cost-effectiveness of screening *BRCA1/2* mutation carriers with breast magnetic resonance imaging, *JAMA* 295:2374–2384, 2006.
42. Lee JM, McMahon PM, Kong CY, et al: Cost-effectiveness of breast MR imaging and screen-film mammography for screening BRCA1 gene mutation carriers, *Radiology* 254:793–800, 2010.
43. Feig S: Cost-effectiveness of mammography, MRI, and ultrasonography for breast cancer screening, *Radiol Clin North Am* 48:879–891, 2010.
44. Kriege M, Brekelmans CT, Boetes C, et al: Efficacy of MRI and mammography for breast-cancer screening in women with a familial or genetic predisposition, *N Engl J Med* 351:427–437, 2004.
45. Warner E, Plewes DB, Hill KA, et al: Surveillance of *BRCA1* and *BRCA2* mutation carriers with magnetic resonance imaging, ultrasound, mammography, and clinical breast examination, *JAMA* 292:1317–1325, 2004.
46. Hagen AI, Kvistad KA, Maehle L, et al: Sensitivity of MRI versus conventional screening in the diagnosis of *BRCA*-associated breast cancer in a national prospective series, *Breast* 16:367–374, 2007.

CHAPTER 5

MRI Features of Ductal Carcinoma in Situ

Virginia M. Molleran

Breast MRIDuctal carcinoma in situ (DCIS) now makes up 20% to 30% of newly diagnosed breast cancers,[1] an increase in detection that is largely attributed to the advent of screening mammography. Before the advent of screening mammography, DCIS made up about 5% of breast cancers. DCIS is defined as intraductal malignancy that does not extend beyond the basement membrane, and therefore—at least theoretically—has no propensity to metastasize. It is not considered an immediate, life-threatening disease. However, it can progress to invasive disease and can also harbor invasive disease that may not be evident with clinical evaluation or conventional imaging. Thus accurate detection and characterization of DCIS may ultimately have a significant impact on breast cancer survival. Magnetic resonance imaging (MRI) is a highly sensitive imaging tool for detecting invasive breast carcinoma, and it is also very effective for identifying DCIS.

Pathology and Natural History of Ductal Carcinoma in Situ

DCIS is a biologically diverse disease. Traditionally, DCIS classification was based on architectural features and divided into two categories based on the presence or absence of comedo necrosis (Figure 5.1).Those without comedo necrosis were further categorized as cribriform, solid, papillary, or micropapillary. However, this categorization is relatively subjective, leading to pathologic inconsistencies and is also not predictive of the potential for recurrence or progression to invasive disease.[2]

Classification based on tumor grade and the presence or absence of necrosis is more predictive of a potential for tumors to recur. Multiple classification schemes based on nuclear grade and the presence or absence of necrosis have been proposed, but investigators have not arrived at a single, universally accepted classification scheme.

High-grade and non–high-grade DCIS behave differently and have different imaging features on mammography. Most (90%) of DCIS detected with mammography is seen as microcalcifications, but the entire lesion may not calcify.[3] Low-grade DCIS is typically associated with amorphous calcifications, whereas high-grade DCIS is more typically associated with pleomorphic and fine linear branching calcifications (Figures 5.2 and 5.3). However, the mammographic features overlap substantially, and the grade of DCIS cannot reliably be determined by its mammographic features.[4] High-grade lesions are more consistently associated with calcifications; low-grade lesions are more likely to be mammographically occult and more likely to be underestimated in extent by image readers.[5] The degree of underestimation has been shown to be less with higher-grade comedo-type DCIS than for lower-grade micropapillary/cribriform type.[6] A masslike appearance is also possible and may be directly caused by tumor or may be caused by periductal fibrosis or elastosis.

Only 30% to 40% of invasive cancer contains calcifications. Because DCIS is a probable precursor to invasive ductal carcinoma, it has been postulated that the majority of DCIS is not calcified and not detected by mammography.[7]

DCIS grading is similar to that for invasive cancer with low, high, and intermediate grades. Low-grade lesions contain monotonous-appearing cells with small nuclei, minimal nuclear pleomorphism, and infrequent mitoses. Cell polarity with respect to the basement membrane is well preserved. High-grade lesions consist of cells with large pleomorphic nuclei and frequent mitoses, and comedo necrosis is frequently present. Intermediate-grade lesions do not have features of either low- or high-grade lesions[5,8] (Figure 5.4). Lesions that are heterogeneous in grade are assigned the highest grade present.

Limited information exists about the natural history of DCIS because most is excised. Studies looking at patients with untreated DCIS (probably initially diagnosed as benign with the diagnosis then changed to DCIS after pathologic reevaluation) show a 30% to 50% rate of progression to invasive cancer.[1] Progression to invasive cancer can occur with all nuclear grades, but low-grade lesions seem to progress more slowly than high-grade lesions.[9] As yet, a reliable method has not been found for differentiating lesions that will become invasive from those that will not. However, molecular and genetic evidence exists that high-grade DCIS probably progresses to high-grade invasive cancer and low-grade DCIS probably progresses to low-grade invasive cancer.[10]

DCIS has an excellent prognosis, with 10-year mortality after excision or mastectomy of 2%.[11] Treatment is mastectomy or lumpectomy, generally with radiation.

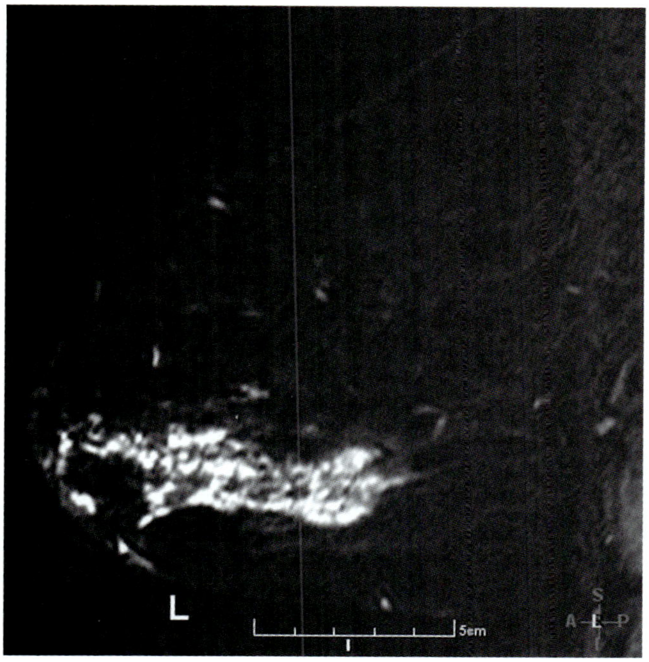

FIGURE 5.1 Sagittal T1-weighted postcontrast subtraction image. High-grade DCIS with comedo necrosis shows as segmental non–mass-like (NME) with clumped internal enhancement pattern.

Adjunctive pharmacotherapy can also be used. In the NSABP B-24 trial of lumpectomy followed by breast irradiation with or without tamoxifen, the drug decreased the local recurrence rate for DCIS (8% with tamoxifen vs. 11.1% without).[9] Controversy exists over the need for sentinel node biopsy because, by definition, DCIS is not invasive and so would not be expected to cause nodal metastases; however, axillary nodal metastases are found in 5% to 15% of patients with DCIS.[12] Presumably, metastases developed after the pathologist missed the foci of invasion.

When DCIS recurs, it recurs as invasive cancer in 50% of cases.[13] The reported range for progression to invasive cancer is 14% to 75%. Factors that increase the likelihood of recurrence include young patient age, presence of risk factors for breast cancer, high tumor grade, presence of necrosis, and large lesion size. Evidence is inconsistent that patients with human epidermal growth factor receptor 2 (HER2)-positive tumors and estrogen receptor (ER)-negative tumors have a poorer prognosis.[14]

The most important risk factor for DCIS recurrence is the presence of positive surgical margins after resection.[15] However, universal agreement has not been reached on adequate margin width. Margin widths of 1 to 3 mm have been variably reported as adequate,[16] with the lowest risk of recurrence with a margin width of 10 mm.[17]

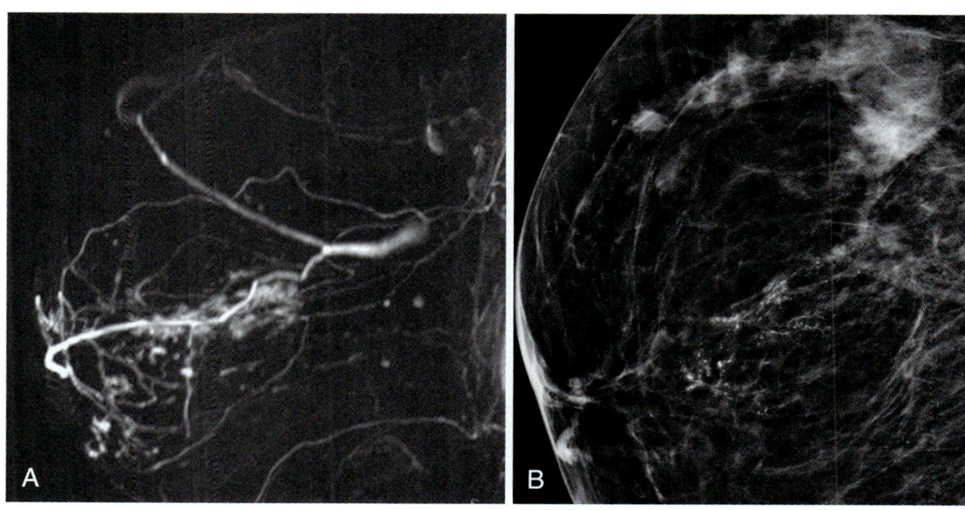

FIGURE 5.2 A-B, A maximum-intensity projection (MIP) MRI image showing branching segmental NME corresponding closely to the distribution of highly suspicious, fine pleomorphic and linear-branching calcifications on mammography.

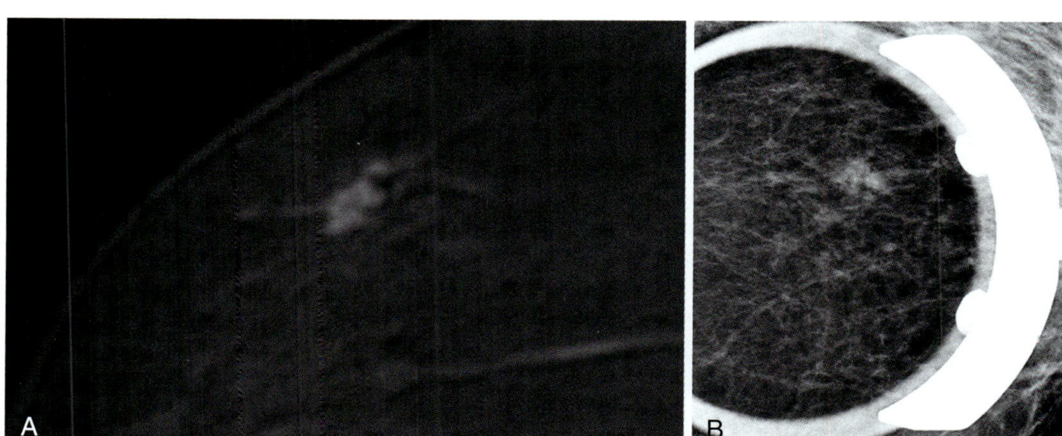

FIGURE 5.3 High-grade DCIS representing as a small, irregular mass on MRI (**A**) and mammography (**B**). Associated faint calcifications were visible mammographically.

MRI Morphologic Features

The most common morphologic feature of DCIS on MRI imaging is non–mass-like enhancement (NME), shown in Figure 5.5. NME is described in the American College of Radiology Breast Imaging Reporting and Data System (BI-RADS) lexicon as enhancement that is not a mass but still is discrete from normal surrounding breast tissue.[18] It is characterized by its distribution and pattern of internal enhancement. In the literature, NME is the reported lesion type in 40% to 82% of DCIS cases,[7,19-25] with most studies showing NME in more than half of all DCIS cases.[7,19,20,22-25] The reported frequencies of distribution types are somewhat variable. This can be attributed to the relatively subjective nature of application of the BI-RADS lexicon descriptors. For example, the same lesion could be described as either a focal area or segmental enhancement by different observers. Although any distribution pattern can be seen, segmental enhancement is the most common.[5,20,23] The most commonly reported pattern of internal enhancement for NME lesions is clumped enhancement (Figure 5.6).[20,23,24] Clumped enhancement can be described as closely associated, rounded areas of enhancement reminiscent of cobblestones. DCIS appears as a mass in 14% to 60% of cases.[7,20,21,23,24] Mass margins are most commonly described as irregular.

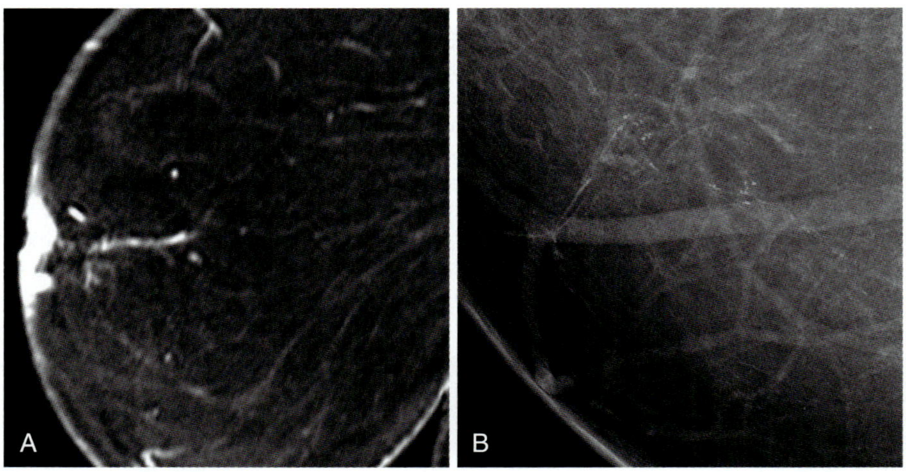

FIGURE 5.4 **A,** Intermediate-grade DCIS with cribriform and solid architecture presenting as very thin linear NME with persistent enhancement on MRI, corresponding in distribution to linearly distributed calcifications seen on mammography (**B**).

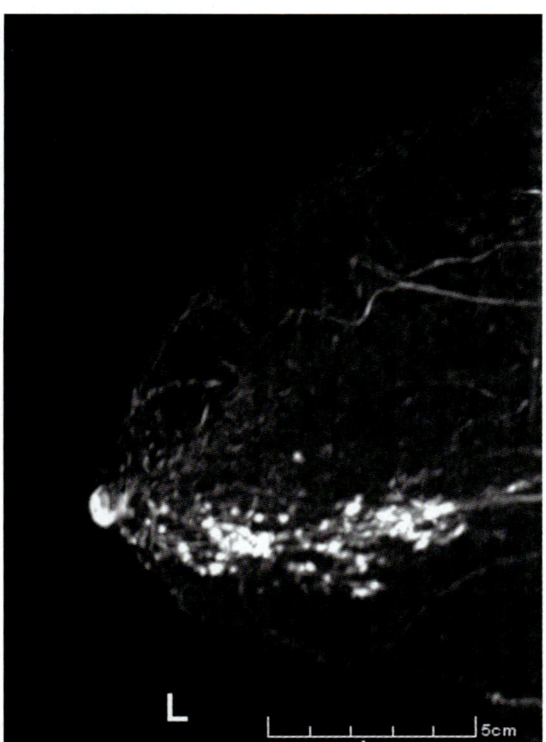

FIGURE 5.5 MRI MIP image shows DCIS as segmental NME with clumped internal enhancement.

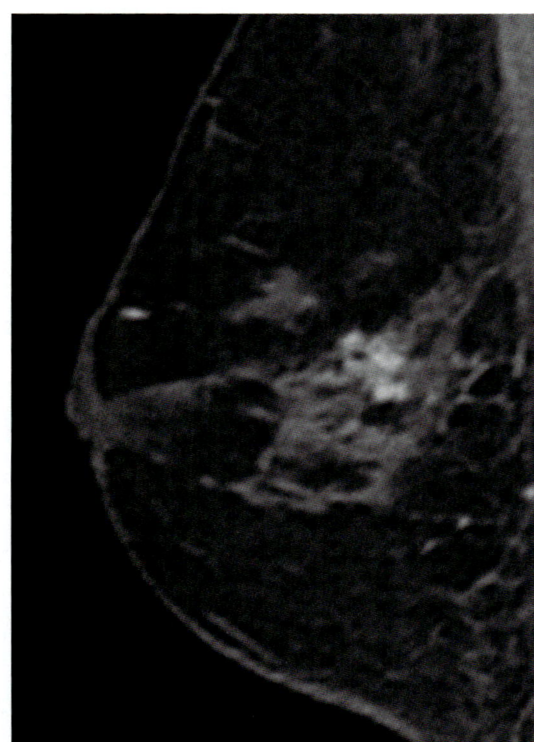

FIGURE 5.6 Intermediate grade DCIS is seen on MRI as a focal area of clumped enhancement.

Clustered Ring Enhancement

Clustered ring enhancement (Figure 5.7) has recently been described as an internal enhancement pattern associated with NME that appears to have a strong correlation with DCIS. Clustered ring enhancement was first described by Tozaki in 2006[26] and consists of conglomerate, small, round, hypointense structures surrounded by enhancement. Histologically, this pattern has been shown to correlate with crowded, DCIS-filled ducts,[26] with the enhancement postulated to correspond to the periductal stroma and duct wall.[27] The reported positive predictive value for malignancy with this finding ranges from 67% to 96%.[27-30] In one study,[27] 28 of 51 malignancies (55%) with clustered ring enhancement were DCIS. In 16 of 23 invasive cancers with clustered ring enhancement, associated DCIS made up 50% or more of the tumor. In another study,[29] clustered ring enhancement was seen in 74% of malignancies presenting as segmental enhancement (positive predictive value, 83%). No clustered ring enhancement was found in six of seven tubular or lobular cancers in the study. However, seven of eight high-risk lesions (atypical ductal hyperplasia and multiple micropapillomas) also showed clustered ring enhancement. The authors postulate that this may be secondary to the lesion's intraductal nature.

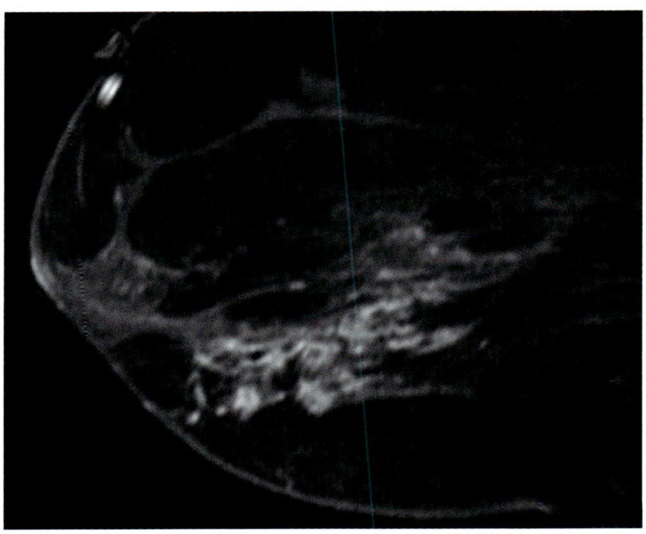

FIGURE 5.7 MRI image showing DCIS with areas of clustered ring enhancement.

Kinetic Features

In terms of kinetic characteristics, DCIS frequently shows features similar to invasive cancer but may have a greater propensity toward slower enhancement and persistent and plateau curves than invasive cancer (Figure 5.8). Van Goethem and coworkers[21] compared 49 cases of pure DCIS with 213 cases of enhancing invasive carcinoma. DCIS showed washout kinetics slightly less frequently than invasive cancer: 53.8% for pure DCIS versus 65.3% for enhancing invasive carcinoma; 60.9% of DCIS cases reached peak enhancement after 3 minutes, whereas most invasive masses showed peak enhancement between 1 and 3 minutes. The only statistically significant kinetic parameter differentiating between DCIS and invasive cancer was signal intensity increase of more than 100%, which was seen in 76.9% of DCIS and 91.1% of invasive cancer. Other studies have demonstrated similar results: 50% to 78% of DCIS cases showed suspicious kinetics with rapid initial uptake of contrast and delayed phase washout- or plateau-curves.[24,25,31] Another study showed a similar distribution of delayed phase curves (57.5% showing washout or plateau curves), but only 25% showed strong initial phase uptake.[22] These results imply that a meaningful proportion of DCIS lesions will show kinetic features *not* typical of malignancy.

Jansen and colleagues[32] correlated the MRI morphologic and kinetic features of 79 cases of pure DCIS with their nuclear grade and mammographic appearance. Most (68%) had rapid initial phase enhancement. Delayed phase curves were variable, with 44% showing washout curves and the remainder somewhat evenly divided between persistent and plateau curves. However, when the cases were grouped according to their mammographic features, delayed-phase curve type and kinetic parameters differed significantly, with the cases that showed masses mammographically much more likely to exhibit washout curves than did the cases showing calcifications mammographically. Cases presenting as mammographic masses also tended to reach peak enhancement earlier than cases presenting as calcifications: 90% of masses showed washout curves (Figure 5.9), and the average time to peak enhancement for masses was

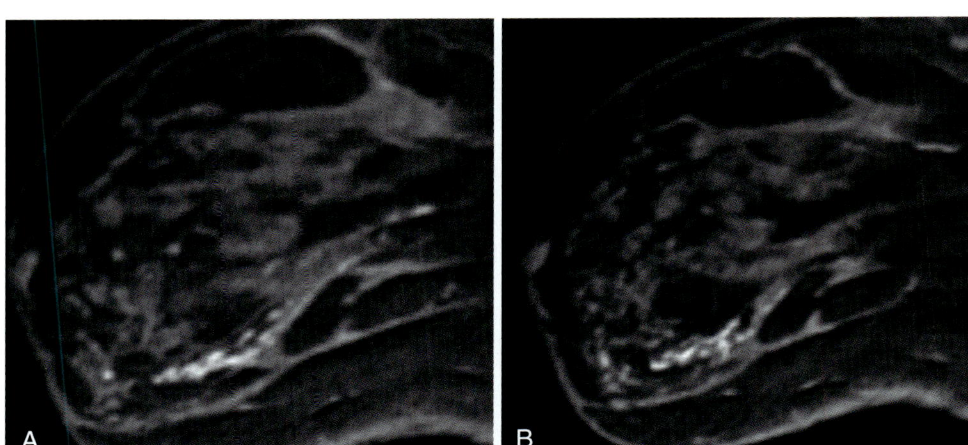

FIGURE 5.8 A and B, Contiguous sagittal T1-weighted post-contrast images. DCIS is seen on MRI as linear NME with persistent enhancement curves.

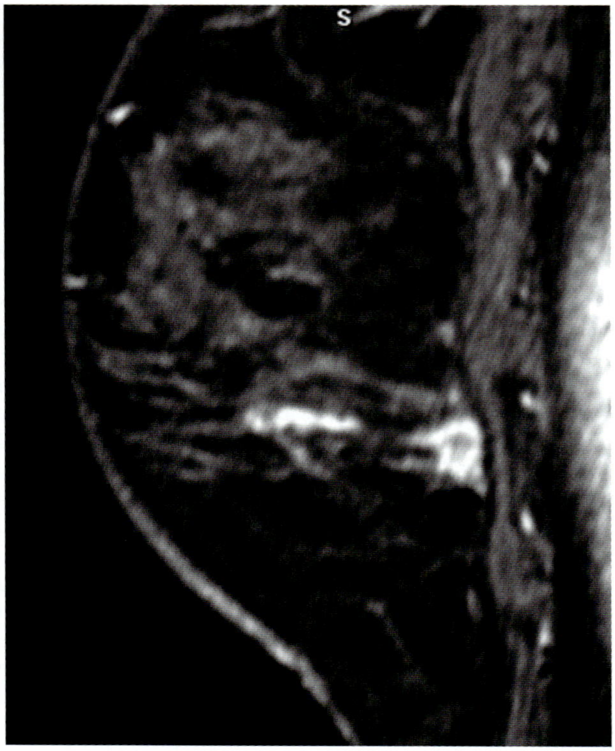

FIGURE 5.9 Linear NME shows on MRI with persistent enhancement adjacent to an irregular rimmed, enhancing mass with washout. Invasive ductal carcinoma with associated DCIS was found at mastectomy.

just under 2 minutes. Forty-five percent of cases with fine linear, fine pleomorphic, or fine linear-branching calcifications showed washout curves, with average time to peak enhancement just under 3.5 minutes. Only 22% of cases presenting as amorphous or indistinct calcifications showed washout curves, and their average time to peak enhancement was 4.4 minutes. Similarly, Vag and colleagues[33] showed a greater tendency for DCIS lesions present as masses on MRI (90.9%) to exhibit washout curves than did cases presenting as NME (38.3%).

In another study, including 403 malignant lesions and 171 benign lesions, Jansen and coworkers[34] compared the kinetic features of benign and malignant masses and NME. Malignant masses were significantly more likely to show faster contrast uptake, shorter time to peak enhancement, and stronger washout curves than benign masses. However, the only statistically significant difference between benign and malignant nonmass lesions was in their signal enhancement ratio (SER), which is a measure of contrast washout relative to the first postcontrast scan. Benign lesions showed a lower average SER (0.76) than the SER of malignant lesions (0.93). Because DCIS shows a greater tendency than invasive cancer to present as NME, it follows that it would have a greater tendency toward less suspicious enhancement than invasive cancer. Although DCIS may show typically malignant kinetic features, particularly when appearing as a mass, these results underscore the importance of not dismissing NME because of benign kinetic features.

Why Does Ductal Carcinoma in Situ Enhance?

Invasive tumors need to create a vascular supply to continue growing. This is probably also true for DCIS, although the mechanism is less clear. In invasive tumors, neoangiogenesis is mediated by vascular endothelial growth factor (VEGF) as well as other angiogenic and antiangiogenic factors.[35] VEGF has been shown to correlate with both increased microvessel density and poorer prognosis in invasive cancer.[36] Tumor angiogenesis is also an independent prognostic factor in breast cancer.[36] An increased number of microvessels has been correlated with more rapid uptake of contrast in breast MRI.[5] Therefore one may postulate that a greater degree of contrast enhancement on MRI would indicate poorer prognosis.

There is no clear relationship between VEGF and microvessel density in DCIS,[36] and in situ tumor angiogenesis may not be the same as angiogenesis seen in invasive tumors.[35] In invasive tumors, the neovascularity is seen interspersed among tumor cells, presumably the result of angiogenic factors produced by the tumor cells. In DCIS, the neovascularity is seen in the surrounding stroma and may be the result of angiogenic factors produced by the stromal cells. The neovascularity in DCIS can occur in two patterns: a ring or cuff of vessels immediately underlying the basement membrane and surrounding the duct or more diffusely dispersed microvessels in the stroma. The diffuse pattern has been associated with high histologic grade and comedo necrosis. The periductal pattern (cuff of vessels) has been shown to increase with progression of the epithelial abnormality (from low grade to high grade) and invasion.[5]

Based on this pattern, one would correctly expect that the enhancement in DCIS predominantly occurs in the surrounding stroma rather than in the ducts themselves. This has been demonstrated by Kanemaki and colleagues,[37] who performed high-resolution MRI imaging of 11 patients with DCIS using a microscopy coil with a resolution of 0.137 mm. Enhanced areas in DCIS correlated with periductal stroma that showed histologic changes such as neovascularization, inflammatory cell infiltrate, and edema. Within enhanced areas, internal hypointense structures correlated with tumor-involved ducts containing tumor, debris, and necrotic material. Sizes of these hypointense structures on imaging correlated with diameters of the ducts seen histologically.

Angiogenesis in DCIS may also occur because of a disruption of the myoepithelial layer in the lesion.[5] Myoepithelial cells not only form part of a physical barrier between the epithelium and stroma but also secrete angiogenesis inhibitors. Jansen[38] has shown, using a mouse model, that gadolinium crosses the basement membrane and accumulates within ducts in DCIS. The authors hypothesize that this may be due to increased permeability of the basement membrane, perhaps caused by protease secretion by cancer cells.

MRI Appearance and Ductal Carcinoma in Situ Grade

High- and low-grade DCIS have both different clinical courses and a tendency toward different features on mammography. Therefore it would be reasonable to expect that their presentation on MRI would be different as well,

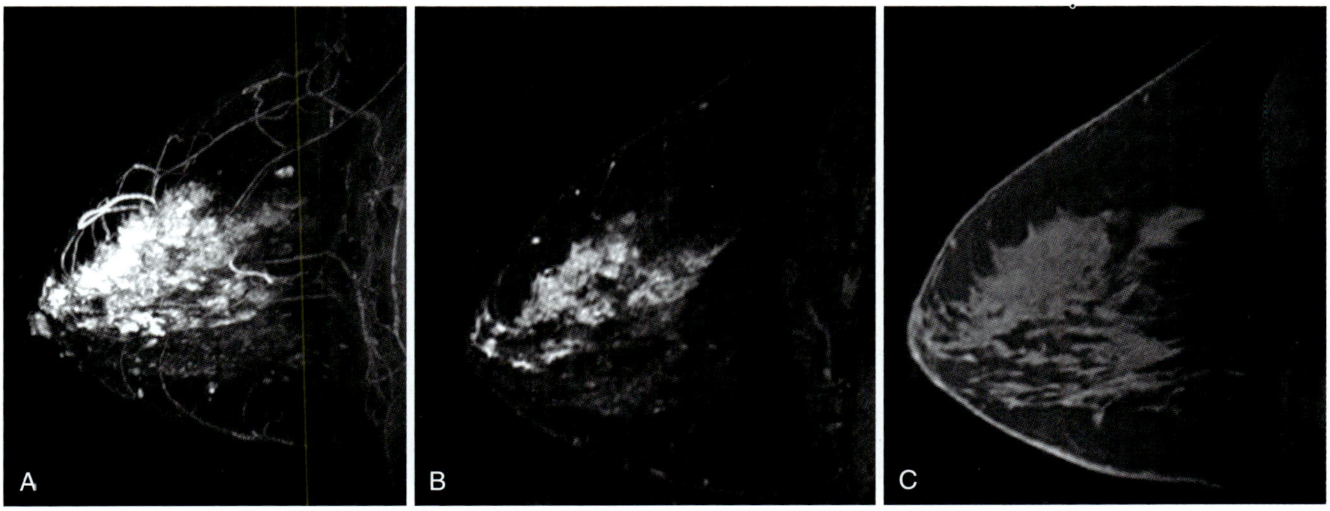

FIGURE 5.10 **A,** In this MIP MRI image, DCIS is seen as regional enhancement. Mammography was negative. This lesion was stable from an MRI performed 9 months earlier. **B,** Subtracted image shows a heterogeneous internal enhancement pattern. **C,** On fat-suppressed precontrast T1-weighted image, there is loss of the normal breast architecture with slightly lower T1 signal.

especially because MRI imaging provides more physiologic information related to contrast enhancement. Results of studies evaluating MRI features based on tumor grade have been mixed. One of the largest studies evaluating this issue[32] showed no correlation between MRI lesion morphology or enhancement parameters and nuclear grade. This study included 79 cases of pure DCIS. A later study of 31 patients with pure DCIS[24] also showed no significant difference in MRI morphology, tumor size, and kinetic characteristics between high-grade and non–high-grade DCIS.

Other studies have shown differences related to tumor grade and other biological markers, with differences in kinetic parameters seen more frequently than differences in morphologic parameters. In a study of 45 cases in 2005, Esserman and coworkers[39] found that lesions with clumped enhancement were more likely than lesions with heterogeneous enhancement to be high-grade lesions. In that study, focal lesions tended to be small, low-grade, ER-positive tumors. Lesions with regional and multiregional distribution and heterogeneous enhancement tended to be ER-positive, and MRI readers were prone to overestimate their size (Figure 5.10). The authors postulate that difficulties with accurate size estimates may be because of the DCIS being scattered and hard to measure pathologically or due to associated proliferative changes such as sclerosing adenosis, atypical hyperplasia, and fibrocystic change. Large homogeneous lesions tended to be high-grade tumors with associated inflammatory changes. Liu and Peng[19] found that high-grade DCIs was more common in nonmass lesions than mass lesions. ER status and HER2 status did not differ significantly between mass and nonmass lesions.

Several studies have shown differences in kinetic parameters.[31,33,36] In a study of 74 cases of pure DCIS, Facius and coworkers[31] found that grade 2 and 3 lesions more often showed an enhancement pattern considered typical of malignancy (rapid initial increase to 100% in the first 90 seconds with delayed phase plateau or washout than grade 1 lesions. Vag and colleagues[33] evaluated 47 cases of pure DCIS and found a trend for lesions with higher nuclear grades to show more suspicious kinetics, but this was not statistically significant.

Probably the most convincing evidence of possible differences in MRI presentation between low- and high-grade lesions comes from a large screening study by Kuhl and coworkers[6] in 2007, which included 167 cases of pure DCIS. They found that MRI had a much greater sensitivity for high-grade DCIS than mammography—98% for MRI versus 52% for mammography. They also found that for low-grade DCIS, "each method detected a sizable number of low-grade DCIS that went undetected by the other imaging method." Eighty-three percent of the DCIS lesions depicted only by mammography were either low or intermediate grade. The sensitivity of mammography decreased with higher nuclear grade. Mammography was more sensitive in detecting high-grade DCIS with necrosis than high-grade DCIS without necrosis; by contrast, the sensitivity of MRI did not depend on the presence or absence of necrosis. Mammography did a better job of detecting smaller DCIS lesions than did MRI.

MRI Sensitivity

In early studies, the reported sensitivity of MRI for DCIS was disappointingly low, with reported sensitivity as low as 20%.[7] MRI was considered unreliable for detecting and assessing the extent of DCIS.[40] However, reported MRI sensitivities for DCIS in more recent literature are higher, ranging from 79% to 97% (Table 5.1), and in most cases, MRI sensitivity was significantly higher than that of mammography. This improvement has been attributed largely to greater emphasis on high spatial resolution over high temporal resolution.[40] Improved spatial resolution allows better differentiation of nonmass lesions with kinetic curves that are not suspicious from background parenchymal enhancement. A higher level of radiologist training and experience certainly contributes to this, as well as the use of MRI computer-aided detection software, which can enhance lesion identification by allowing better three-dimensional and kinetic evaluation.

Diffusion-Weighted MRI

Diffusion-weighted imaging is a relatively new MRI technique that quantifies the diffusion of water molecules in tissues. This diffusion is affected by microenvironmental factors, including tissue cellularity and the presence and extent of intact restrictive cell membranes. Water molecules can more freely diffuse in less cellular tissues or in tissues in which the cell membranes have been disrupted. More dense cellular tissues, such as malignant tumors, allow less diffusion (Figure 5.11). Diffusion-weighted imaging is a noncontrast technique relying on applied gradients to cause phase shifts that vary with position. As diffusing water molecules travel farther from their point of origin, they become increasingly out of phase, resulting in signal loss. As a result, tissues with less restricted diffusion will lose signal, and tissues with more restricted diffusion will have higher signal intensity.

From the diffusion-weighted images, an apparent diffusion coefficient (ADC) map can be calculated. ADC is a measure of the average area covered by a molecule per unit time. The ADC will be lower for tissues with more restricted diffusion, and, thus, malignancies will have lower ADC values than benign tissues. Information obtained from diffusion-weighted imaging has the potential to increase the specificity of breast MRI.

Studies have confirmed a lower ADC in invasive breast carcinoma than in normal tissue.[46-49] However, diffusion-weighted imaging may not be expected to perform as well in DCIS, in which there is less cellularity (particularly in low-grade tumors) and more interspersed normal tissue. DCIS tends to have ADC values that lie between those of invasive cancers and normal tissues.[46,47,49] There has been interest in using diffusion-weighted imaging to identify either less aggressive, low-grade DCIS (and thus spare patients from unnecessary treatment) or more aggressive, high-grade lesions. In a pilot study involving 22 cases of DCIS, Iima and colleagues[46] found that the mean ADCs for high- and intermediate-grade DCIS were significantly lower than those for low-grade lesions, and the mean ADC for low-grade DCIS was lower than that for normal breast tissue. Rahbar and coworkers[50] found that non–high-grade DCIS exhibited greater diffusion-weighted signal intensity than high-grade DCIS, but they found no difference in ADC values.

Conclusion

MRI is a highly sensitive imaging modality for detecting DCIS. DCIS is a heterogeneous disease with a spectrum of clinical behaviors ranging from high-grade lesions that show fairly rapid progression to invasive disease to low-grade lesions that, if left untreated, may never become

Table 5.1 Reported Sensitivities of MRI for Detecting Ductal Carcinoma in Situ

Reference	Year	Number	Sensitivity of MRI	Sensitivity of Mammography
Marcotte-Bloch et al.[23]	2011	32/33	97%	NS
Tozacki[44]	2011	148/156	95%	NS
Chan et al.[24]	2010	27/31	87%	74%
Santamaria et al.[22]	2008	63/86	73%	93%
Uematsu et al.[45]	2008	23/24	96%	58%
Kim et al.[43]	2007	68/72	94%	86%
Kuhl et al.[6]	2007	153/167	92%	56%
Rosen et al.[20]	2007	55/64	86%	NS
Bazzocchi et al.[42]	2006	26/33	79%	NA*
Menell et al.[7]	2005	29/33	88%	27%
Van Goethem et al.[21]	2005	40/49	82%	61%
Berg et al.[41]	2004	34/38	89%	55%

NS, not stated.
Note: Number is the number of cases of DCIS detected with MRI/total number of DCIS cases.
*All DCIS cases were obtained from mammographically detected calcifications.

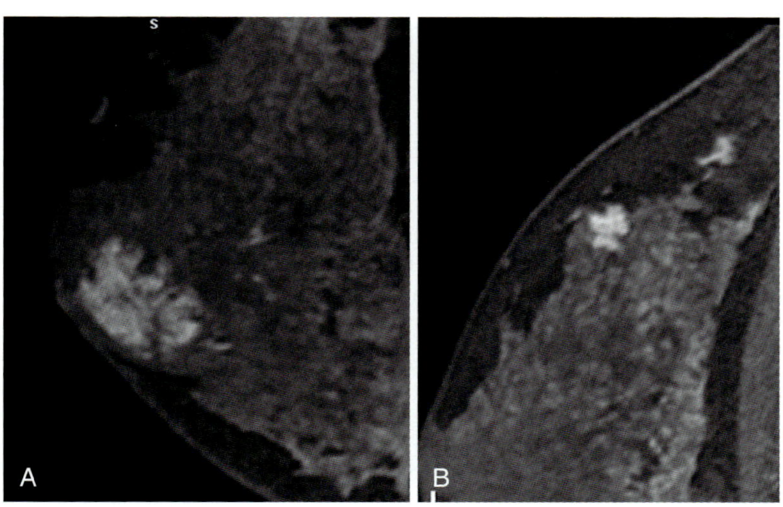

FIGURE 5.11 Sagittal T1-weighted post-contrast images of the right (A) and left (B) of a 21-year-old female shows a malignant phyllodes tumor. MRI was performed because of a family history of a paternal grandmother with breast cancer at age 21 and showed a small irregular mass in the left breast (**B**). MRI-guided biopsy showed DCIS.

clinically evident. The MRI features of DCIS reflect its intraductal nature with NME, with segmental distribution being its most common presentation. Enhancement kinetics are more variable, with a greater propensity to show kinetic patterns more typical of benign pathology than invasive disease. So far, definitive imaging differences between high- and low-grade DCIS lesions have not been found, and further studies leading to the ability to preoperatively determine tumor grade and aggressiveness would be useful because they could differentiate lesions likely to progress to invasive cancers from those that may never become invasive, thereby sparing the patient unnecessary therapy. Advanced MRI imaging techniques such as diffusion-weighted imaging also may contribute significantly to characterizing DCIS.

References

1. Jansen SA: Ductal carcinoma in situ: detection, diagnosis, and characterization with magnetic resonance imaging, *Semin Ultrasound CT M* 306–318, 2011.
2. Tsikitis VL, Chung MA: Biology of ductal carcinoma in situ classification based on biologic potential, *Am J Clin Oncol* 29:305–310, 2006.
3. Kuhl CK: Why do purely intraductal cancers enhance on breast MR images? *Radiology* 253:281–283, 2009.
4. Slanetz PJ, Giardino AA, Oyama T, et al: Mammographic appearance of ductal carcinoma in situ does not reliably predict histologic subtype, *Breast J* 7:417–421, 2001.
5. Takayuki Y, Naoko M, Mika W, et al: Radiologic-pathologic correlation of ductal carcinoma in situ, *RadioGraphics* 30:1183–1198, 2010.
6. Kuhl CK, Schrading S, Bieling HB, et al: MRI for diagnosis of pure ductal carcinoma in situ: a prospective observational study, *Lancet* 370:485–492, 2007.
7. Menell JH, Morris EA, Dershaw DD, Abramson AF, Brogi E, Liberman L: Determination of the presence and extent of pure ductal carcinoma in situ by mammography and magnetic resonance imaging, *Breast J* 11:382–390, 2005.
8. Mossa-Basha M, Fundaro GM, Shah BA, Ali S, Pantelic MV: Ductal carcinoma in situ of the breast: MR imaging findings with histopathologic correlation, *RadioGraphics* 30:1673–1687, 2010.
9. Patani N, Khaled Y, Al Reefy S, Mokbel K: Ductal carcinoma in-situ: an update for clinical practice, *Surg Oncol* 20:e23–e31, 2011.
10. Bombonati A, Sgroi DC: The molecular pathology of breast cancer progression, *J Pathol* 223:307–317, 2011.
11. Virnig BA, Tuttle TM, Shamilyan T, Kane RL, et al: Ductal carcinoma in situ of the breast: A systemic review of incidence, treatment and outcome, *J Natl Cancer Inst* 102:170–178, 2010.
12. Amersi F, Hansen NM: The benefits and limitations of sentinel lymph node biopsy, *Curr Treat Options Oncol* 7:141–151, 2006.
13. Kuerer HM, et al: Ductal carcinoma in situ: state of the science and roadmap to advance the field, *J Clin Oncol* 27:279–288, 2009.
14. Shamliyan T, Wang SY, Virnig BA, et al: Association between patient and tumor characteristics with clinical outcomes in women with ductal carcinoma in situ, *J Natl Cancer Inst Monogr* 41:121–129, 2010.
15. Wang SY, Shamliyan T, Virnig BA, et al: Tumor characteristics as predictors of local recurrence after treatment of ductal carcinoma in situ: a meta-analysis, *Breast Cancer Res Treat* 127:1–14, 2011.
16. Newman LA: Local control of ductal carcinoma in situ based on tumor and patient characteristics: the surgeon's perspective, *J Natl Cancer Inst Monographs* 152–157, 2010.
17. Pinder SE, Ellis IO: The diagnosis and management of pre-invasive breast disease: ductal carcinoma in situ (DCIS) and atypical ductal hyperplasia(ADH)–current definitions and classification, *Breast Cancer Res* 5:254–257, 2003.
18. Ikeda DM, Hylton NM, Kuhl CK: *Breast imaging reporting and data system, BiRADS: magnetic resonance imaging*, Reston, Va, 2003, American College of Radiology.
19. Liu H, Peng W: MRI morphological classification of ductal carcinoma in situ (DCIS) correlating with different biological behavior, *Eur J Radiol* 81:214–217, 2012.
20. Rosen EL, Smith-Foley SA, DeMartini WB, Eby PR, Peacock S: Lehman CD. BI-RADS MRI enhancement characteristics of ductal carcinoma in situ, *Breast J* 13:545–550, 2007.
21. Van Goethem M, Schelfout K, Kersschot E, et al: Comparison of MRI features of different grades of DCIS and invasive carcinoma of the breast, *JBR-BTR* 88:225–232, 2005.
22. Santamaria G, Velasco M, Farrus B, Zanon G, Fernandez PL Preoperative MRI of pure intraductal breast carcinoma—a valuable adjunct to mammography in assessing cancer extent, *Breast* 17:186–194, 2008.
23. Marcotte-Bloch C, Balu-Maestro C, Chamorey E, et al: MRI for the size assessment of pure ductal carcinoma in situ (DCIS): a prospective study of 33 patients, *Eur J Radiol* 77:462–467, 2011.
24. Chan S, Chen JH, Agrawal G, et al: Characterization of pure ductal carcinoma in situ on dynamic contrast-enhanced MR imaging: do non high grade and high grade show different imaging features?, *J Oncol* Jan 2010.
25. Neubauer H, Li M, Kuehne-Heid R, Schneider A, Kaiser WA: High grade and non-high grade ductal carcinoma *in situ* on dynamic MR mammography: characteristic findings for signal increase and morphological pattern of enhancement, *Br J Radiol* 76:3–12, 2003.
26. Tozaki M: Fukuda K. High-spatial-resolution MRI of non-masslike breast lesions: interpretation model based on BI-RADS MRI descriptors, *Am J Roentgenol* 187:330–337, 2006.
27. Uematsu T, Kasami M: High-spatial-resolution 3-T breast MRI of non-masslike enhancement lesions: an analysis of their features as significant predictors of malignancy, *Am J Roentgenol* 198:1223–1230, 2012.
28. Sakamoto N, Tozaki M, Higa K, et al: Categorization of non-mass-like breast lesions detected by MRI, *Breast Cancer* 15:241–246, 2008.
29. Yuen S, Uematsu T, Masako K, Uchida Y, Nishimura T: Segmental enhancement on breast MR images: differential diagnosis and diagnostic strategy, *Eur Radiol* 18:2067–2075, 2008.
30. Tozaki M, Igarashi T, Fukuda K: Breast MRI using the vibe sequence: clustered ring enhancement in the differential diagnosis of lesions showing non-masslike enhancement, *Am J Roentgenol* 187:313–321, 2006.
31. Facius M, Renz DM, Neubauer H, et al: Characteristics of ductal carcinoma in situ in magnetic resonance imaging, *Clin Imaging* 31:394–400, 2007.
32. Jansen SA, Newstead GM, Abe H, Shimauchi A, Schmidt RA, Karczmar GS: Pure ductal carcinoma in situ: kinetic and morphologic mr characteristics compared with mammographic appearance and nuclear grade, *Radiology* 245:684–691, 2007.
33. Vag T, Baltzer PA, Dietzel M, et al: Kinetic characteristics of ductal carcinoma in situ (DCIS) in dynamic breast MRI using computer-assisted analysis, *Acta Radiol* 51:955–995, Nov 2010.
34. Jansen SA, Shimauchi A, Zak L, Fan X, Karczmar GS, Newstead GM: The diverse pathology and kinetics of mass, nonmass, and focus enhancement on MR imaging of the breast, *J Magn Reson Imaging* 33:1382–1389, 2011.
35. Rice A, Quinn CM: Angiogenesis, thrombospondin, and ductal carcinoma in situ of the breast, *J Clin Pathol* 55:569–574, 2002
36. Oshida K, Nagashima T, Ueda T, et al: Pharmacokinetic analysis of ductal carcinoma in situ of the breast using dynamic MR mammography, *Eur Radiol* 15:1353–1360, 2005.
37. Kanemaki Y, Kurihara Y, Okamoto K, et al: Ductal carcinoma in situ: correlations between high-resolution magnetic resonance imaging and histopathology, *Radiat Med* 25:1–7, 2007.
38. Jansen SA, Paunesku P, Fan X, et al: Ductal carcinoma in situ: x-ray fluorescence microscopy and dynamic contrast-enhanced MR imaging reveals gadolinium uptake within neoplastic mammary ducts in a murine model, *Radiology* 253:399–406, 2009.
39. Esserman LJ, Kumar AS, Herrera AF, et al: Magnetic resonance imaging captures the biology of ductal carcinoma in situ, *J Clin Oncol* 24: 4603–4610, 2006.
40. Lehman CD: Magnetic resonance imaging in the evaluation of ductal carcinoma in situ, *J Natl Cancer Inst Monographs* 150–151, 2010.
41. Berg WA, Gutierrez L, Ness Aiver MS, et al: Diagnostic accuracy of mammography, clinical examination, US, and MR imaging in preoperative assessment of breast cancer, *Radiology* 233:830–849, 2004.
42. Bazzocchi M, Zuiani C, Panizza P, et al: Contrast-enhanced breast MRI in patients with suspicious microcalcifications on mammography: results of a multicenter trial, *Am J Roentgenol* 186:1723–1732, 2006.
43. Kim DY, Moon WK, Cho N, et al: MRI of the breast for the detection and assessment of the size of ductal carcinoma in situ, *Korean J Radiol* 8:32–39, 2007.
44. Tozaki M: BI-RADS-MRI terminology and evaluation of intraductal carcinoma and ductal carcinoma in situ, *Breast Cancer* 20:13–20, 2013.

45. Uematsu T, Yuen S, Kasami M, Uchida Y: Comparison of magnetic resonance imaging, multidetector row computed tomography, ultrasonography, and mammography for tumor extension of breast cancer, *Breast Cancer Res Treat* 112:461–474, 2008.
46. Iima M, Le Bihan D, Okumura R, et al: Apparent diffusion coefficient as an MR imaging biomarker of low-risk ductal carcinoma in situ: a pilot study, *Radiology* 260:364–372, 2011.
47. Partridge SC, DeMartini WB, Kurland BF, Eby PR, White SW, Lehman LD: Quantitative diffusion-weighted imaging as an adjunct to conventional breast MRI for improved positive predictive value, *Am J Roentgenol* 193:1716–1722, 2009.
48. Kul S, Cansu A, Alhan E, Dinc H, Gunes G, Reis A: Contribution of diffusion-weighted imaging to dynamic contrast-enhanced MRI in the characterization of breast tumors, *Am Roentgenol* 196:210–217, 2011.
49. Park MJ, Cha ES, Kang BJ, Ihn YK, Baik JH: The role of diffusion-weighted imaging and the apparent diffusion coefficient (ADC) values for breast tumors, *Korean J Radiol* 8:390–396, 2007.
50. Rahbar HR, Partridge SC, Eby PR, et al: Characterization of ductal carcinoma in situ on diffusion-weighted breast MRI, *Eur Radiol* 21: 2011–2019, 2011.

CHAPTER 6

MRI Features of Invasive Disease

Virginia M. Molleran

Breast magnetic resonance imaging (MRI) has become an important part of the work-up of patients with newly diagnosed breast cancers. Although no large studies have proved a survival advantage, and questions remain as to whether preoperative MRI has reduced re-excision and recurrence rates, the potential benefit of preoperative MRI cannot be questioned. MRI can identify foci of invasive disease with greater sensitivity than mammography or sonography, allowing identification of multicentric and multifocal disease that would otherwise go undetected. Identifying these additional foci may lead to a more extensive lumpectomy than originally planned, or even mastectomy. MRI may also demonstrate axillary lymphadenopathy and chest wall invasion, which can have an impact on surgical management. MRI is also the most accurate modality for monitoring patients undergoing neoadjuvant chemotherapy.

Ductal carcinoma makes up about 85% of all breast cancers. Invasive lobular carcinoma constitutes another 5% to 15%. Special types of breast cancer and sarcoma make up the remainder. These include tubular, medullary, and mucinous carcinomas. Inflammatory carcinoma does not represent a distinct histologic subtype of breast carcinoma, but it is distinguished by its clinical presentation and because its treatment differs from that of other breast cancers. Recognition of these special types of breast cancer may have implications in the management of breast cancer. The mammographic and sonographic features of these special types of breast cancer have been well characterized, but their MRI features are not as widely known. MRI may allow more accurate distinction of the various types of breast cancer than that provided by conventional imaging because it adds physiologic information. This chapter discusses the MRI features of several special types of breast cancer.

MRI of Invasive Lobular Carcinoma

Invasive lobular carcinoma constitutes 5% to 15% of breast cancers. It is characterized by an insidious growth pattern, with uniform, small, round tumor cells, typically infiltrating in single file. This growth pattern is probably the result of a lack of e-cadherin expression, a gene involved in cell-cell cohesion.[1] Lack of e-cadherin expression is one way that invasive lobular carcinoma (ILC) is differentiated histologically from invasive ductal carcinoma (IDC). ILC does not cause a significant desmoplastic reaction and is less commonly associated with calcifications than is IDC. As such, ILC is typically harder to detect during a physical exam, being more likely to present as palpable thickening or skin or nipple retraction than as a discrete palpable mass.[2]

On mammography, lobular carcinoma tends to be iso- or hypodense to breast tissue, limiting its visibility. Although the most common presentation on mammography is a spiculated or ill-defined mass,[3] it is more likely than IDC to present as an asymmetry or architectural distortion.[4] Round or circumscribed masses are uncommon, seen in only 1% to 3% of cases.[3] It is not uncommon for findings to be present on one view only, most commonly the craniocaudal view because of its better compression.[3] Another characteristic finding on mammography is that of a "shrinking" breast. It is thought that the sheet-like infiltrating pattern of the tumor reduces the breast's natural elasticity, allowing for less spreading of the tissue during mammographic compression.[5] Clinically, however, the breast may remain symmetric in size with respect to the other side. Microcalcifications also are uncommon, being reported in 1% to 28% of cases,[11] presumably owing to the absence of associated ductal carcinoma in situ (DCIS).

These factors all contribute to a decreased sensitivity of mammography, and ILC is a well-known cause of false-negative mammography results. The reported sensitivity of mammography ranges from 34% to 92%.[7] But even when mammography detects tumors, it tends to underestimate their size.[8]

Ultrasound has a higher sensitivity for ILC than mammography, ranging from 68% to 98%.[7,9] Imaged by ultrasound, ILC most commonly appears as an irregular, hypoechoic mass with ill-defined or spiculated margins and associated acoustic shadowing.[3] The tumor may also appear as shadowing without a discrete mass because of the sheet-like infiltrative nature of the tumor.

Because it can be more difficult to detect both clinically and on imaging than other cancers, ILC is more frequently locally advanced at diagnosis and is generally a larger tumor at the time of presentation than is IDC.[1] It also has a higher incidence of multifocality and multicentricity than does IDC.[3] Patients with ILC are more likely to have positive surgical margins after lumpectomy,[10] and although ILC often manifests with larger tumors, overall patient survival

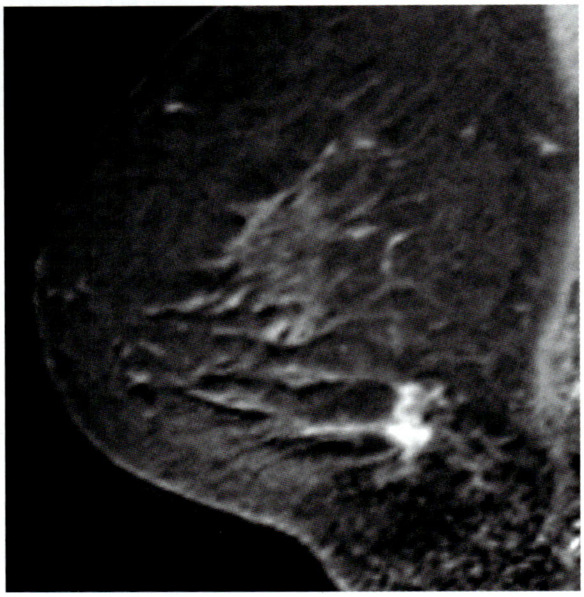

FIGURE 6.1 Invasive lobular carcinoma appears as an irregular mass with slow early phase enhancement and persistent delayed phase kinetics.

is similar to or slightly better than that of patients with IDC.[1] Despite its more infiltrative growth pattern, ILC is very similar to IDC in its MRI appearance (Figure 6.1 through Figure 6.5). The most common MRI presentation is an irregularly shaped mass with irregular or spiculated margins.[8,9,11,12] Round masses are rarely described: In a meta-analysis by Mann and colleagues,[8] only 1 out of 143 masses was described as round. Absence of smooth margins was a feature found to be significantly associated with ILC by Stivalet and coworkers[9]; however, a study by Levrini and colleagues[11] found smooth margins in 5 of 13 masses. Mass internal enhancement is most often described as heterogeneous.[12,13] Two studies comparing the morphologic features of ILC with those of IDC on MRI found no significant difference in the distribution of morphologic descriptors between the two.[4,12]

Some investigators have described a *stranding* pattern of tumor enhancement associated with ILC. Qayyum and coworkers[5] described a pattern of multiple, small, enhancing foci with or without interconnecting enhancing strands. This pattern was seen in 62% of their cases and correlated with the histopathologic finding of tumor clusters separated by either normal breast tissue or tumor cells infiltrating in single file between more nodular tumor foci. In 8%, enhancing septa were seen without a dominant focus. A similar pattern of multiple small enhancing foci separated by enhancing strands was reported in a later study by Schelfout and colleagues[14] and seen in 12% of cases. This pattern is concordant with the single file and sheetlike pattern of infiltrative growth seen with ILC. Another common pattern described by Schelfout was a dominant lesion surrounded by multiple small enhancing foci.

In terms of kinetic features, two early studies reported a later peak enhancement for ILC cases with wash-out seen only in a minority of cases.[8] In a later study by Dietzel and coworkers[15] again comparing IDC to ILC, almost all ILCs and IDCs showed intermediate or strong wash-in, but delayed phase wash-out was more common with IDC, present in 72.6% of IDC cases versus 57.4% of ILC cases. Mann and colleagues[4] also compared enhancement kinetics between ILC and IDC. They found that the maximum relative enhancement and the fraction of voxels that showed rapid enhancement were similar between the two groups. However, in the ILC group, a smaller proportion of the tumor showed delayed phase wash-out curves than in the IDC group, and a larger proportion of the tumor showed persistent delayed phase curves. Accordingly, when visual inspection, rather than computer-aided detection (CAD), was used to assess kinetics, wash-out was more frequently seen, but involved a smaller proportion of the tumor in ILC than in IDC. They concluded that ILC enhances slower than IDC, reaching peak enhancement later, but there is no significant difference in the peak enhancement.

ILC has a greater propensity to be multifocal or multicentric than IDC (see Figure 6.5). Additionally, it can be difficult to detect on conventional imaging. These factors make MRI an indispensable tool in preoperative assessment of ILC. As previously discussed, MRI more accurately determines tumor size in lobular carcinoma than does mammography.[6,16] In a meta-analysis by Mann and coworkers,[8] additional ipsilateral malignant lesions were detected only on MRI in 32% of patients with histologically proven ILC. Overall, MRI findings changed management in 28% of cases. In another study of 57 patients with ILC,[17] MRI changed management in 49%, resulting in more extensive surgery in 40% and less extensive surgery in 9%. In a larger study of 267 patients with ILC, investigators reported reduced reexcision rates in patients undergoing breast conservation therapy with preoperative MRI (9%) compared to re-excision rates in those with no preoperative MRI (27%).[18]

Mucinous Carcinoma

Mucinous carcinoma of the breast is an uncommon variety of breast cancer accounting for 1% to 7% of all breast cancers and typically seen in an older age group. Its characteristic feature is production of abundant extracellular mucin, resulting in a histologic appearance of islands of tumor cells floating on pools of mucin. However, the tumor can frequently have a mixed histologic pattern, with variable amounts and distribution of IDC NOS (not otherwise specified). In these cases the tumor is described as *mixed mucinous carcinoma*. The term *pure mucinous carcinoma* is used when less than 10% of the tumor is made up of IDC.[19]

The distinction between pure mucinous carcinoma and mixed mucinous carcinoma is important because pure mucinous carcinoma has a lower likelihood of axillary lymph node metastases and an overall better prognosis than the mixed type. The 10-year survival rate for pure mucinous carcinoma ranges from 87% to 90.4%, and that for mixed mucinous carcinoma ranges from 54% to 66%.[20]

The imaging features of mucinous carcinoma depend on the amount of extracellular mucin present and whether it is pure or mixed with IDC NOS.[20-23] Pure mucinous carcinomas with abundant extracellular mucin are more likely to appear on mammography as a mass with circumscribed

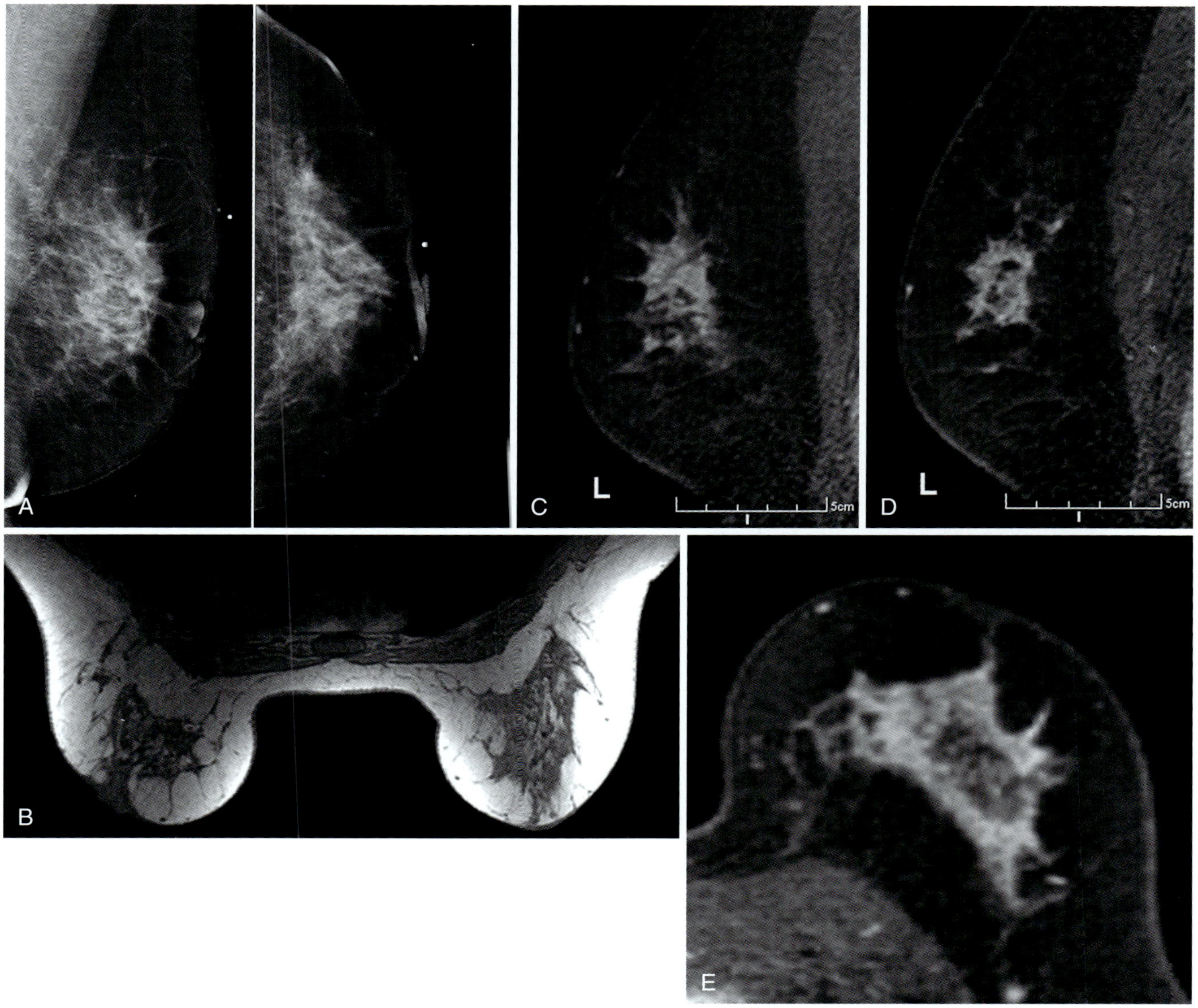

FIGURE 6.2 Invasive lobular carcinoma is illustrated in a 47-year-old woman who presented with left nipple retraction and a palpable left breast mass. **A**, Mammography shows mild nipple retraction on the left but is otherwise negative. **B**, Axial non-fat–suppressed precontrast MRI image shows nipple retraction without other abnormality. **C** and **D**, Sagittal postcontrast MRI images show a large area of NME in regional distribution without discrete mass or architectural distortion. The lesion demonstrated rapid enhancement with plateau and wash-out curves, but predominantly plateau curves. **E**, Axial post-contrast MRI image shows a large area of NME in regional distribution.

or microlobulated margins, whereas mixed tumors usually have indistinct or spiculated margins. Calcifications are uncommon. On ultrasound, mucinous carcinomas may be isoechoic or hypoechoic. Complex mixed cystic and solid masses are frequent. There may be associated acoustic enhancement. This finding is more commonly seen in tumors with abundant mucin.

Several studies have described the MRI features of mucinous carcinoma.[20,24-27] The most characteristic MRI feature of mucinous carcinoma is high T2 signal intensity caused by the high water content of the mucin (Figure 6.6). The tumor may contain areas of iso-intense T2 signal related to fibrous septations and bands or related to areas hemorrhage and necrosis.[20] More solid components of the tumor may also show lower T2 signal intensity.[27] The predominant lesion type is a mass. Mass shape is most frequently lobular and less often round or oval. Mass margins are most frequently smooth but can be irregular.

The internal enhancement pattern depends on the distribution of the cellular elements. A rim enhancement pattern is frequently seen and has been attributed to a peripheral distribution of cellular elements.[26] Otherwise, internal enhancement tends to be heterogeneous and can be attributed to the heterogeneous distribution of cellular elements and mucin in the tumor. Dark internal septations have been described related to thick fibrous septa.[20,26]

Another typical feature of mucinous carcinoma on MRI is slow or persistent enhancement kinetics. This is due to the longer time it takes for contrast to diffuse through the mucin compared with its diffusion in more cellular tumors or in tumors with more fibrous stroma.[27] Rapid enhancement with wash-out can also be seen, although this is less common. In one study,[20] tumors with higher cellular grade tended to have stronger enhancement, and lower-grade tumors tended to have mild enhancement.

On diffusion-weighted imaging, the apparent diffusion coefficient (ADC) of pure mucinous tumors has been shown to be higher than that of IDC NOS and that of benign tissues.[28,29] This is not surprising in light of the generally low cellularity and mucin content of pure mucinous carcinomas. Woodhams and colleagues[28] found that mixed mucinous carcinomas had ADC values between those of IDC and pure mucinous carcinomas, although there were only two cases of mixed mucinous carcinoma in that study. Hatakenaka[29] found a significant difference between the ADCs of mucinous tumors and ADCs of fibroadenomas, which is important because other MRI features, such as high T2 signal and tendency toward persistent enhancement, can be similar between mucinous tumors and fibroadenomas. Thus diffusion-weighted imaging may aid in imaging differentiation between benign fibroadenomas and mucinous carcinomas.

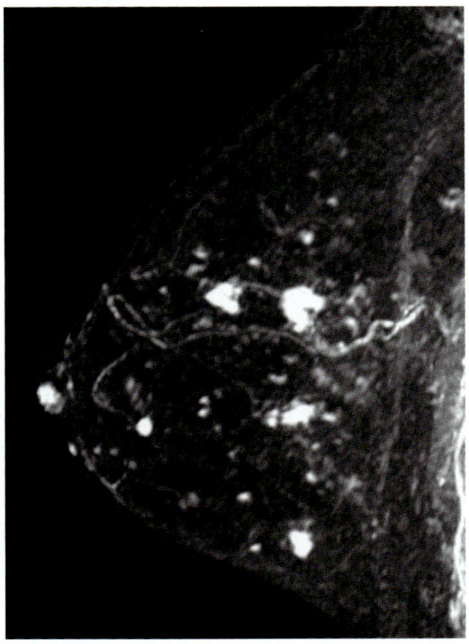

FIGURE 6.3 Multifocal invasive lobular carcinoma is illustrated in a saggital maximum-intensity projection (MIP) MRI image showing multiple irregular enhancing masses. MRI-guided biopsy for the two largest lesions showed invasive lobular carcinoma.

Medullary Carcinoma

Medullary carcinoma is rare, accounting for 5% to 7% of all breast cancers.[30] It has an increased incidence in young women, making up 11% of breast cancers in women receiving the diagnosis of breast cancer at age 35 or younger.[19] It also has an increased incidence in women who are breast and ovarian cancer susceptibility (*BRCA1*)-gene–positive. True medullary carcinoma has a better prognosis than invasive ductal carcinoma, having a 10-year survival rate of 92%.[31]

The World Health Organization criteria for the histologic diagnosis of medullary carcinoma includes "syncytial growth pattern (>75%), diffuse moderate to marked lymphocytoplasmacytic infiltrate, moderate to marked nuclear pleomorphism, and complete histologic circumscription."[19] Medullary carcinoma does not infiltrate the surrounding tissues, growing with a "pushing" margin, sometimes with encapsulation, resulting in a tumor with a circumscribed appearance histologically. At gross evaluation, its features can mimic those of a fibroadenoma.[32] There is no glandular structure and scant stroma is present.[30] Lymphocytoplasmacytic infiltrate is a prominent feature, and can be within the tumor or in its surroundings. The tumor is often quite large at presentation.

Lesions that exhibit some, but not all of these features were formerly considered to be atypical medullary carcinomas. Now these tumors are referred to as IDC with

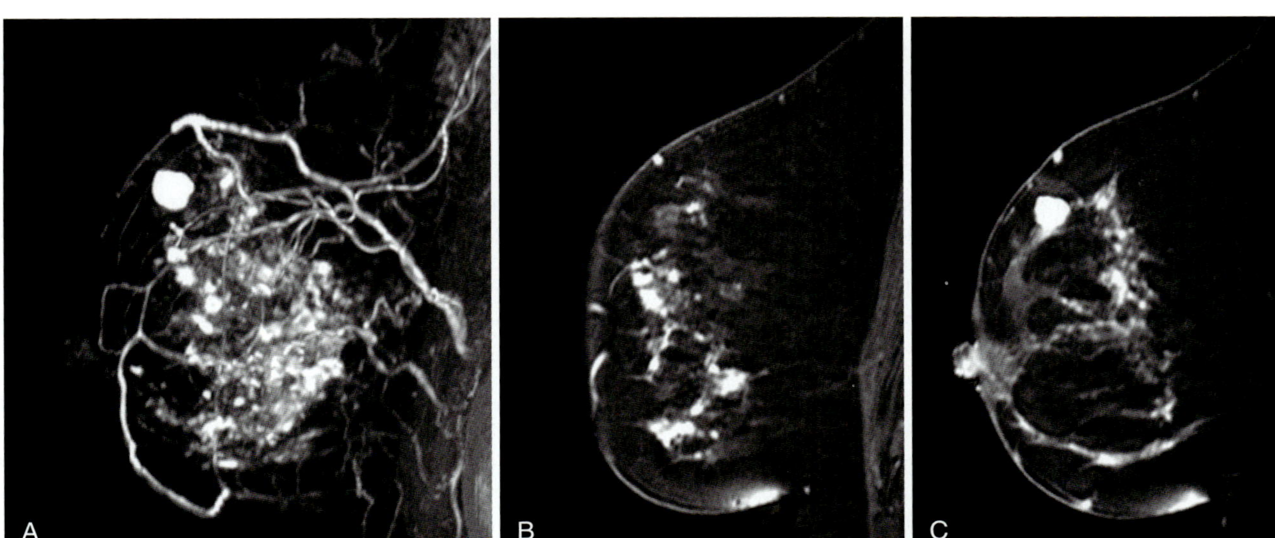

FIGURE 6.4 Postcontrast MIP image (**A**) and sagittal postcontrast MRI images (**B** and **C**) show diffuse distribution of multiple irregular masses and a smooth lobular mass (**C**), representing multicentric invasive lobular carcinoma.

medullary features. The histologic differentiation between typical medullary carcinoma and IDC with medullary features is important because these atypical tumors do not exhibit the same good prognosis.

The mammographic and sonographic features of medullary carcinoma can also mimic those of fibroadenomas. On mammography, medullary carcinoma usually appears as a noncalcified mass, frequently of high density, with circumscribed, indistinct, or obscured margins.[33-35] On ultrasound, medullary carcinomas present as hypoechoic masses associated with acoustic enhancement, shadowing, or no posterior acoustic features. Margins may be lobular, circumscribed, or indistinct but tend not to be spiculated.[33-35] In comparison with IDC with medullary features, typical medullary carcinoma is more frequently seen as a circumscribed mass on mammography.[31,34] In one study,[34] two thirds of typical medullary carcinomas had circumscribed margins and the remainder had partially indistinct margins. Only 1 of 15 typical medullary carcinomas contained calcifications compared with 4 of 17 cases of IDC with medullary features.

By histologic definition, medullary carcinoma is a circumscribed mass. However, on imaging, it frequently presents with indistinct margins. This has been attributed to surrounding lymphoplasmacytic infiltrates.[31]

Two studies have specifically described the MRI appearance of medullary carcinoma. Tominaga and colleagues[30] compared the MRI findings in eight cases of medullary carcinoma with their histopathologic appearance. All eight cases were masses with lobular shape and smooth margins. All were iso-intense on precontrast T1-weighted images and iso- or slightly hyperintense on T2-weighted images. All showed plateau or wash-out kinetic curves. The tumors all showed peripheral enhancement in the late phase, which the authors thought suggested prominent surrounding inflammatory changes. Four tumors had homogeneous internal enhancement, all of which had a uniform distribution of tumor cells without necrosis. Four lesions had heterogenous internal enhancement with "small non-enhanced spots" (Figure 6.7). All of these tumors had necrotic areas.

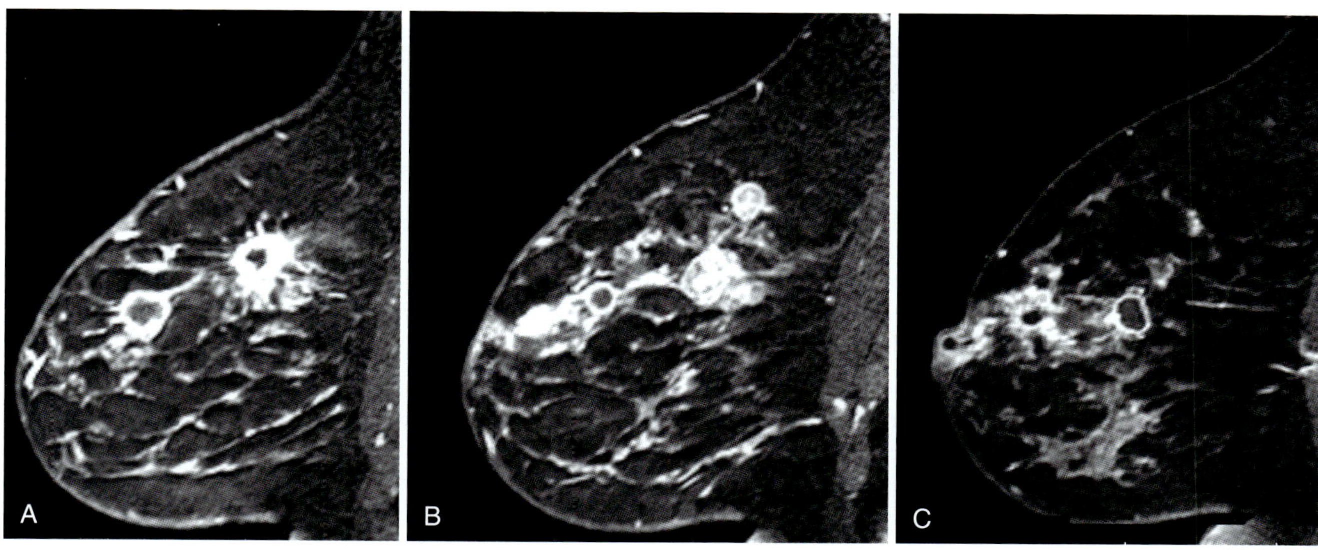

FIGURE 6.5 **A** through **C**, Sagittal postcontrast MRI images show multiple rim-enhancing masses in the upper left breast in linear distribution, with involvement of the nipple (**C**) representing multifocal unvasive lobular carcinoma

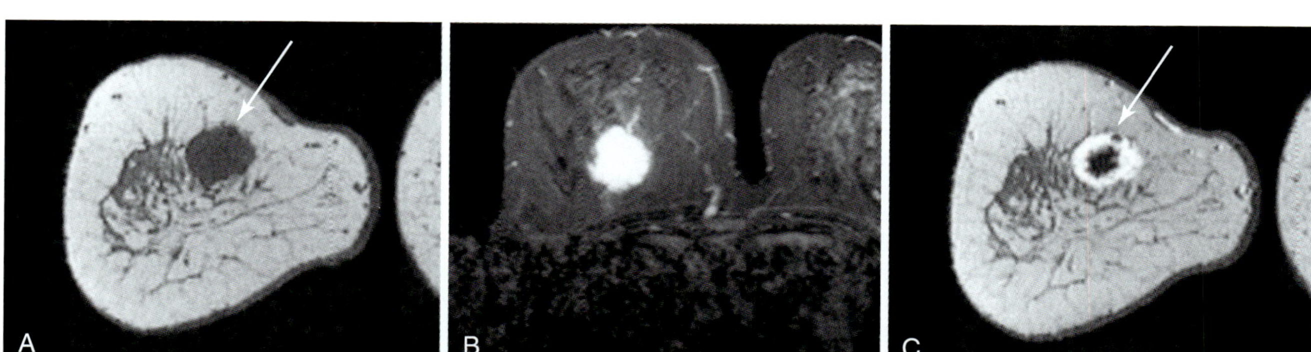

FIGURE 6.6 Pure mucinous carcinoma is shown in MRI scans. Precontrast T1- and T2-weighted images (**A** and **B**) show a round mass (*arrow*) with mildly irregular margins and uniformly high T2 signal. After contrast administration (**C**), rim enhancement is seen with persistent delayed phase kinetics. At histology, the tumor cells were noted to be predominantly at the periphery of the tumor, corresponding to the rim enhancement pattern. *(From Okafuji T, Yabuuchi H, Sakai S, et al. MR imaging of pure mucinous carcinoma of the breast,* Eur J Radiol *60:405–413, 2006.)*

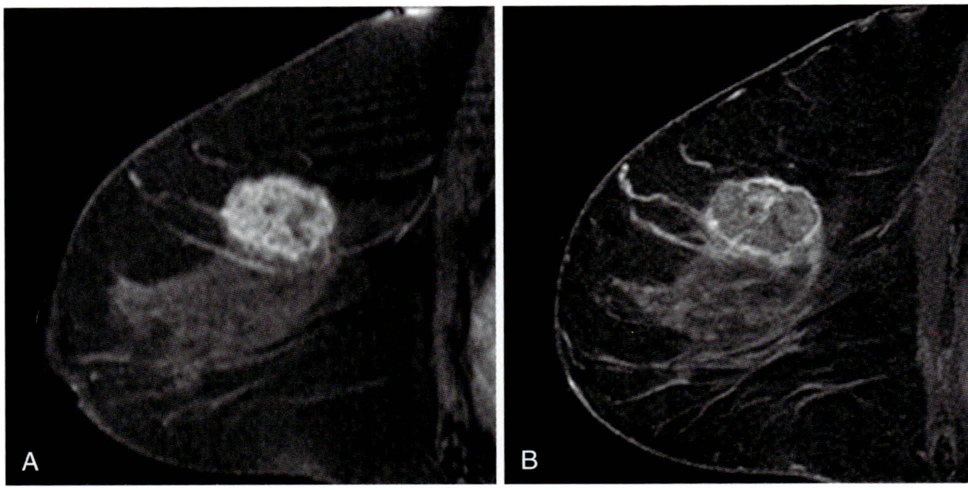

FIGURE 6.7 Medullary carcinoma is shown in MRI scans. Postcontrast sagittal images obtained 40 seconds after contrast injection (**A**) and 8 minutes after contrast injection (**B**) show a heterogeneously enhancing lobular mass with smooth margins. Rim enhancement is more evident on the 8-minute postcontrast image. Small central areas of nonenhancement are visible. At histology, there were small necrotic areas within the tumor. *(From Tominaga J, Hama H, Kimura N, et al. MR imaging of medullary carcinoma of the breast,* Eur J Radiol *70:525-529, 2009.)*

More recently, Jeong and coworkers[33] described the MRI features of 15 medullary carcinomas. All 15 lesions were masses on MRI. Two were irregular masses with irregular margins, and the rest were oval or lobular masses with smooth margins. All lesions were iso- or hypointense on precontrast T1-weighted images, and iso- or hyperintense on T2-weighted images. Thirteen of 15 lesions showed rim enhancement with or without internal septations. Internal septations on MRI correlated with fibroepithelial septations at histology. Nine of 15 lesions showed a hypointense rim on T2-weighted images. The authors believe that this might have been caused by a peripheral fibrous capsule. At histology, the two irregular masses had intense lymphocytic reaction or secondary nodules around the tumor, causing the appearance of a microlobulated border.

Papillary Carcinoma

Papillary lesions of the breast represent a family of lesions that have in common a frondlike growth pattern with epithelium supported by a fibro-vascular stroma. Papillary lesions of the breast include benign papillomas, papillary DCIS, and papillary carcinoma. The presence or absence of myoepithelial cells lining the basement membrane of the frondlike projections differentiates benign papillomas, in which they are present, from papillary carcinoma, in which they are absent.

Papillary carcinoma can be invasive or noninvasive. The noninvasive forms were previously described as intracystic or intraductal, depending on whether a cystic component was identified. However, the "cystic" form likely represents an intraductal lesion growing within an obstructed and cystically dilated duct. In both cases, there is a central mass encased by a thickened fibrous wall. The term *encapsulated papillary carcinoma* is now favored to describe both lesion types.[36] Classically, the fibrous wall contains myoepithelial cells, supporting the classification as a noninvasive lesion. However, myoepithelial cells may be absent in a large proportion (in 85% of cases), leading some investigators to consider these lesions to be indolent invasive lesions.[37] Special stains such as p63, calponin, smooth muscle actin, and CD10 can be used to assess for the presence or absence of myoepithelial cells.[36] There can be associated foci of typical invasive carcinoma, usually ductal carcinoma. These are most commonly located at the periphery of the lesion and can also infiltrate beyond the fibrous capsule.[38]

The imaging features of papillary lesions reflect the intraductal nature of the lesion. These lesions commonly present as a retro-areolar round, oval, or lobulated mass. Mammographically, the mass margins may be circumscribed or indistinct. Spiculation is uncommon. There may be associated clustered calcifications. On ultrasound, single or multiple masses may be seen. Masses are usually hypoechoic and may be solid or complex, with a cystic component. Masses commonly show posterior acoustic enhancement.[39] The imaging features of papillary carcinoma overlap with those of benign papillomas and there are no imaging features that can reliably differentiate between benign and malignant papillary lesions.[40] Hemorrhage is a frequent feature of papillary lesions and may be caused by torsion of the stalk and infarction of the solid components. This can lead to hemorrhage within the cyst fluid. The fibrovascular core may contain large vessels that may be apparent on Doppler ultrasound.[41]

Clinically, papillary carcinomas are rare, accounting for fewer than 2% of all breast carcinomas. They typically occur in an older patient population than the typical patient population with ductal carcinomas. Patients commonly present with bloody nipple discharge, which is present in 5% to 25%.[37]

The literature regarding the MRI appearance of papillary carcinoma is scant and generally limited to case reports. A multi-cystic appearance with marked enhancement of the cyst wall, intralesion septations, and mural nodules has been described, as well as intracystic hemorrhage causing fluid-fluid levels on precontrast images[42] (Figure 6.8). Multifocal areas of high precontrast T1 signal owing to hemorrhage have also been described.[19] The largest series was reported by Linda and colleagues[24] and included eight cases of intracystic and intraductal papillary carcinoma and five cases

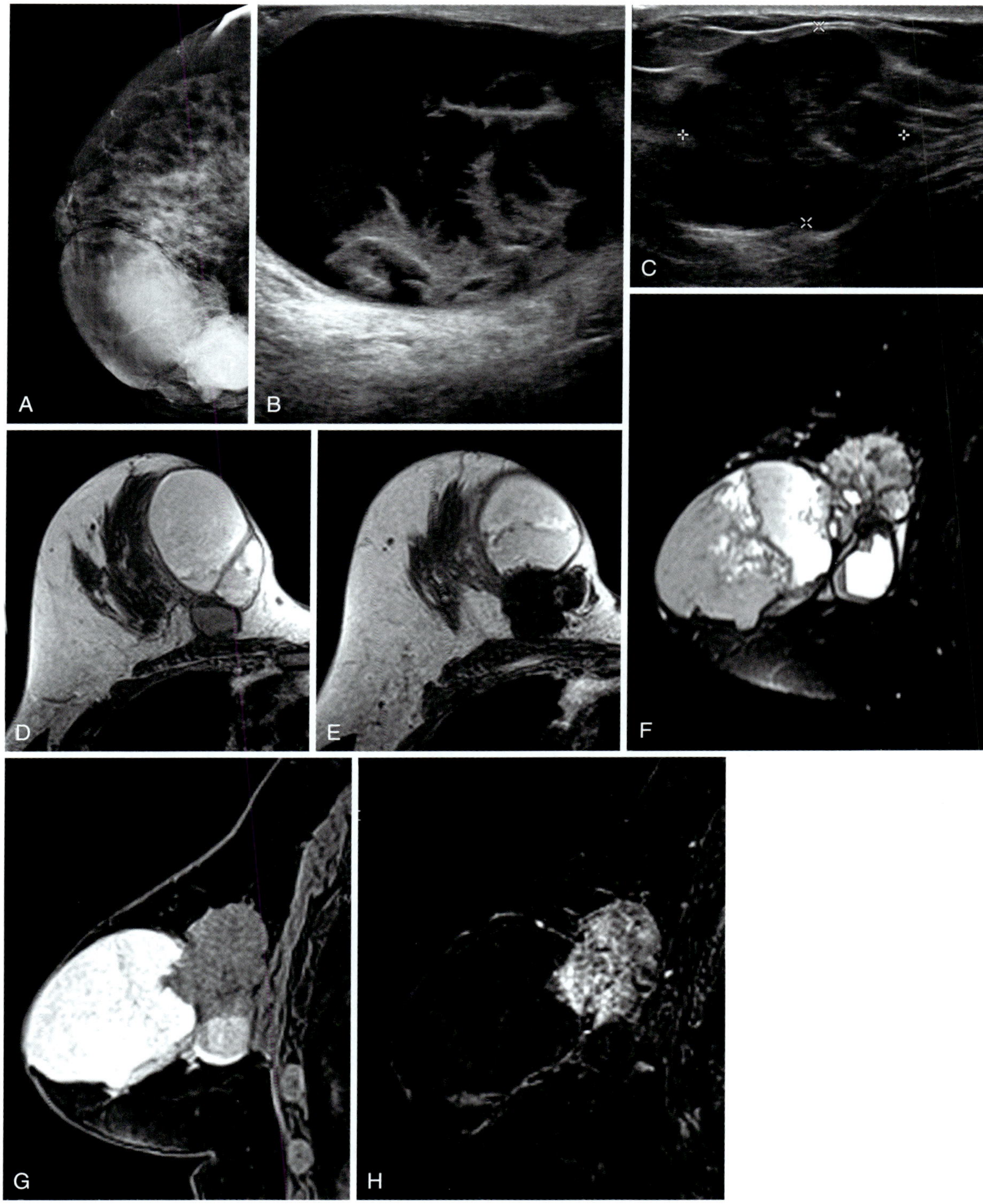

FIGURE 6.8 Papillary carcinoma is seen in a 59-year-old woman presenting with a large, longstanding, palpable lump. There was bluish discoloration of the overlying skin. **A,** Mammography of the right breast, craniocaudal view shows a multilobular mass in the inner right breast with a large well-circumscribed component anteriorly, and a more lobular hyperdense component posteriorly associated with suspicious calcifications. Ultrasound of the anterior component (**B**) shows a circumscribed complex mass with an internal frondlike solid component. Ultrasound of the posterior component (**C**) shows a predominantly solid mass with ill-defined, lobular margins. Axial non-fat suppressed precontrast T1-weighted MRI images (**D** and **E**) show a multiloculated lesion with predominantly high–signal-intensity fluid anteriorly and a low–signal-intensity solid mass posteriorly. Sagittal T2-weighted image (**F**) shows fluid-fluid levels within the lesion. Sagittal fat-suppressed precontrast T1-weighted MRI image (**G**) better shows the solid component and high–signal-intensity fluid within the lesion. Sagittal postcontrast subtraction MRI image (**H**) shows the enhancing solid mass posteriorly and nonenhancing cystic component anteriorly. The frondlike solid component seen on ultrasound did not show significant enhancement. The enhancing solid portion extends into the posterior aspect of the cystic component. The patient underwent mastectomy showing an 8.5-cm intracystic papillary carcinoma anteriorly and a 4.5-cm invasive papillary carcinoma posteriorly, invading into the posterior wall of the cyst.

of invasive papillary carcinoma. They found that the morphologic and kinetic features of papillary carcinoma were somewhat variable. Three of four intracystic tumors were detectable on MRI as round or oval masses with well-defined borders. Intraductal papillary carcinomas were more likely to be seen as irregular masses, with two of four described as irregular in shape, and one described as *dendritic* in shape. No intracystic or intraductal tumors had wash-out, and out of all eight intracystic or intraductal lesions, only one case showed more than 100% enhancement in the first postcontrast minute. Invasive papillary carcinomas were also more likely to appear as irregular or *dendritic* masses, and three of four lesions detectable with MRI had ill-defined borders. Three of four detectable invasive papillary carcinomas had greater than 100% early enhancement and three of four had wash-out. Invasive papillary carcinomas were also more likely to show inhomogeneous internal enhancement or rim enhancement than intraductal or intracystic lesions.

Triple-Negative Breast Cancers

Triple-negative breast cancers do not express estrogen receptor (ER) or progesterone receptor (PR), and do not overexpress or amplify the type-2 human epidermal growth factor receptor (*HER2*) gene. As this is a definition of exclusion, triple-negative cancers probably represent a somewhat heterogeneous population of cancers. Recent studies in genetic profiling have identified four distinct subtypes of breast cancer: luminal A, luminal B, *HER2*-enriched, and the basal type.[43] The luminal A and B types are hormone receptor–positive and tend to have a better prognosis than the other subtypes. The *HER2*-enriched and basal-like types are more biologically aggressive. There is no consensus as to how to define a basal-like cancer, but triple-negative cancer is considered a surrogate for the basal subtype.

Triple-negative cancers make up about 7% to 15% of all breast cancers.[44] They have a higher incidence in premenopausal African-American women[45] and are also associated with a younger age at patient presentation and with obesity.[46] They make up about 70% of breast cancers diagnosed in women who are *BRCA*-1 positive.[44]

Triple-negative cancers are biologically aggressive tumors. They show aggressive histologic features, tending to be high-grade tumors with a high mitotic index.[47] In general, triple-negative cancers have a poor prognosis. They are unresponsive to the usual endocrine therapy but are highly responsive to conventional chemotherapy. They have a propensity to metastasize early to the brain and lung but are less likely to metastasize to bone. Triple-negative cancers tend to recur early, usually within 2 to 3 years. However, after 5 years there is a relatively low risk of distant metastases.[46]

On mammography, triple-negative cancer is much more commonly seen as a mass than as calcifications, architectural distortion, or focal asymmetry. Calcifications are less commonly seen than with ER-positive and *HER2*-positive tumors.[48] Mass shape tends to be round, oval, or lobular more commonly than irregular.[44,45,49,50] Mass margins are more frequently circumscribed and less commonly spiculated than in ER-positive and *HER2*-positive tumors.[49,50] In one study, in which triple-negative breast cancer was compared with ER-positive and *HER2*-positive tumors,[49] triple-negative breast cancer was less likely to have associated DCIS. The authors note that the mammographic features suggest "a more rapid pattern of carcinogenesis that leads directly to invasive cancer with no major in situ component or precancerous stage."

On MRI, triple-negative cancers present much more commonly as masses than as nonmass enhancement (NME), with masses seen in 77% to 95% of cases[51-53] and NME seen in 5% to 23% (Figure 6.9). Masses are round in 10% to 47%, lobular in 8% to 41%, and irregular in 15% to 21% of cases.[51-53] In two studies, wash-out was seen in 90% and 95% of cases.[51,52] In a third study, wash-out was seen in 50% of cases.[53] Rim enhancement is also a common feature, and has been reported in 50% to 80% of cases.[51-53] Uematsu and colleagues[53] found that masses with smooth borders were more likely to have rim enhancement and very high T2 signal than were masses with irregular borders. Rim enhancement is a feature associated with a poor prognosis.

Another MRI feature commonly reported in triple-negative cancer is central high T2 signal on precontrast images. This has been reported in 34% to 65% of cases.[51-53] In one study, in which pathologic and imaging features were correlated,[53] very high T2 signal correlated with areas of tumor necrosis, which is a poor-prognostic indicator. Conversely, all ER-positive, PR-positive, *HER2*-negative tumors that had very high T2 signal were mucinous carcinomas. Intratumoral necrosis has also been associated with a poor response to neoadjuvant chemotherapy.[54]

Uematsu and coworkers[53] compared the MRI findings of triple-negative cancers with those of ER-positive, PR-positive, and *HER2*-negative. Mass features significantly associated with triple-negative breast cancer were smooth margins, rim enhancement, persistent enhancement, and very high T2 signal. Youk and colleagues[51] compared triple-negative breast cancer with ER-positive and *HER2*-positive tumors. Triple-negative tumors were more significantly associated with round or oval mass shape, smooth margins, and rim enhancement than were ER-positive or *HER2*-positive tumors. The proportions were as follows[51]:

- Round or oval mass shape: triple-negative breast cancer, 77%; ER-positive, 38%; *HER2*-positive, 27%
- Smooth margins: triple-negative breast cancer, 71%; ER-positive, 6%; *HER2*-positive, 1%
- Rim enhancement: triple-negative breast cancer, 50%; ER-positive, 9%; *HER2*-positive, 7%

It would be expected that diffusion weighted imaging would show ADC values for triple-negative breast cancers to be lower than for other breast cancers, given their tendency to be more aggressive tumors. However, Youk and colleagues[51] found that the mean ADC value for triple-negative breast cancer was significantly higher than for ER-positive and *HER2*-positive tumors. The authors thought that this was probably secondary to tumor necrosis. Shin and colleages[55] and Tozaki and Hoshi[56] both found a significantly higher choline content for triple-negative breast cancer than for cancers that were not triple-negative.

Inflammatory Breast Cancer

Inflammatory breast cancer (IBC) is the most aggressive and lethal form of breast cancer. It is rare, accounting for 1% to 6% of all breast cancers. It is defined mainly by its clinical appearance, typically consisting of rapid development of

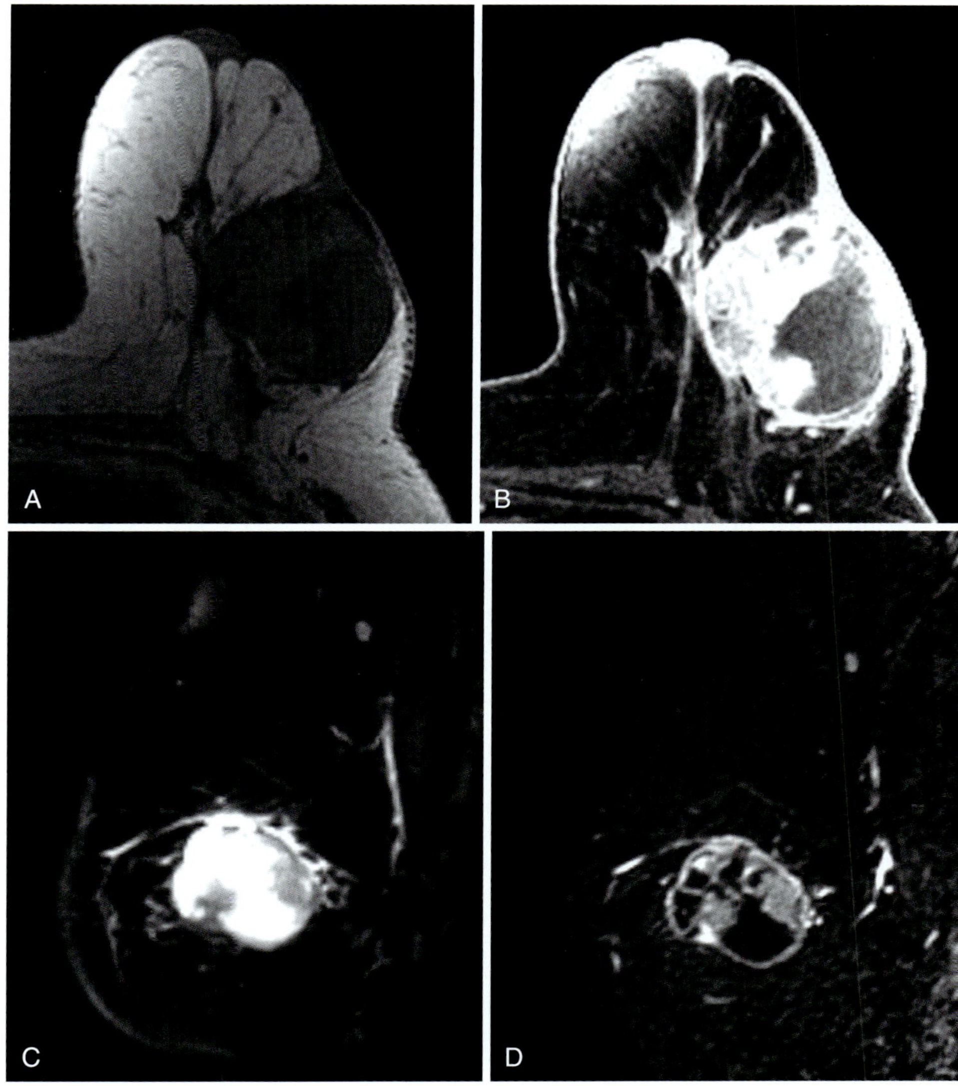

FIGURE 6.9 Triple-negative cancer is seen in MRI images from a 76-year-old woman presenting with a large fungating mass in the left breast. Precontrast (**A**) and postcontrast (**B**) axial images show a large mass with smooth margins, central necrosis, and peripheral nodular enhancement. The enhancing portions of the tumor showed wash-out delayed phase kinetics. On T2-weighted images (**C**), the lesion showed very high internal T2 signal with peripheral areas of lower signal that corresponded to nodular areas of enhancement on postcontrast images. Sagittal postcontrast subtraction image **(D)** shows heterogeneous internal enhancement of the tumor with non-enhancing necrotic areas.

breast enlargement, edema, and tenderness, associated with widespread skin erythema and warmth. The skin may have a peau d'orange appearance. A palpable lump may or may not be present. The symptoms usually have been present for less than 3 months at the time of patient presentation. Axillary adenopathy is also a frequent clinical finding. IBC is not a true inflammatory process, and therefore there is no fever or elevated white blood cell count. However, the symptoms are identical to those seen in mastitis. Risk factors for IBC include African-American race, high body mass index, and young age at presentation.[58]

The differential diagnosis also includes locally advanced breast cancer with skin involvement, which is distinguished from IBC by the clinical history of a longstanding palpable lump. Rarely, other malignancies such as lymphoma can have a similar clinical presentation. Postradiation changes and edema secondary to congestive heart failure are other causes of skin thickening and edema, although these can usually be differentiated by the clinical history.

The diagnosis of inflammatory cancer is made by punch biopsy of the skin showing tumor emboli in dermal lymphatics. However, punch biopsy may be negative in 25% or more of cases.[58] Some patients may have all the pathologic features of IBC, with tumor emboli in dermal lymphatic, but no clinical symptoms. This is considered occult IBC.

The prognosis of inflammatory carcinoma is poor, with an average survival of 12 to 36 months.[59] Fifty-five percent to 85% of patients have metastases to the axillary or supraclavicular nodes.[58] Twenty percent of patients have distant metastases at the time of diagnosis.[57] The treatment for IBC is neoadjuvant chemotherapy, followed by mastectomy and chest wall radiation.

No single histopathologic tumor subtype is associated with inflammatory cancer. Any histopathologic subtype can be seen, but the most common type is poorly differentiated invasive ductal carcinoma.[56] The tumor frequently grows with a diffusely infiltrative pattern, without a distinct intraductal component.[58] The histologic hallmark of inflammatory cancer is the presence of prominent tumor emboli within subdermal lymphatic vessels. These tumor emboli cause lymphatic obstruction, which is responsible for the symptoms. Subdermal lymphatic tumor emboli can also be seen in locally advanced breast cancer, but the emboli are not as large or as numerous.[58]

The role of breast imaging in IBC is to guide biopsy, stage locoregional disease, and monitor response to neoadjuvant chemotherapy.[60] MRI is the most sensitive imaging modality for detecting the primary breast parenchymal lesion in IBC.[59,61]

Mammography may be significantly limited in inflammatory breast carcinoma. Breast tenderness and swelling can significantly limit the ability to compress the breast, and some patients may not tolerate mammography at all. Breast edema leads to diffusely increased density of the breast, which can obscure masses and other signs of cancer. As a result, mammography is less sensitive than other modalities in detecting the underlying cancer.[57,59,61] Mammography generally shows an enlarged breast with diffuse skin and trabecular thickening and overall increased density. There may be evidence of the underlying cancer such as a mass, architectural distortion, and calcifications, although calcifications are less commonly seen in IBC than in nonIBC.[62] Axillary adenopathy is also commonly present.

Ultrasound is more sensitive than mammography in detecting an underlying primary breast parenchymal lesion but may also be limited by breast edema, which can cause diffusely increased echogenicity of the breast tissue. Ultrasound is also useful in evaluating for lymphadenopathy, not only in the axilla but also in the supraclavicular, infraclavicular, and internal mammary nodal basins.

Skin thickening is a hallmark of the disease. Normal breast skin thickness is 0.5 to 2 mm.[63] The skin may also enhance in IBC cases, but skin enhancement is not pathognomic of inflammatory cancer. Skin enhancement may also be seen in other conditions, including mastitis, postradiation change, postsurgical change, and locally advanced cancer with skin involvement. Normal skin may show mild, thin enhancement.[63] Skin enhancement was described as heterogeneous in 84% of patients and nodular or irregular in 44% in one study.[59] The term *punched-out* sign has been used to describe focal areas of rapid enhancement in the skin, with the remainder of the skin showing slow, continuous enhancement.[64] Presumably, these focal areas of enhancement represent foci of tumor within the skin. In another study, the likelihood of skin enhancement increased with skin thickness.[65] The presence of skin enhancement seems to correlate with the identification of dermal lymphatic tumor emboli pathologically. Lee and colleagues[57] found skin enhancement in all patients with pathologic proof of tumor emboli in the dermal lymphatics, although the numbers in this study were small.

Edema is another common finding with IBC, identified as ill-defined areas of high signal intensity on T2-weighted images. Edema may involve the skin, breast parenchyma, chest wall, or prepectoral soft tissues.[58,64,66] Parenchymal edema may be diffuse or may be limited to the peritumoral tissues. The breast is usually enlarged compared with the opposite side, but occasionally may be smaller owing to loss of normal elasticity.[65]

The morphologic features of the primary tumor reflect its aggressive nature. The primary tumor may present as one or more masses or as NME. Masses are very commonly multiple, with one study reporting multiple masses in 90% of cases presenting as masses, and more than seven masses present in 40%.[38] The masses may be confluent, and one study describes the appearance of the tumor as "innumerable tiny contiguous enhancing nodules interconnected by NME" in more than 50% of cases.[61] In the same study, masses most commonly had irregular margins and heterogeneous internal enhancement. Multicentric disease is more common than multifocal or unifocal disease on MRI.[59,61] Wash-out or plateau delayed phase curves are seen in 85% to 100%.[59,61,65-68]

When the tumor presents as NME, a diffuse or multiregional distribution is common (Figures 6-10 and 6-11),and is more common than a segmental distribution.[64,66,67] In two studies reporting the frequencies of linear and ductal distributions, there were no cases of either.[64,67] A reticular/dendritic pattern was seen in 9% of all cases of presenting as NME in one study.[64] This pattern has been described as abnormally thickened and distorted parenchymal strands, reminiscent of irregular septal thickening in the lungs at high-resolution chest computed tomography (CT).[69] In one study, NME was present to some extent in all cases and was seen surrounding masses in cases presenting primarily as masses.[64] Thickening and pathologic enhancement of Cooper's ligaments have also been described.[64]

The most important differential diagnostic consideration for IBC is nonpuerperal mastitis, which can have exactly the same presentationas IBC. Renz and coworkers[68] compared the MRI findings in 48 patients with IBC with MRI findings in 42 patients with acute mastitis. They found no statistically significant difference between IBC and acute mastitis in morphology of masses and NME, incidence of breast enlargement, or incidence of diffuse skin thickening. However, there was a difference in kinetic features. IBC was more likely to have rapid enhancement and washout, whereas most cases of acute mastitis showed plateau curves. More masses with a greater average size were detected with IBC. Masses in acute mastitis more likely to be high in T2 signal intensity secondary to abscess formation. NME was more likely to be subareolar in acute mastitis because of the ascending nature of the infection from the nipple but more likely to be central or dorsal in IBC. The punched-out sign was more frequent in inflammatory breast cancer than in acute mastitis. Axillary lymph nodes were more likely to have a malignant appearance with IBC.

Locally advanced breast cancer should also be differentiated from IBC because their treatments differ. Patients with locally advanced breast cancer are potential candidates for breast conservation after neoadjuvant chemotherapy, whereas patients with IBC require mastectomy. Renz and colleagues[64] compared the MRI findings in 48 patients with IBC to MRI findings in 52 patients with locally advanced breast cancer. They found no difference in mass shape, margin type, incidence of tumor necrosis, or enhancement characteristics between the two groups. The number of masses in any given patient was greater with IBC, but average tumor size was greater with locally advanced breast cancer. The punched-out sign in the skin was seen with a greater frequency in IBC, and associated NME was more extensive with IBC than with locally advanced breast cancer. In a similar comparison, Girardi et al[67] found that IBC most commonly presented as NME and locally advanced breast cancer most commonly presented as a mass. NME was most commonly diffuse with IBC and most commonly segmental with locally advanced breast cancer. A "reticular dendritic"

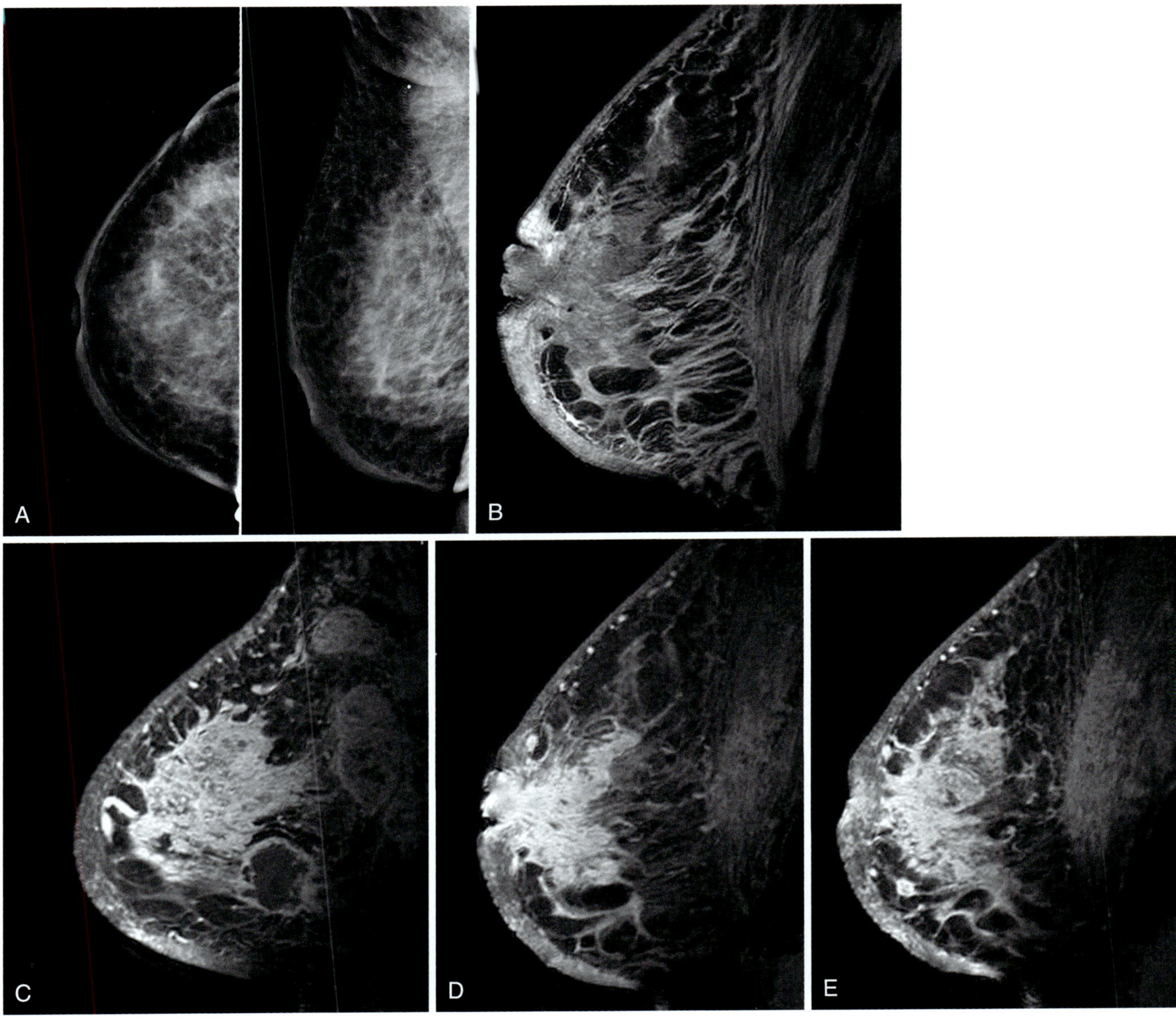

FIGURE 6.10 Inflammatory carcinoma is seen in a 57-year-old woman presenting with diffuse right breast enlargement and skin thickening as well as matted right axillary lymph nodes. **A,** Mammography of the right breast shows nipple retraction with diffuse skin and trabecular thickening but without a discrete mass. **B,** Sagittal T2-weighted MRI image shows linear areas of increased T2 signal throughout the breast, extending all the way to the pectoralis muscle. Increased T2 signal is seen in the pectoralis muscle as well and is consistent with edema. Note that the area of tumor in the subareolar region is lower in T2-signal intensity. **C** through **E,** Sagittal postcontrast MRI images show diffuse NME and skin enhancement. A necrotic mass is present in the lower outer breast (**C**) on MRI but not visible mammographically. Additionally, multiple enlarged and heterogeneously enhancing lymph nodes are seen in the axillary region consistent with nodal metastasis (**C**). Thickening and localized enhancement of the pectoralis muscle is evident and consistent with tumor involvement (**D, E**). Nipple retraction is also evident (**D**). The tumor showed predominantly rapid enhancement with wash-out delayed phase kinetics.

appearance of masses was more frequent with IBC than with locally advanced breast cancer. However, the only statistically significant difference between the two groups was in the incidence of breast edema, being more common in IBC than in locally advanced breast cancer.

Conclusion

Although special types of breast cancer make up only a small percentage of newly diagnosed cancers, they can have imaging and clinical features that distinguish them from the most commonly seen type of breast cancer, infiltrating ductal carcinoma. Mucinous and medullary carcinomas can have an appearance that mimics benign lesions on mammography and ultrasound. However, in the case of medullary carcinoma, the internal enhancement pattern would indicate the malignant nature of the lesion. Conversely, mucinous carcinomas can have an appearance more suggestive of a benign lesion on MRI, with slow enhancement and high T2 signal. Awareness of this appearance may help prevent misdiagnosis of a mucinous carcinoma as a benign lesion.

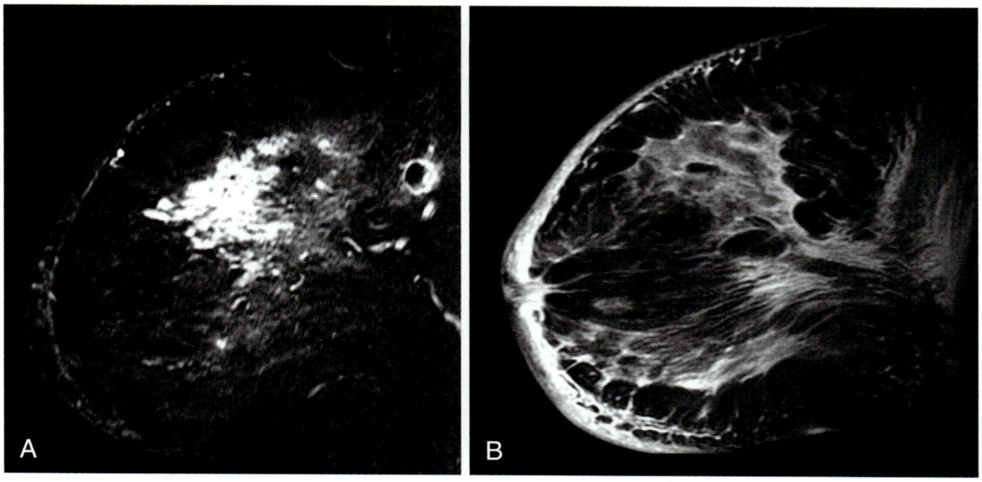

FIGURE 6.11 Inflammatory carcinoma is shown in MRI of a 43-year-old African-American woman with right breast IDC 12 years earlier who presented with diffuse right breast skin redness and inflammation, without pain or palpable mass. Her symptoms did not improve with antibiotics. Biopsy showed triple-negative IDC. **A,** Sagittal postcontrast subtraction image shows regional NME as well as diffuse skin thickening and enhancement. An enlarged necrotic lymph is seen in the axillary region. **B,** T2-weighted sagittal image shows patchy increased signal throughout the skin and breast parenchyma consistent with edema. Edema is also seen along the pectoralis muscle border and within the muscle.

Triple-negative cancer is defined based on its molecular profile, rather than by a specific histologic appearance. These tumors can also have a benign appearance on conventional imaging. However, their internal enhancement pattern, with a tendency toward central necrosis and rim enhancement, can indicate their aggressive nature.

Lobular carcinoma is distinguished by its tendency toward multifocality and multicentricity and a tendency toward a more benign pattern of internal enhancement. Thus additional lesions seen on breast MRI in patients with lobular carcinomas may need to be managed with a higher degree of suspicion than those seen in other patients.

In the case of IBC, MRI may allow much better assessment of size and location of the index lesion than conventional imaging and is also the best modality for imaging follow-up after chemotherapy.

References

1. Mann RM: The effectiveness of MR imaging in the assessment of invasive lobular carcinoma of the breast, *Magn Reson Imaging Clin North Am* 18:259–276, 2010.
2. Harvey JA: Unusual breast cancers: useful clues to expanding the differential diagnosis, *Radiology* 242:683–694, 2007.
3. Lopez JK, Bassett LW: Invasive lobular carcinoma of the breast: spectrum of mammographic, US, and MR imaging findings, *Radiographics* 29:165–176, 2009.
4. Mann RM, Veltman J, Huisman H, Boetes C: Comparison of enhancement characteristics between invasive lobular carcinoma and invasive ductal carcinoma, *J Magn Reson Imaging* 34:293–300, 2011.
5. Qayyum A, Birdwell RL, Daniel BL, et al: MR Imaging features of infiltrating lobular carcinoma of the breast: histopathologic correlation, *AJR Am J Roentgenol* 178:1227–1232, 2002.
6. Mann RM, Veltman J, Barentsz JO, et al: The value of MRI compared to mammography in the assessment of tumor extent in invasive lobular carcinoma of the breast, *Eur J Surg Oncol* 34:135–142, 2008.
7. Michael M, Garzoli E, Reiner CS: Mammography, sonography and MRI for detection and characterization of invasive lobular carcinoma of the breast, *Breast Dis* 30:21–30, 2008.
8. Mann RM, Hoogeveen YL, Blickman JG, Boetes C: MRI compared to conventional diagnostic work-up in the detection and evaluation of invasive lobular carcinoma of the breast: a review of existing literature, *Breast Cancer Res Treat* 107:1–14, 2008.
9. Stivalet A, Luciani A, Pigneur F, et al: Invasive lobular carcinoma of the breast: MRI pathological correlation following bilateral total mastectomy, *Acta Radiol* 53:367–375, 2012.
10. Apple SK, Lopez JK, Basset LW: Invasive lobular carcinoma. In Bassett LW, Mahoney MC, Apple SK, D'orsi CJ, editors: *Breast imaging*, Philadelphia, PA, 2011, Elsevier, pp 483–501.
11. Levrini G, Mori CA, Vacondio R, Borasi G, Nicoli F: MRI patterns of invasive lobular cancer: T1 and T2 features, *Radiol Med* 113:1110–1125, 2008.
12. Kim SH, Cha ES, Park CS, et al: Imaging features of invasive lobular carcinoma: comparison with invasive ductal carcinoma, *Jpn J Radiol* 29:475–482, 2011.
13. Yeh ED, Slanetz PJ, Edmister WB, Talele A, Monticciolo D, Kopans DB: Invasive lobular carcinoma: spectrum of enhancement and morphology on magnetic resonance imaging, *Breast J* 9:13–18, 2003.
14. Schelfout K, Van Goethem M, Kersschot E, et al: Preoperative breast MRI in patients with invasive lobular breast cancer, *Eur Radiol* 14:1209–1216, 2004.
15. Dietzel M, Baltzer PA, Vag T, et al: Magnetic resonance mammography of invasive lobular versus ductal carcinoma: systematic comparison of 811 patients reveals high diagnostic accuracy irrespective of typing, *J Comput Assist Tomogr* 34:587–595, 2010.
16. McGhan LJ, Wasif N, Gray RJ, et al: Use of preoperative magnetic resonance imaging for invasive lobular cancer: good, better, but maybe not the best? *Ann Surg Oncol* 17:255–262, 2010.
17. Caramella T, Chapellier C, Ettore F, et al: Value of MRI in the surgical planning of invasive lobular breast carcinoma: a prospective and a retrospective study of 57 cases: comparison with physical examination, conventional imaging, and histology, *Clin Imaging* 31:155–161, 2007.
18. Mann RM, Loo CE, Wobbes T, et al: The impact of preoperative breast MRI on the re-excision rate in invasive lobular carcinoma of the breast, *Breast Cancer Res Treat* 119:415–422, 2010.
19. Yoo JL, Woo OH, Kim YK, et al: Can MR imaging contribute in characterizing well-circumscribed breast carcinomas? *Radiographics* 30: 1689–1702, 2010.
20. Monzawa S, Yokokawa M, Sakuma T, et al: Mucinous carcinoma of the breast: MRI features of pure and mixed forms with histopathologic correlation, *AJR Am J Roentgenol* 192:W125–W131, 2009.
21. Memis A, Ozdemir N, Parildar M, Ustun EE, Erhan Y: Mucinous (colloid) breast cancer: mammographic and US features with histologic correlation, *Eur J Radiol* 35:39–43, 2000.
22. Chopra S, Evans AJ, Pinder SE, et al: Pure mucinous breast cancer-mammographic and ultrasound findings, *Clin Radiol* 51:421–424, 1996.
23. Lam WWM, Chu WCW, Tse GM, Ma TK: Sonographic appearance of mucinous carcinoma of the breast, *AJR Am J Roentgenol* 182: 1069–1074, 2004.

24. Linda A, Londero V, Mazzarella F, Zuiani C, Bazzocchi M: Rare breast neoplasms: is there any peculiar feature on magnetic resonance mammography? *Radiol Med* 112(6):850–862, 2007.
25. Yuen S, Uematsu T, Kasami M, et al: Breast carcinomas with strong high-signal intensity on T2-weighted MR images: pathological characteristics and differential diagnosis, *J Magn Reson Imaging* 25:502–510, 2007.
26. Okafuji T, Yabuuchi H, Sakai S, et al: MR imaging features of pure mucinous carcinoma of the breast, *Eur J Radiol* 60:405–413, 2006.
27. Kawashima M, Tamaki Y, Nonaka T, et al: MR imaging of mucinous carcinoma of the breast, *AJR Am J Roentgenol* 179 179–183, 2002.
28. Woodhams R, Kakita S, Hata H, et al: Diffusion-weighted imaging of mucinous carcinoma of the breast: evaluation of apparent diffusion coefficient and signal intensity in correlation with histologic findings, *AJR Am J Roentgenol* 193:260–266, 2009.
29. Hatakenaka M, Soeda H, Yabuuchi H, et al: Apparent diffusion coefficients of breast tumors: clinical application, *Magn Reson Med Sci* 7:23–29, 2008.
30. Tominaga J, Hama H, Kimura N, Takahashi S: MR imaging of medullary carcinoma of the breast, *Eur J Radiol* 70:525–529, 2009.
31. Liberman L, LaTrenta LR, Samli B, Morris EA, Abramson AF, Dershaw DD: Overdiagnosis of medullary carcinoma: a mammographic-pathologic correlative study, *Radiology* 201:443–446, 1996.
32. Linda A, Zuiani C, Girometti R, et al: Unusual malignant tumors of the breast: MRI features and pathologic correlation, *Eur J Radiol* 75:178–184, 2010.
33. Jeong SJ, Lim HS, Lee JS, et al: Medullary carcinoma of the breast: MRI findings, *AJR Am J Roentgenol* 198:W482–W487 2012.
34. Yilmaz E, Lebe B, Balci P, Sal S, Canda T: Comparison of mammographic and sonographic findings in typical and atypical medullary carcinomas of the breast, *Clin Radiol* 57:640–645, 2002.
35. Meyer JE, Amin E, Lindfors KK, Lipman JC, Stomper PC, Genest D: Medullary carcinoma of the breast: mammographic and US appearance, *Radiology* 170(1 Pt 1):79–82, 1989.
36. Rodríguez MC, Secades AL, Angulo JM: Best cases from the AFIP: intracystic papillary carcinoma of the breast, *Radiographics* 30: 2017–2021, 2010.
37. Rakha EA, Gandhi N, Climent F, van Deurzen CH, et al: Encapsulated papillary carcinoma of the breast: an invasive tumor with excellent prognosis, *Am J Surg Pathol* 35:1093–1103, 2011.
38. Pal SK, Lau SK, Kruper L, et al: Papillary carcinoma of the breast: an overview, *Breast Cancer Res Treat* 122:637–645, 2010.
39. Liberman L, Feng TL, Susnik B: Case 35: Intracystic papillary carcinoma with invasion, *Radiology* 219:781, 2001.
40. Lam WWM, Chu WCW, Tang APY, Tse G, Ma TKF: Role of radiologic features in the management of papillary lesions of the breast, *AJR Am J Roentgenol* 186:1322–1327, 2006.
41. Eiada R, Chong J, Kulkarni S, Goldberg F, Muradali D: Papillary lesions of the breast: MRI, ultrasound, and mammographic appearances, *AJR Am J Roentgenol* 198:264–271, 2012.
42. Soo MS, Williford ME, Walsh R, Bentley RC, Kornguth PJ: Papillary carcinoma of the breast: imaging findings, *AJR Am J Roentgenol* 164: 321–326, 1995.
43. Martincich L, Deantoni V, Bertotto I, et al: Correlations between diffusion-weighted imaging and breast cancer biomarkers, *Eur Radiol* 22:1519–1528, 2012.
44. Boisserie-Lacroix M, Mac Grogan G, Debled M, et al: Radiological features of triple-negative breast cancers (73 cases), *Diagn Interv Imaging* 93:183–190, 2012.
45. Krizmanich-Conniff KM, Paramagul C, Patterson SK, et al: Triple receptor-negative breast cancer: imaging and clinical characteristics, *AJR Am J Roentgenol* 199:458–464, 2012.
46. Eiermann W, Bergh J, Cardoso F, et al: Triple negative breast cancer: proposals for a pragmatic definition and implications for patient management and trial design, *Breast* 21:20–26, 2012.
47. Chen JH, Agrawal G, Feig B, et al: Triple-negative breast cancer: MRI features in 29 patients, *Ann Oncol* 18:2042–2043, 2007.
48. Ko ES, Lee BH, Kim HA, Noh WC, Kim MS, Lee SA: Triple-negative breast cancer: correlation between imaging and pathological findings, *Eur Radiol* 20:1111–1117, 2010.
49. Yang WT, Dryden M, Broglio K, et al: Mammographic features of triple receptor-negative primary breast cancers in young premenopausal women, *Breast Cancer Res Treat* 111:405–410, 2008.
50. Wang Y, Ikeda DM, Narasimhan B, et al: Estrogen receptor–negative invasive breast cancer: imaging features of tumors with and without human epidermal growth factor receptor type 2 overexpression, *Radiology* 246:367–375, 2008.
51. Youk JH, Son EJ, Chung J, Kim JA, Kim EK: Triple-negative invasive breast cancer on dynamic contrast-enhanced and diffusion-weighted MR imaging: comparison with other breast cancer subtypes, *Eur Radiol* 22:1724–1734, 2012.
52. Dogan BE, Gonzalez-Angulo AM, Gilcrease M, Dryden MJ, Yang WT: Multimodality imaging of triple receptor-negative tumors with mammography, ultrasound, and MRI, *AJR Am J Roentgenol* 194:1160–1166, 2010.
53. Uematsu T, Kasami M, Yuen S: Triple-negative breast cancer: correlation between MR imaging and pathologic findings, *Radiology* 250: 638–647, 2009.
54. Kawashima H, Inokuchi M, Furukawa H, Kitamura S: Triple-negative breast cancer: are the imaging findings different between responders and nonresponders to neoadjuvant chemotherapy? *Acad Radiol* 18:963–969, 2011.
55. Shin HJ, Baek HM, Cha JH, Kim HH: Evaluation of breast cancer using proton MR spectroscopy: total choline peak integral and signal-to-noise ratio as prognostic indicators, *AJR Am J Roentgenol* 198:W488–W497, 2012.
56. Tozaki M, Hoshi K: 1H MR spectroscopy of invasive ductal carcinoma: correlations with FDG PET and histologic prognostic factors, *AJR Am J Roentgenol* 194:1384–1390, 2010.
57. Lee KW, Chung SY, Yang I, et al: Inflammatory breast cancer: imaging findings, *Clin Imaging* 29:22–25, 2005.
58. Robertson FM, Bondy M, Yang W, et al: Inflammatory breast cancer: The disease, the biology, the treatment, *CA Cancer J Clin* 60:351–375, 2010.
59. Yang WT, Le-Petross HT, Macapinlac H, et al: Inflammatory breast cancer: PET/CT, MRI, mammography, and sonography findings, *Breast Cancer Res Treat* 109:417–426, 2008.
60. Le-Petross CH, Bidaut L, Yang WT: Evolving role of imaging modalities in inflammatory breast cancer, *Semin Oncol* 35:51–63, 2008.
61. Le-Petross HT, Cristofanilli M, Carkaci S, et al: MRI features of inflammatory breast cancer, *AJR Am J Roentgenol* 197:W769–W776, 2011.
62. Alunni JP: Imaging inflammatory breast cancer, *Diagn Interv Imaging* 93:95–103, 2012.
63. Kalli S, Freer PE, Rafferty EA: Lesions of the skin and superficial tissue at breast MR imaging, *Radiographics* 30:1891–1913, 2010.
64. Renz DM, Baltzer PA, Böttcher J, et al: Inflammatory breast carcinoma in magnetic resonance imaging: a comparison with locally advanced breast cancer, *Acad Radiol* 15:209–221, 2008.
65. Kalli S, Freer PE, Rafferty EA: Lesions of the skin and superficial tissue at breast MR imaging, *Radiographics* 30:1891–1913, 2010.
66. Carbognin G, Calciolari C, Girardi V, Camera L, Pollini G: Pozzi Mucelli R. Inflammatory breast cancer: MR imaging findings, *Radiol Med* 115:70–82, 2010.
67. Girardi V, Carbognin G, Camera L, et al: Inflammatory breast carcinoma and locally advanced breast carcinoma: characterization with MR imaging, *Radiol Med* 116:71–83, 2011.
68. Renz DM, Baltzer PA, Böttcher J, et al: Magnetic resonance imaging of inflammatory breast carcinoma and acute mastitis. A comparative study, *Eur Radiol* 18:2370–2380, 2008.
69. Molleran V, Mahoney MC: The BI-RADS breast magnetic resonance imaging lexicon, *Magn Reson Imaging Clin North Am* 18:171–185, 2012.

CHAPTER 7

Benign Findings in Breast MRI

Su-Ju Lee
Mary C. Mahoney

The current practice of breast imaging calls for using breast magnetic resonance imaging (MRI) only on high-risk patients with appropriate indications to maximize cancer detection yield and minimize the false-positive rate. Even with careful selection of patients, radiologists usually encounter benign findings more frequently than malignant lesions when interpreting breast MRI. It is important for radiologists to be familiar with these benign findings because it will enable them to select lesions for biopsy with improved specificity and to better assess radiologic-pathologic concordance of biopsy results. Some benign lesions, however, are simply indistinguishable from malignancy on imaging, and biopsy is necessary for histologic diagnosis. This chapter describes the MRI appearances of common and uncommon benign findings.

Benign Cystic Lesions

Duct Ectasia

Duct ectasia is a nonspecific dilation of the major subareolar ducts, with occasional involvement of smaller ducts. It has been found in women of all ages, and its etiology is unknown. Some consider all inflammatory processes as the initiating event, leading to destruction of the elastic network of the duct with subsequent duct ectasia and periductal fibrosis. Others suggest that duct dilation is the primary event, caused by obstruction of the ducts leading to secondary inflammation owing to leakage of duct contents.[1]

Most patients are asymptomatic. Some may present with spontaneous and intermittent clear to yellow nipple discharge. Mammographically, the calcified proteinaceous secretions within dilated ducts appear as bilateral symmetric rodlike "secretory calcifications." Ultrasonography will demonstrate dilated ducts filled with anechoic fluid, without or with debris.[1]

On MRI, ectatic ducts are usually incidental findings. They appear as non-enhancing, fluid-filled, often branching, tubular structures converging toward the nipple.[2] The contents of the ducts may show signal intensities similar to that of water, hypointense on T1-weighted images and hyperintense on T2-weighted sequences. More often, the fluid is hyperintense in signal on T1-weighted images because of proteinaceous or hemorrhagic contents (Figure 7.1, *A*). Because of such signal hyperintensity on precontrast images, postcontrast subtraction images are usually needed to confirm absence of contrast enhancement (Figure 7.1, *B*). Focal enhancement within the duct lumen would raise concern for intraductal papilloma or carcinoma.

Fibrocystic Changes

Fibrocystic change (FCC) refers to a constellation of benign breast changes that represent normal but exaggerated, hormonally mediated breast tissue response. The histologic findings include cyst formation, apocrine metaplasia, mild epithelial hyperplasia, stromal fibrosis, and mild adenosis. It is common in younger women, affecting one third of females 20 to 45 years of age. There is no increased risk for the subsequent development of breast carcinoma in women with non-proliferative FCC.[3] The risk of developing carcinoma is increased to 1.5 to 2 times when FCC is associated with moderate or florid ductal hyperplasia and increased 5 times with the presence of atypia.[1]

FCCs do not have specific mammographic or sonographic findings other than cyst formation. FCC has a wide spectrum of morphologic and kinetic features on MRI. It may appear as prominent nonmasslike enhancement in regional, focal, or segmental distribution[4] (Figures 7-2 and 7-3). A focal (nodular) form of FCC may appear as a mass with spiculated or smooth margins (Figures 7-4 and 7-5). The degree of initial enhancement ranges from slow to rapid, and the kinetic curves may vary between washout, plateau, or persistent enhancement during the delayed phase. In a small series of 11 cases studied by Chen and colleagues,[5] 62% of FCC showed early rapid enhancement with delayed washout, mimicking carcinoma.

Simple and Inflammatory Cysts

Cysts may be an isolated finding or may be seen as a component of FCCs on breast imaging. Simple cysts appear as circumscribed round or oval structures that are signal hyperintense on T2-weighted images and without contrast enhancement on postcontrast T1-weighted sequences (Figure 7.6). Cysts associated with inflammation will show a thickened enhancing wall on postcontrast images (Figure 7.7).

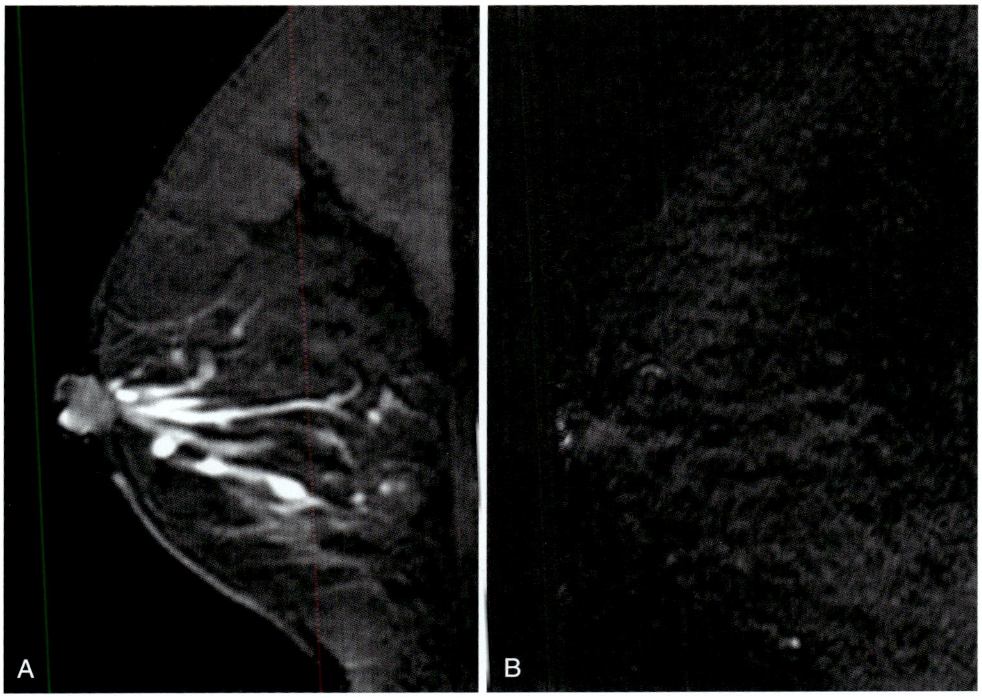

FIGURE 7.1 Duct ectasia is seen in a 61-year-old breast and ovarian cancer susceptibility (*BRCA*) gene–positive woman undergoing high-risk screening MRI. **A,** T1-weighted fat-suppressed noncontrast image shows dilated retroareolar ducts containing high signal intensity proteinaceous fluid. **B,** Postcontrast subtraction image is needed to confirm the absence of contrast enhancement within the dilated ducts.

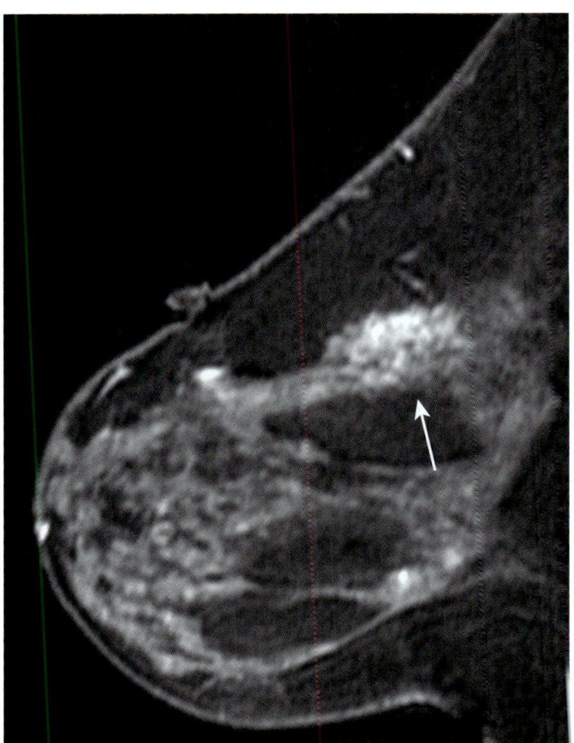

FIGURE 7.2 FCCs are seen in a 42-year-old woman with a recent diagnosis of right breast carcinoma. Sagittal T1-weighted fat-suppressed postcontrast MRI image shows regional clumped nonmasslike enhancement (*arrow*) in the ipsilateral breast. Enhancement kinetics are rapid and persistent. Biopsy revealed fibrocystic changes.

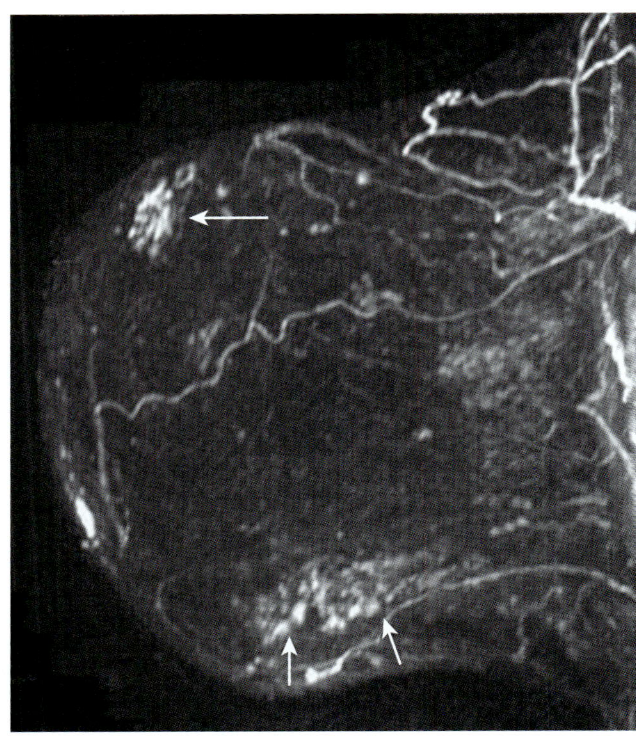

FIGURE 7.3 FCCs are seen in a 36-year-old woman with strong family history of premenopausal breast cancer. On screening MRI, T1-weighted fat-suppressed postcontrast maximum-intensity projection (MIP) image shows clumped nonmasslike enhancement in focal (*single arrow*) and segmental (*double arrows*) distributions. Enhancement kinetics are slow and persistent. Biopsies of both lesions yielded fibrocystic changes.

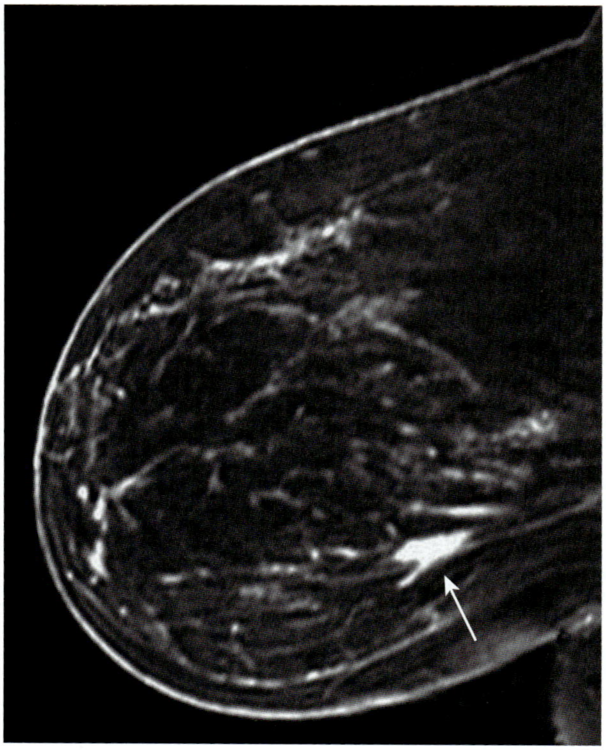

FIGURE 7.4 Focal (nodular) FCCs are seen in a 47-year-old woman with strong family history of premenopausal breast cancer. Sagittal T1-weighted fat-suppressed postcontrast MRI image shows an oblong 0.9 × 1.8 cm mass with irregular margins at 6 o'clock (*arrow*). The mass shows heterogeneous enhancement with rapid and persistent kinetics. Biopsy yielded fibrocystic changes.

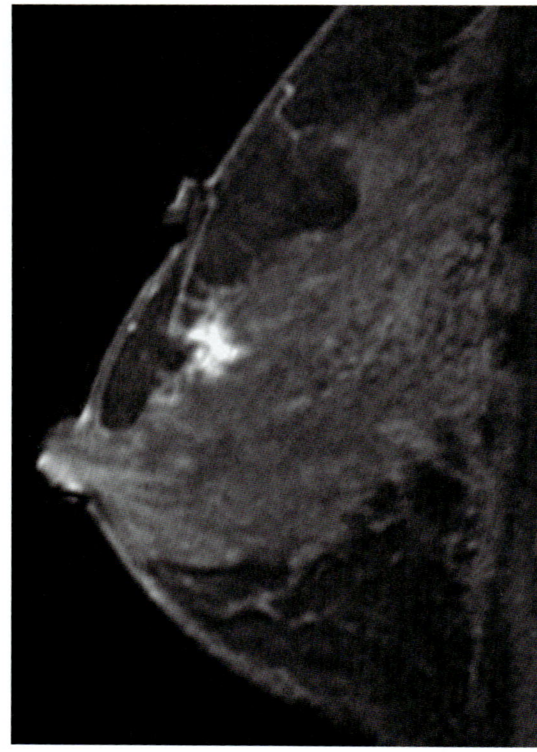

FIGURE 7.5 Focal (nodular) FCCs are seen in a 36-year-old woman with a palpable mass in the right breast, negative dense mammogram and sonogram. Sagittal T1-weighted fat-suppressed postcontrast MRI image shows a 1 cm irregular mass with heterogeneous enhancement and rapid and persistent enhancement kinetics. MRI-guided biopsy showed fibrocystic changes.

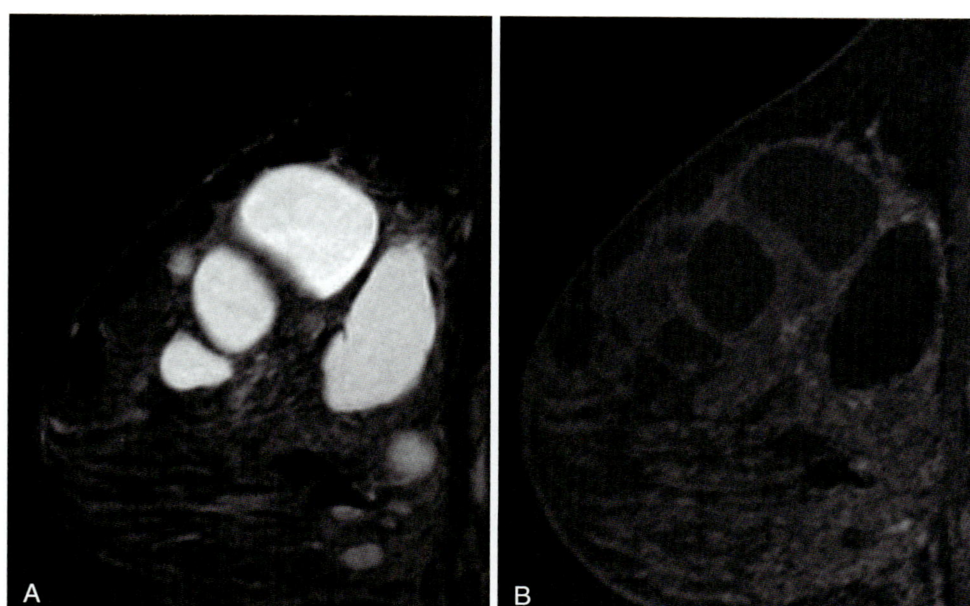

FIGURE 7.6 Simple cysts are seen in a 42-year-old woman with family history of premenopausal breast cancer in mother and sister. **A,** Screening breast MRI shows multiple cysts that are signal hyperintense on fat-suppressed T2-weighted sequence. **B,** There is no enhancement of the walls or contents of the cysts on the postcontrast fat-suppressed T1-weighted image.

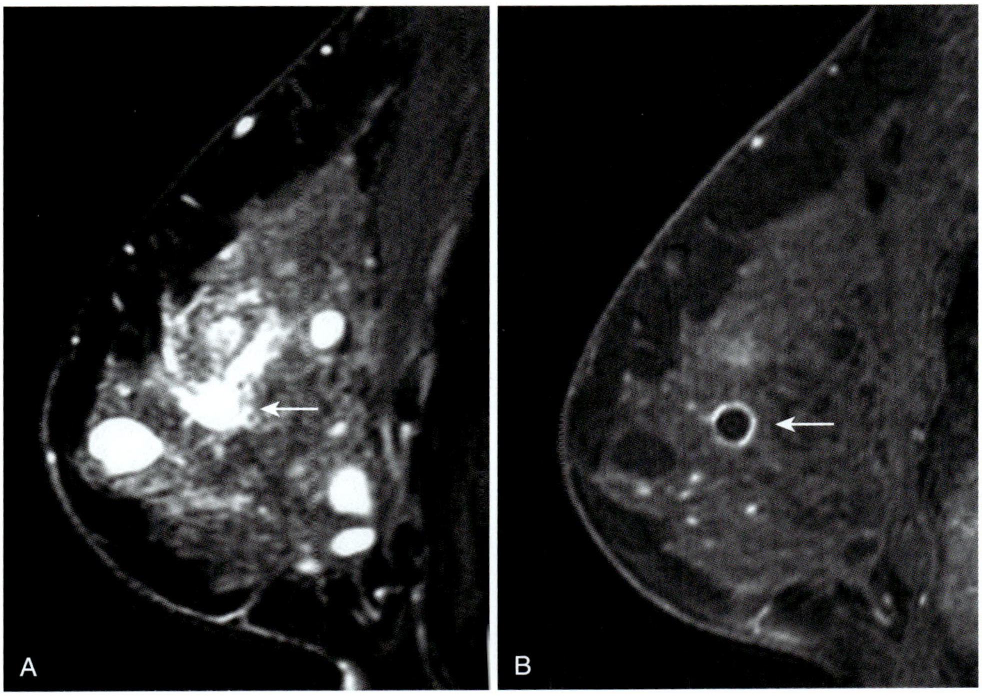

FIGURE 7.7 An inflammatory cyst is seen in a 49-year-old woman with a history of lumpectomy for tubular carcinoma of the right breast who underwent 6-month postoperative follow-up MRI. **A,** Sagittal fat-suppressed T2-weighted image shows a lesion with irregular margins (*arrow*) as well as multiple hyperintense cysts. **B,** Corresponding fat-suppressed T1-weighted image shows the lesion to be an inflammatory cyst with an enhancing thick wall and nonenhancing fluid content (*arrow*).

Benign Proliferative Lesions

Sclerosing Adenosis

Sclerosing adenosis is a benign proliferative lesion composed of distorted epithelial, myoepithelial, and stromal elements in a lobulocentric pattern. It may form a distinct nodule, hence the term *nodular sclerosing adenosis* or *adenosis tumor*.[3]

Sclerosing adenosis is usually asymptomatic and is often an incidental microscopic finding in breast tissue removed for another indication. The nodular form may cause a palpable mass. Mammographically, sclerosing adenosis may present as clustered, round, or punctate microcalcifications; a focal asymmetry; architectural distortion; or a spiculated mass. The combination of these features may mimic carcinoma. Its sonographic appearance is also nonspecific, including masses with circumscribed, indistinct, or microlobulated margins.[1]

On MRI, sclerosing adenosis may present as ductal enhancement or as homogeneously enhancing masses that are oval or round with lobulated or angular margins.[6,7] According to Oztekin and coworkers[7], it shows intermediate signal intensity on T1- and T2- weighted images, with rapid initial enhancement and delayed persistent or washout kinetics. At our institution, both plateau and washout kinetics have been observed in biopsy-proved sclerosing adenosis. Figure 7.8 illustrates an example of nodular sclerosing adenosis showing as a mass.

Radial Sclerosing Lesion

Radial scar is a benign sclerosing breast lesion of unknown cause, characterized by a central fibroelastotic core with radiating ducts and lobules exhibiting various proliferative changes. The term *complex sclerosing lesion* is used in cases in which the lesion is larger than 1 cm or composed of several closely contiguous fibroelastotic areas.[3] Rosen prefers the term *radial sclerosing lesions* for both entities.[8] Radial sclerosing lesions are considered high-risk lesions because of their association with carcinomas. This entity will be covered in Chapter 8.

Usual Ductal Hyperplasia

Ductal hyperplasia of usual type, or usual ductal hyperplasia (UDH), is a benign epithelial proliferation in a duct or lobule beyond the usual double cell layer, but no more than three to four cell layers above the basement membrane. It is a response to hormonal stimulation and imbalance. The term can be misleading, because this lesion usually occurs within the terminal ductal lobular unit (TDLU).[3]

UDH is clinically silent and almost always detected on screening mammography as microcalcifications or a mass. It does not have specific sonographic presentation. No systematic review of the MRI appearance of UDH is available in the literature. Published images demonstrate either foci or nonmasslike enhancement (stippled or clumped) in a linear, ductal, or regional distribution (Figure 7.9). Some biopsy-proved cases at our institution showed UDH as a subcentimeter mass (Figure 7.10). Delayed enhancement kinetics may be persistent, plateau, or mixed with some washout.

Columnar Cell Changes/Flat Epithelial Atypia

Columnar cell changes refer to a condition in which the normal epithelial cell layer of the TDLU is replaced by one or two layers of taller columnar epithelial cells that have basal nuclei and apical cytoplasmic snouts. When these columnar cells show cellular stratification with more than two cell layers, the entity is described as columnar cell hyperplasia. Columnar cell change with atypia and columnar cell hyperplasia with atypia are collectively referred to as

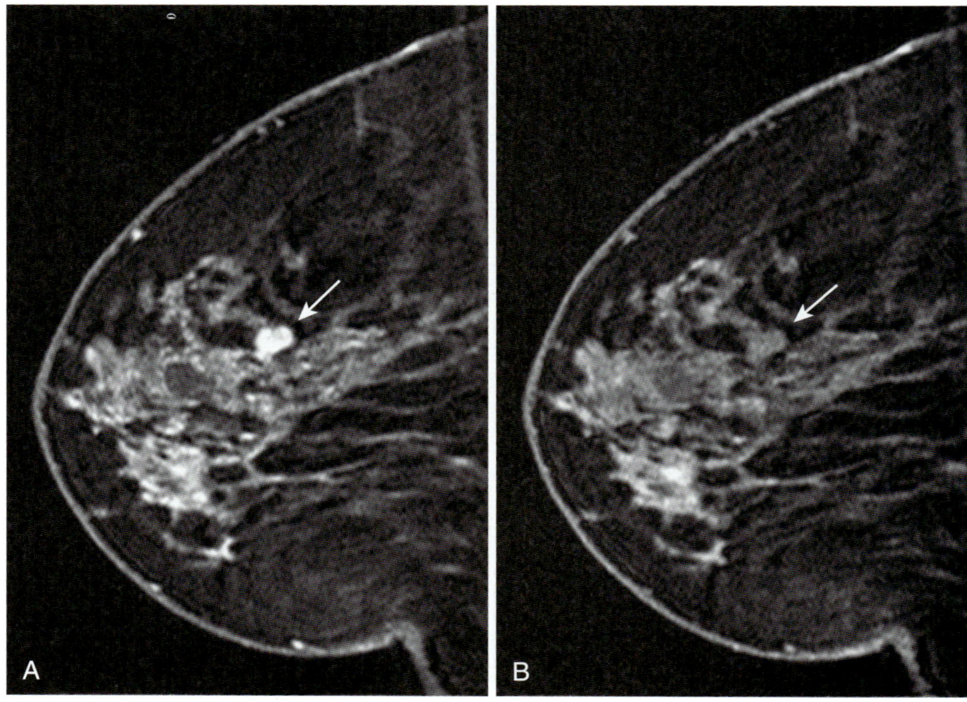

FIGURE 7.8 Nodular sclerosing adenosis is seen in a 42-year-old woman with a family history of breast cancer undergoing screening breast MRI. **A,** Sagittal T1-weighted postcontrast image with subtraction shows a 1-cm lobular mass (*arrow*) with irregular margins and homogeneous enhancement. **B,** T1-weighted, fat-suppressed precontrast image shows the mass (*arrow*) to be isointense in signal to normal parenchyma. The lesion exhibits a medium rate of initial enhancement with delayed plateau kinetics. Biopsy revealed nodular sclerosing adenosis.

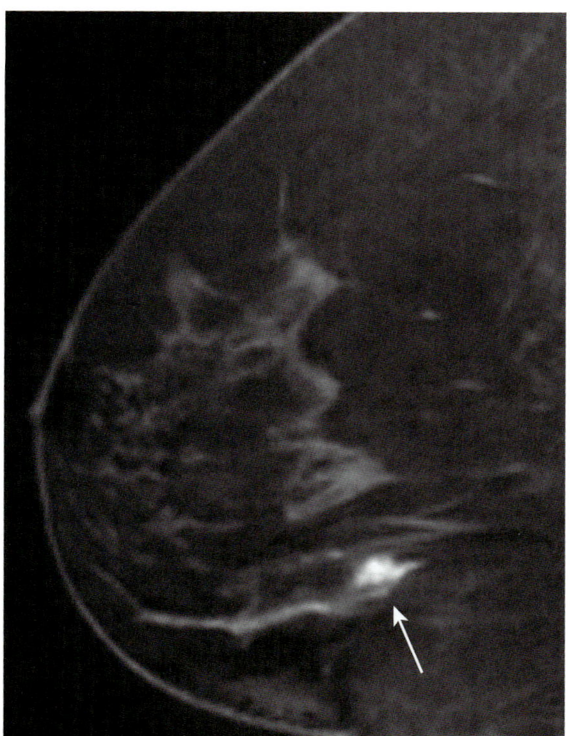

FIGURE 7.9 UDH is seen in a 58-year-old woman with a history of remote right mastectomy for breast cancer. Screening mammogram shows a developing focal asymmetry in the inferior breast. On MRI for problem solving, sagittal T1-weighted fat-suppressed postcontrast image shows focal clumped nonmasslike enhancement (*arrow*). Biopsy yielded usual ductal hyperplasia.

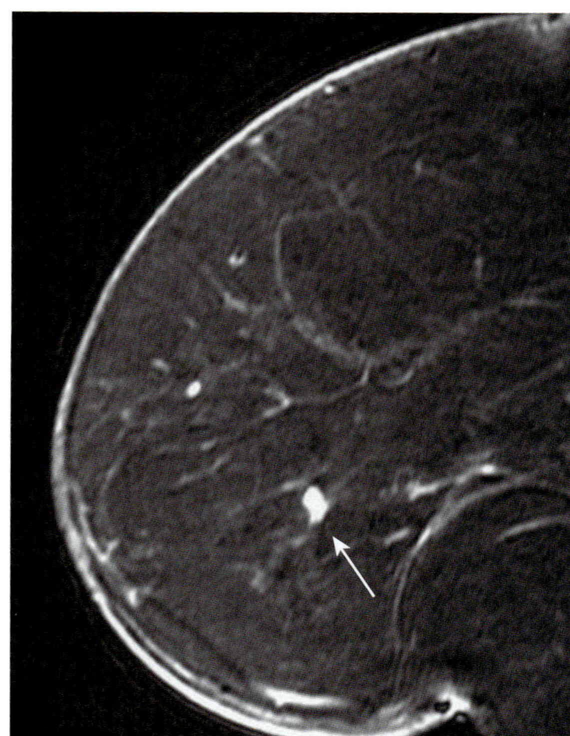

FIGURE 7.10 UDH is seen in a 52-year-old woman with a history of left breast cancer, after left mastectomy and right reduction mammoplasty, undergoing high-risk screening MRI. Sagittal T1-weighted fat-suppressed postcontrast image shows a small oval mass with slightly irregular inferior margins (*arrow*). It exhibits rapid enhancement with mixed plateau and washout kinetics. Biopsy revealed usual ductal hyperplasia.

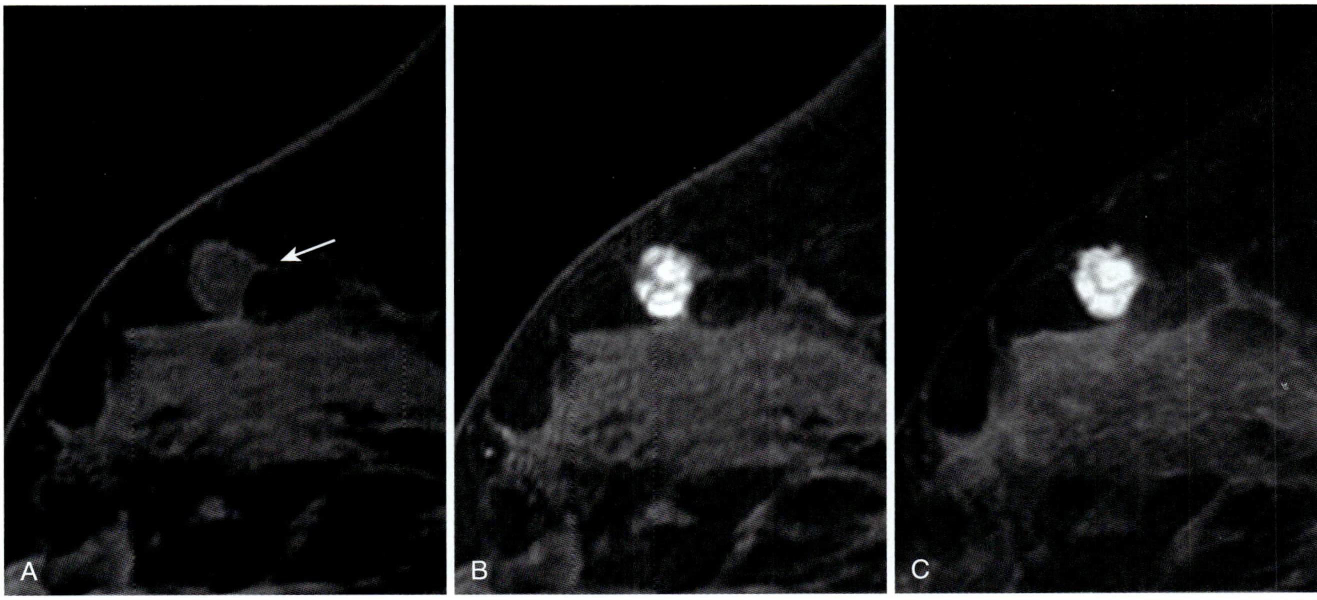

FIGURE 7.11 Fibroadenoma is seen in a 35-year-old woman with a strong family history of breast cancer undergoing high-risk screening breast MRI. **A**, Sagittal T1-weighted fat-suppressed noncontrast image of the right breast shows a mass hypointense in signal to the adjacent parenchyma (*arrow*). **B**, Sagittal T1-weighted fat-suppressed postcontrast image shows smooth lobular margins and internal nonenhancing septations. **C**, The dark septations are also visible on a sagittal T2-weighted fat-suppressed image. The mass showed initial rapid and delayed persistent enhancement pattern. Biopsy was performed because of patient preference and revealed a fibroadenoma.

flat epithelial atypia (FEA).[3] Because of its frequent association with carcinomas, FEA is regarded as a high-risk lesion. This entity will be discussed in detail in Chapter 8.

Atypical Ductal Hyperplasia

Atypical ductal hyperplasia (ADH) defines a group of proliferative lesions that have some, but not all, of the features of ductal carcinoma in situ (DCIS), either by lack of a major defining cytologic feature of carcinoma or by having the features to lesser extent than true DCIS.[3] ADH is associated with a 4 to 5 times relative risk of development of breast cancer within 10 to 15 years. It will be covered in Chapter 8.

Lobular Neoplasia

Atypical lobular hyperplasia (ALH) and lobular carcinoma in situ (LCIS) are relatively uncommon lesions, collectively identified as lobular neoplasia. These lesions are considered to be generalized risk factors for subsequent breast cancer, with a relative risk of 4 to 5 times for ALH and 8 to 10 times for LCIS.[3] Lobular neoplasias are high-risk lesions that will be discussed in detail in Chapter 8.

Fibroepithelial Tumors

Fibroadenoma

Fibroadenoma is a benign hyperplastic fibroepithelial tumor characterized by concurrent proliferation of both glandular and stromal elements in varying proportions. It is the most common breast mass encountered in women younger than 35 years of age and the most common solid mass in women of all ages.[1] Juvenile (cellular) fibroadenoma is a variant of fibroadenoma that occasionally occurs in adolescents who present with a rapidly growing, well-defined mass that may reach 20 cm in size. The macroscopic and histologic appearances are similar to fibroadenomas, although the stroma may be more cellular. This makes differentiation from phyllodes tumor challenging in some cases.[3]

A patient with a fibroadenoma usually presents with a mobile, painless, palpable mass. Mammographically, it appears as a circumscribed round, oval, or lobular mass that is iso- or hypodense to the parenchyma. Coarse calcifications, when present, may be diagnostic. Sonographically, it appears as a mass that is iso- or hypoechoic to fat, with a parallel orientation to the skin. Atypical findings include microlobulated or indistinct margins and acoustic shadowing due to internal calcification.[1] In keeping with their histologic heterogeneity, fibroadenomas have been shown to have widely varied MRI appearances. On MRI, a fibroadenoma typically appears as an oval mass with smooth margins. It may have a lobular shape. On T1-weighted images, it is iso- or hypointense to normal parenchyma. On T2-weighted images, its signal intensity varies with the amount of myxoid (high signal) and fibrous (low signal) components. The fibrous component increases with increasing age. The degree of contrast enhancement varies with its degree of sclerosis and cellularity.[9]

Nunes and coworkers[10] described low-signal internal septations that are seen on T2- or enhanced T1- weighted images, representing dense collagen bands, as 89% to 93% specific for the diagnosis of fibroadenoma. The specificity increased slightly when internal septations were seen in combination with features of smooth margins or lobular shape.[10] Figure 7.11 illustrates a fibroadenoma with these classic features. However, such septations are observed in only 40% to 64% of fibroadenomas on MRI.[9,10] Furthermore, they have recently been described in benign and malignant phyllodes tumors and mucinous carcinoma and may be of limited value for diagnosing fibroadenoma when considered alone.[11-13]

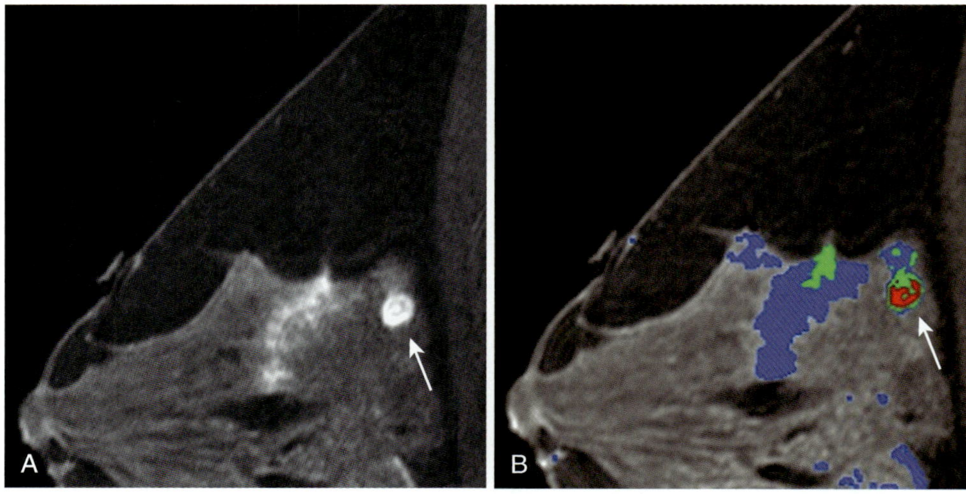

FIGURE 7.12 Fibroadenoma is seen in a 33-year-old woman with a strong family history of premenopausal breast cancer undergoing high-risk screening breast MRI. **A,** Sagittal T1-weighted fat-suppressed postcontrast image of the right breast shows a 1-cm mass (*arrow*) with smooth margins and heterogeneous enhancement. **B,** The mass has rapid and washout enhancement kinetics based on color overlay (*red, arrow*). Core needle biopsy revealed a fibroadenoma. Surgical excision, performed because of washout kinetics, confirmed the diagnosis of a fibroadenoma.

Fibroadenomas usually enhance homogeneously, with heterogeneous enhancement seen with increasing sclerosis. The most common enhancement kinetics of fibroadenoma is rapid (early phase) and persistent (delayed phase). However, some fibroadenomas are known to show rapid early enhancement with delayed washout kinetics, mimicking malignancy[11] (Figure 7.12).

When a fibroadenoma is suspected on MRI, review of the mammogram and sonogram may help in confirming the diagnosis. However, biopsy should be considered in cases in which a presumed fibroadenoma demonstrates interval growth or atypical features on conventional imaging.

Phyllodes Tumor

Phyllodes tumor is a rare neoplasm with a reported incidence of less than 1% of all female breast tumors. This tumor is similar to fibroadenoma in that it is a fibroepithelial lesion with both epithelial and stromal proliferations. However, phyllodes tumor has a much greater stromal cellularity than a fibroadenoma. Phyllodes tumors are high-risk lesions and will be covered in Chapter 8.

Papillary Lesions

Papillary lesions of the breast may be classified as solitary intraductal papillomas, multiple intraductal (peripheral) papillomas, atypia-DCIS within a papilloma, micropapillary DCIS, and papillary carcinoma.[3,14] Benign papillary lesions include solitary and multiple intraductal papillomas and papillomas with atypia. These are high-risk lesions and will be discussed in detail in Chapter 8.

Mesenchymal Lesions

Pseudoangiomatous Stromal Hyperplasia

Pseudoangiomatous stromal hyperplasia (PASH) is an uncommon benign proliferation of fibrous stroma, containing slitlike pseudovascular spaces lined by myofibroblasts. PASH usually occurs in premenopausal women, probably resulting from an aberrant response to hormonal stimuli. Less commonly, it may occur in postmenopausal females on hormone replacement therapy or as an incidental component of gynecomastia in males. It is considered a neoplastic process because of its ability to recur. However, it is not known to be premalignant.[1]

PASH is usually an incidental microscopic finding in breast biopsies with no mammographic correlate. When symptomatic, a patient with PASH may present with a painless, mobile mass (nodular PASH), frequently misdiagnosed as a fibroadenoma.[1] It can become very large gradually or rapidly (tumoral PASH) or extensively infiltrative (diffuse PASH), causing dramatic asymmetric enlargement of the involved breast. As a mass, PASH may or may not have a discernible capsule. Rarely, skin necrosis can develop over a rapidly growing lesion.[15-22]

Mammographically, nodular PASH may appear as a circumscribed or partially circumscribed mass, or as a developing focal asymmetry.[15] Several authors have reported it as a mass with indistinct, obscured, or spiculated margins.[16,17] No cases of architectural distortion or calcifications were identified.

Sonographically, PASHs usually appear as hypoechoic masses with rare cystic components, and they are often mistaken for fibroadenomas. A less common presentation is an echogenic area containing central linear hypoechoic areas or cysts.[15] Multiple tiny cystic spaces within dense stroma have been reported in tumoral and diffuse forms of PASH.[18,19] Abundant color flow on Doppler, indicating hyperemia in a diffuse PASH, has been observed.[20] Teh and colleagues[18] reported the presence of fine hyperechoic lines in a "lace-like" pattern, corresponding with the dense collagen strands in tumoral PASH. The posterior acoustic features vary from moderate acoustic enhancement to mild shadowing.[1]

As expected with its various forms, PASH has a variable MRI appearance. In the series of Jones and associates,[15] most lesions present as clumped nonmasslike enhancement, in focal or segmental distributions (Figure 7.13). Nodular PASH may appear as a small irregular mass (Figure 7.14).

Only sporadic single case reports are available on the MRI appearance of tumoral or diffuse PASH. Tumoral

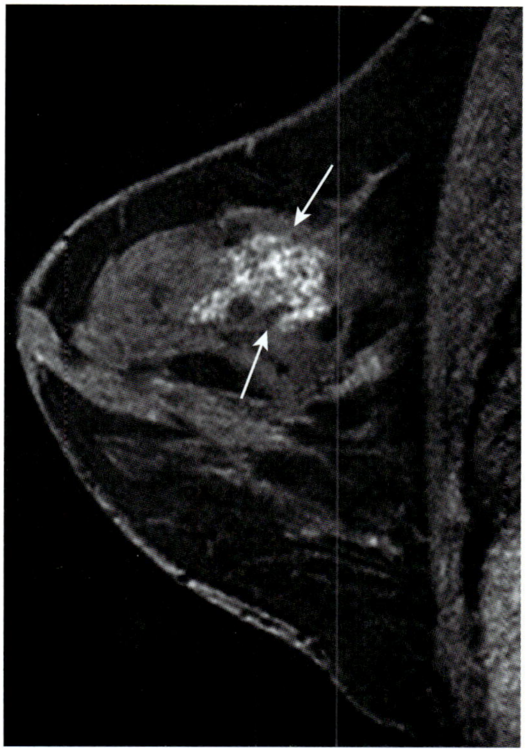

FIGURE 7.13 Pseudoangiomatous stromal hyperplasia is seen in a 35-year-old woman with a prior left mastectomy for rhabdomyosarcoma. Sagittal three-dimensional (3-D) gadolinium-enhanced fast spoiled gradient-echo MR image of right breast, obtained immediately after gadolinium administration, shows an area of nonmasslike clumped enhancement in the upper breast (*between arrows*). The finding shows persistent enhancement. MRI-guided biopsy showed pseudoangiomatous stromal hyperplasia. *(Reprinted with permission from the* American Journal of Roentgenology. *From Jones KN, Glazebrook KN, Reynolds C: Pseudoangiomatous stromal hyperplasia: Imaging findings with pathologic and clinical correlation,* AJR Am J Roentgenol *195:1036-1042, 2010).*

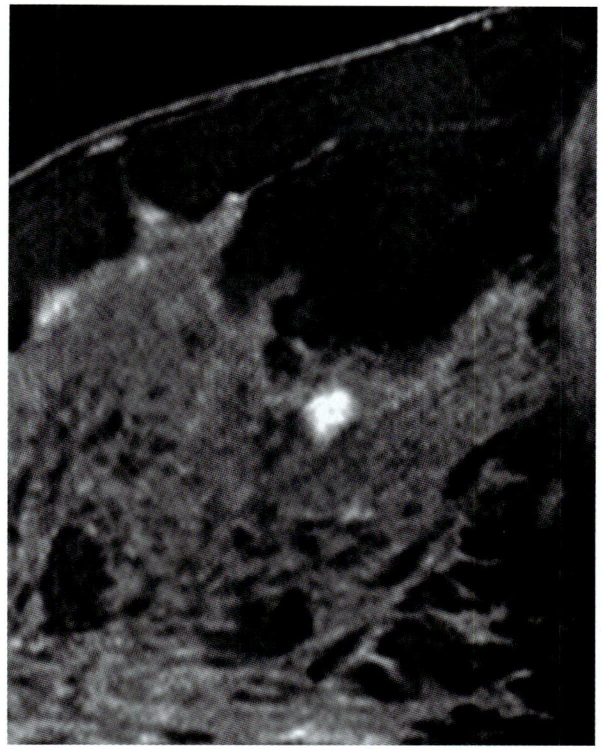

FIGURE 7.14 Nodular PASH is seen in a 43-year-old woman with a family history of premenopausal breast cancer undergoing high-risk screening breast MRI. Sagittal T1-weighted fat-suppressed immediate postcontrast image of the right breast shows a 1.1-cm mass with ill-defined margins and intense enhancement. It showed rapid initial enhancement with delayed washout kinetics. Biopsy revealed pseudoangiomatous stromal hyperplasia.

PASH appears as a large circumscribed mass or a mass without a discernible capsule.[18,19] On T1-weighted sequences, the mass shows intermediate signals with interspersed cysts of lower signals. On T2-weighted sequences, high-signal cysts mixed with low- to intermediate-signal stroma are reported.[18,22] According to Teh and coworkers,[18] hyperintense fine reticular "lacelike" networks on T2-weighted images, thought to correspond to collagen strands, may be a distinguishing MRI feature for tumoral PASH. Enhancement appears heterogeneous on published images, with delayed persistent kinetics (Figure 7.15).

Two cases of bilateral diffuse PASH with similar MRI characteristics were found in the English literature.[20,22] Baskin and associates[22] reported T2 prolongation of prominent stroma between glands on fat-suppressed T2-weighted spin echo images and diffuse prominent enhancement of individual glands throughout the breast. Time-intensity curves show initial rapid and delayed persistent enhancement kinetics.

Most reports describe delayed persistent enhancement kinetics in PASH, especially in the tumoral or diffuse form. However, in cases of PASH presenting as small irregular masses, plateau or washout delayed kinetics have also been observed (see Figure 7.14).[15]

PASH is not premalignant, but may recur locally after excision in 12.5% of cases.[23] Although it was not known to be associated with malignancy previously, Drinka and colleagues[24] recently identified *proliferative PASH* in 2.4% of 79 PASH cases they studied, with atypical ductal and atypical lobular hyperplasia found in 25.6% and infiltrating carcinoma in 11% of proliferative PASH. Hence, they recommend thorough histologic evaluation of biopsy specimen demonstrating PASH, with clinical and radiologic follow-up.[24] The recommended treatment is wide local excision to prevent local recurrence. Rarely, diffuse PASH may necessitate mastectomy for symptomatic and cosmetic indications.[18,19]

Stromal Fibrosis

Stromal fibrosis is a benign lesion characterized by proliferation of fibrous stroma with obliteration and atrophy of mammary ducts and lobules. It has been described by various terms such as *focal fibrous disease*, *fibrous tumor*, *focal fibrosis*, and *fibrous mastopathy*. The diagnosis has become more frequently encountered with increased use of screening mammography, sonography, and breast MRI. Stromal fibrosis may represent 2.1% to 9% of lesions found in image-guided core biopsy.[25]

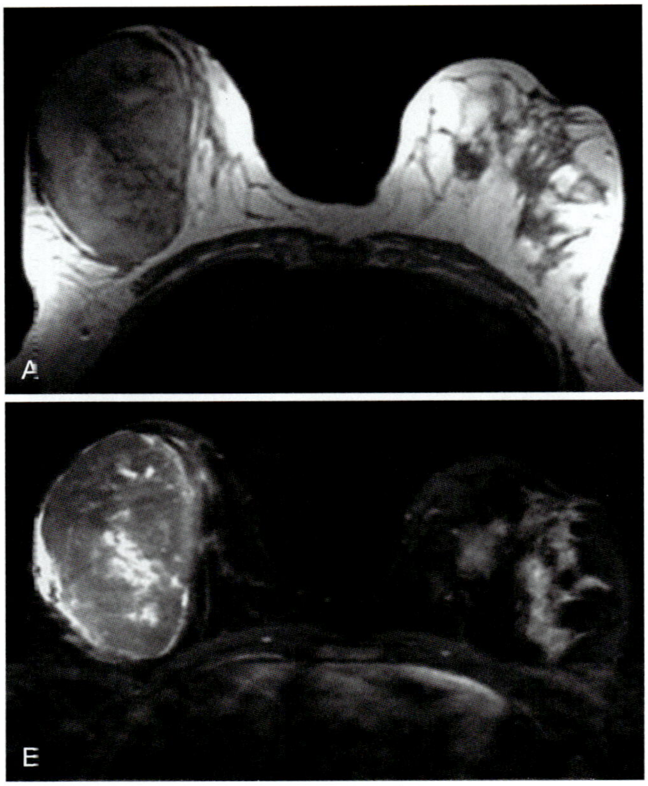

FIGURE 7.15 PASH is shown in tumoral form. **A,** An ovoid well-circumscribed mass is seen in the outer quadrant of the right breast with heterogeneous enhancement after contrast administration. **B,** A short TI inversion recovery (STIR) image shows an intermediate signal intensity lesion with high signal intensity lines within the mass. Enhancement kinetics showed a gradual signal intensity increase. *(From Iglesias A, Arias M, Santiago P, et al.: Benign breast lesions that simulate malignancy: magnetic resonance imaging with radiologic-pathologic correlation,* Curr Probl Diagn Radiol *36:66-82, 2007).*

Clinically, a palpable mass may be found in a patient or the lesion may be seen as a screening mammographic abnormality in an asymptomatic woman. Its mammographic findings are nonspecific, including spiculated mass, architectural distortion, or a benign-appearing circumscribed mass.[1] Sonographically, it may be highly echogenic, similar to normal fibroglandular tissue, or it may present as a circumscribed or spiculated hypoechoic mass. Biopsy is often needed for diagnosis.

Lee and Mahoney[26] studied 40 cases of biopsy-proved, pure stromal fibrosis on breast MRI. More than half of the lesions presented as masses (Figure 7.16), 87% of which were less than 1 cm in size (Figure 7.17). Some appeared as foci or areas of nonmasslike enhancement (Figure 7.18). Although extremely variable, the most common appearance of nonmass lesions was clumped enhancement in linear distribution.

Most lesions were iso- to hypointense to normal parenchyma on T1-weighted images, and variable in signal intensity on T2-weighted sequences, depending on the water content of the lesion. The enhancement kinetics also varied but usually showed medium or rapid initial contrast uptake, with plateau or washout delayed curves. On histopathology, ectatic vessels were found within most of the lesions, which may explain the degree of contrast enhancement on MRI.[26]

Mammary Fibromatosis

Mammary fibromatosis is a rare benign stromal tumor of the breast that accounts for less than 0.2% of all breast tumors. It was initially reported in a patient with Gardner syndrome but may occur sporadically or after trauma or surgery. Most cases were reported in women, with rare cases in men.

Mammary fibromatosis mimics malignancy, both clinically and by imaging. Clinically, it presents as a suspicious palpable mass, which may be associated with skin retraction

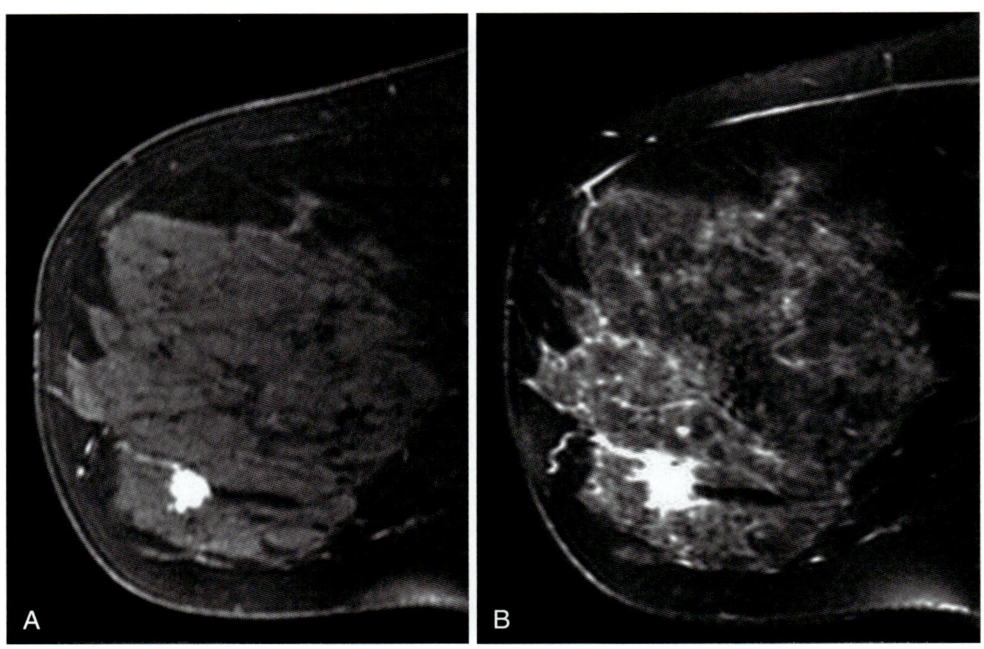

FIGURE 7.16 Stromal fibrosis is seen in a 60-year-old woman with a recent diagnosis of ductal carcinoma in situ (DCIS) of the left breast undergoing staging MRI. **A,** Sagittal T1-weighted postcontrast image shows a lobular mass with irregular margins and intense homogeneous contrast enhancement with initial rapid and delayed washout and plateau kinetics. It was mildly signal hypointense on the corresponding noncontrast image (not shown). **B,** Sagittal T2-weighted fat-suppressed image shows signal hyperintensity of the lesion. Core needle biopsy and subsequent surgical excision revealed stromal fibrosis.

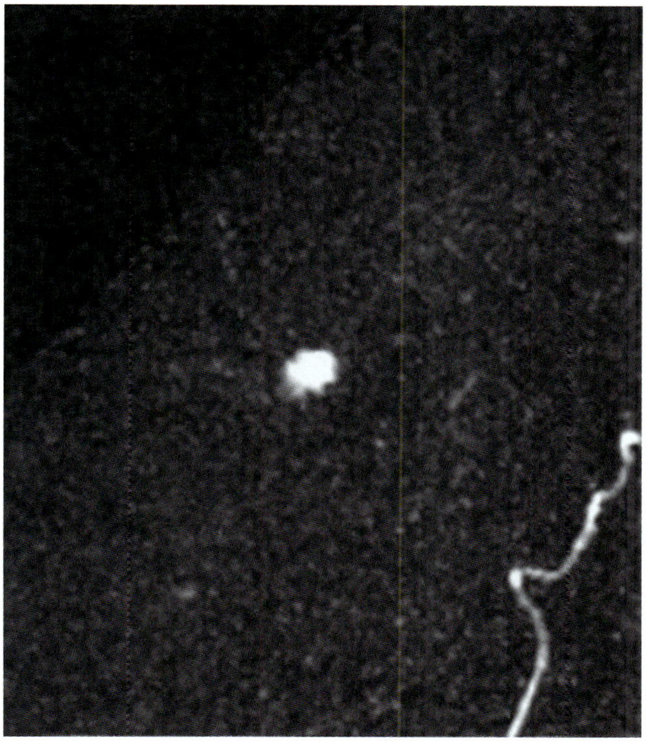

FIGURE 7.17 Stromal fibrosis is seen in a 57-year-old woman who presented for follow-up of an MRI-identified lesion at another institution. Sagittal fat-suppressed T1-weighted postcontrast image shows a 9-mm round mass with irregular margins and homogenous enhancement. Time intensity curve showed initial medium rate of enhancement and delayed plateau kinetics. Biopsy revealed stromal fibrosis.

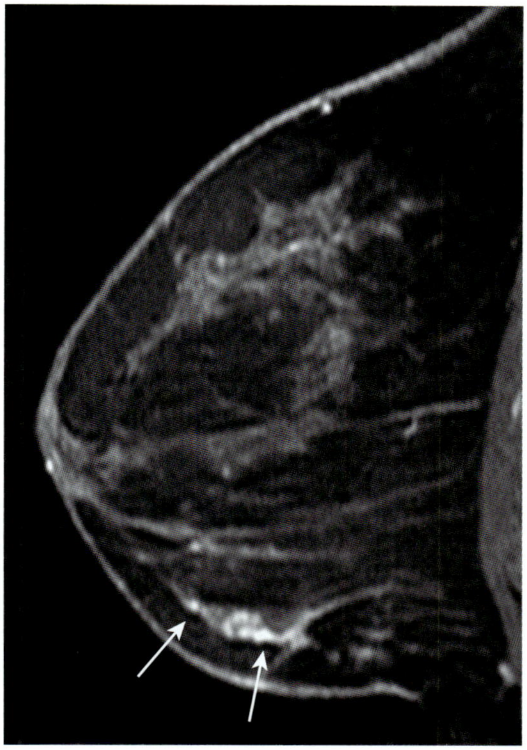

FIGURE 7.18 Stromal fibrosis is seen in a 41-year-old woman with a strong family history of breast cancer undergoing high-risk screening breast MRI. Sagittal T1-weighted fat-suppressed postcontrast image shows stippled and clumped nonmasslike enhancement in a linear distribution in the inferior breast (*arrows*). MRI-guided biopsy revealed stromal fibrosis.

and fixation to the chest wall. It appears as a spiculated mass on mammogram. On ultrasound, it usually appears as an irregular solid hypoechoic mass with spiculated or microlobulated margins and tethering of Cooper ligaments. It may be locally aggressive, involving the pectoralis or intercostal muscles.[27]

On MRI, mammary fibromatosis typically appears as an irregular mass isointense to muscle on T1-weighted images and variably hyperintense on T2-weighted sequences. It typically shows benign persistent enhancement curves in the delayed phase (Figure 7.19), although plateau and washout kinetics have been reported. MRI is the best imaging modality for evaluation of chest wall invasion and extent of disease. The recommended treatment is complete surgical resection with clear margins. Although benign, it is locally aggressive with a high recurrence rate of up to 29%.[27]

Granular Cell Tumor

Granular cell tumor (GCT) is a tumor of Schwann cell origin that may occur at any body site, involving the breast in 6% to 8% of cases. It is an uncommon but important entity because of its tendency to mimic breast carcinoma on clinical and imaging presentations.

Clinically, a patient with GCT usually presents with a palpable firm lump, occasionally associated with skin fixation and thickening and nipple retraction. It has a widely varied mammographic appearance, ranging from a focal asymmetry to a mass with ill-defined or spiculated margins. Its sonographic features also vary widely from benign-appearing masses with circumscribed margins and acoustic enhancement to malignant-appearing masses with spiculated margins and acoustic shadowing. Histologically GCTs with circumscribed margins exhibit scant fibrous stroma, whereas the ones with spiculated margins have a background of dense fibrous stroma.[28]

There are few reports of the MRI appearance of GCT. It has been described as a mass with either smooth or spiculated margins. It is low in signal intensity on T1-weighted images, hypointense to glandular tissue or isointense to skeletal muscle.[21,29,30] The reported T2 signal intensities and enhancement patterns of GCT are widely variable. On T2-weighted sequences, its signal intensity is described as hypointense to muscle,[30] isointense to glandular tissue,[21,29] or demonstrating a high–signal-intensity rim.[31] It may enhance homogenously[30-32] or heterogeneously, particularly pronounced at its margin.[21,29] GCTs show medium or rapid rate of contrast enhancement during early phase, with either persistent[29,32] or washout kinetics[21,30] in the late phase. Figures 7-20 and 7-21 are examples of GCTs identified on MRI.

It is impossible to establish a diagnosis of GCT without biopsy. Despite its diagnostic challenges, GCT is usually benign and carries an excellent prognosis. However, approximately 2% of GCTs are malignant. Malignant GCT can metastasize widely and have a grave prognosis. Wide local excision is the treatment of choice for both benign and malignant GCTs.

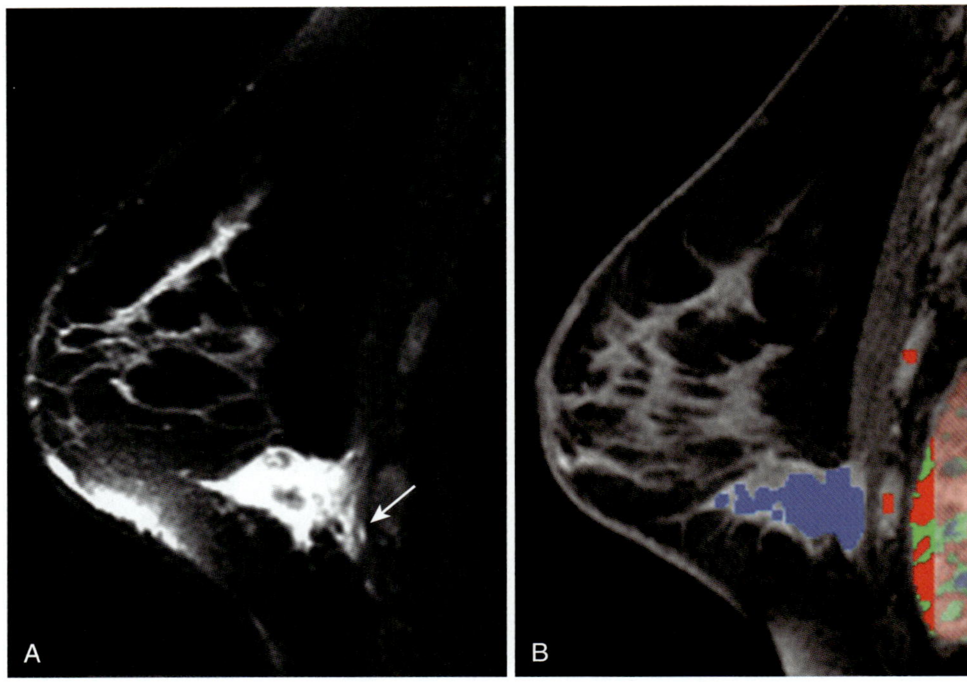

FIGURE 7.19 Fibromatosis is seen in a 28-year-old woman with a palpable mass in the inferior left breast. **A,** T2-weighted image shows a predominantly hyperintense mass invading the pectoralis muscle (*arrow*). **B,** Computer-aided detection (CADstream, Confirma, Inc.) image shows progressive enhancement (*blue*) of fibromatosis. *(Reprinted with permission from the* American Journal of Roentgenology. *From Glazebrook KN, Renolds CA: Mammary Fibromatosis,* AJR Am J Roentgenol *193:856-860, 2009)*

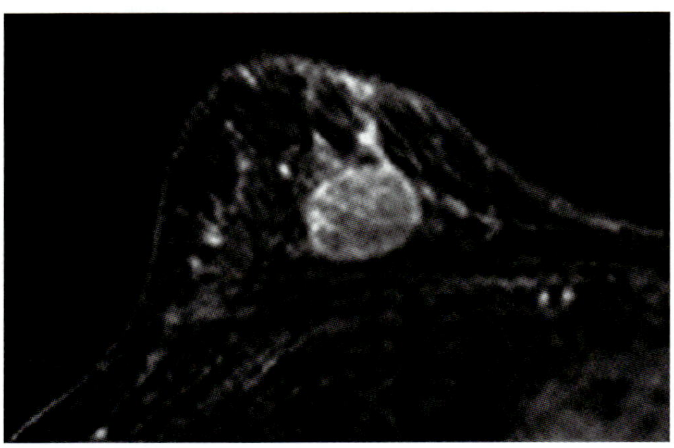

FIGURE 7.20 A GCT is shown in an axial postcontrast subtraction MRI image. It appears as a focal ovoid mass with fine irregular borders and intense enhancement, especially at the borders. *(From Iglesias A, Arias M, Santiago P, et al.: Benign breast lesions that simulate malignancy: magnetic resonance imaging with radiologic-pathologic correlation,* Curr Probl Diagn Radiol *36:66-82, 2007.)*

Long-term surveillance is recommended for large tumors, rapid growth, local recurrence, and multiple lesions, owing to the slight, but real, malignant potential of GCTs.[28]

Diabetic Mastopathy

Diabetic mastopathy is a condition in which stromal proliferation forms fibrous masses, predominantly in female patients with long-standing insulin-dependent (type 1) diabetes mellitus. Rarely, it may occur in males or in type 2 diabetic patients. The interval between the onset of diabetes and presentation of the breast lesion is reportedly about 20 years. It is known by various names, including *diabetic fibrous mastopathy*, *mastopathy in insulin-dependent diabetes*, *diabetic fibrous breast disease*, and *diabetic sclerosing lymphocytic lobulitis of the breast*.[33]

The pathogenesis of diabetic mastopathy is not completely understood. It probably represents an immune reaction to the abnormal accumulation of altered extracellular matrix in the breast, secondary to prolonged hyperglycemia. The characteristic pathology findings include dense keloid-like fibrosis enclosing "epithelioid fibroblasts," lymphocytic ductitis and lobulitis, and perilobular and perivascular lymphocytic infiltration. The lymphocytic infiltrate is composed predominantly of B cells. The increased expression of HLA-DR4 antigen in involved lobular epithelium and the association with other autoimmune diseases support the presumed autoimmune pathogenesis.[33,34]

Clinically, patients usually present with a nontender, palpable, firm to hard mass in one or both breasts. Mammography may reveal a heterogeneously dense parenchymal pattern, focal asymmetry, or a mass with obscured, indistinct, or spiculated margins. Ultrasound shows a heterogeneously hypoechoic mass with ill-defined margins and marked posterior acoustic shadowing. There is absence of color flow signals on Doppler study. Diabetic mastopathy may mimic breast cancer on clinical, mammographic, and ultrasound examinations because of the extensive fibrosis.[35] Tissue sampling is necessary for diagnosis and to exclude a malignancy. Treatment options are either excision or close follow-up, depending on the individual circumstances.

Diabetic mastopathy is isointense to glandular tissue on breast MRI, but a mass can often be appreciated on the non–fat-suppressed T1-weighted image.[1] Wong and colleagues[35] and Tuncbilek and coworkers[36] reported no discernible enhancing mass on postcontrast MRI. Wong and colleagues described nonspecific patchy or diffuse stromal enhancement, and Tuncbilek and associates reported homogeneous, low enhancement and glandular distortion. Figure 7.22 illustrates a published case of diabetic mastopathy.

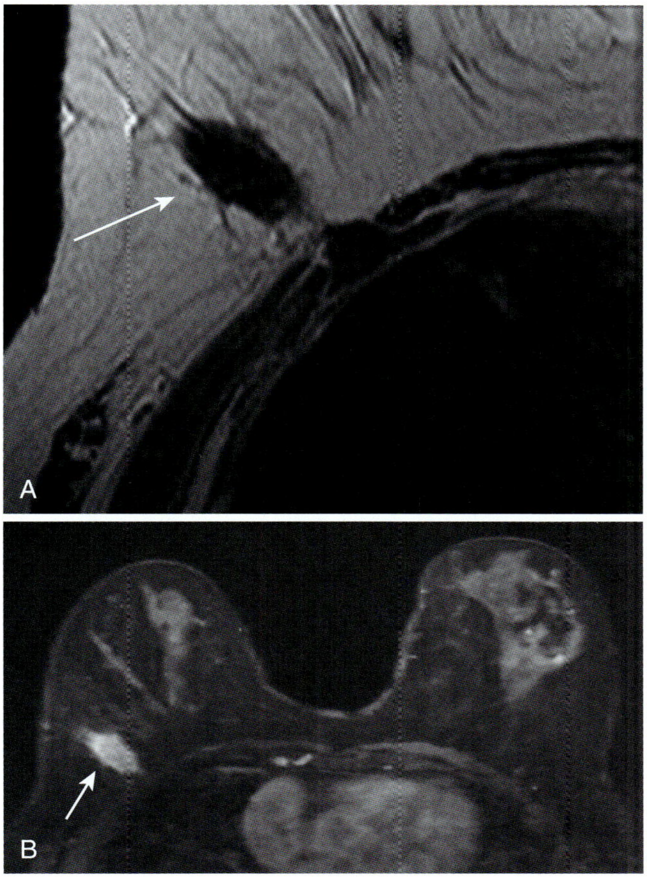

FIGURE 7.21 A GCT is shown. **A,** Axial T2-weighted image, without fat saturation, demonstrates the extremely low signal—hypointense to muscle—throughout the lesion. **B,** Axial fat-saturated postcontrast T1-weighted image shows avid predominantly homogeneous enhancement throughout the GCT, without areas of necrosis, cystic degeneration, or rim-type pattern. The enhancement kinetics were initial rapid and delayed washout. *(From Maki DD, Horne D, Damore II LJ, Jones C: Magnetic resonance appearance of granular cell tumor of the breast,* Clin Imaging *33:395-397, 2009).*

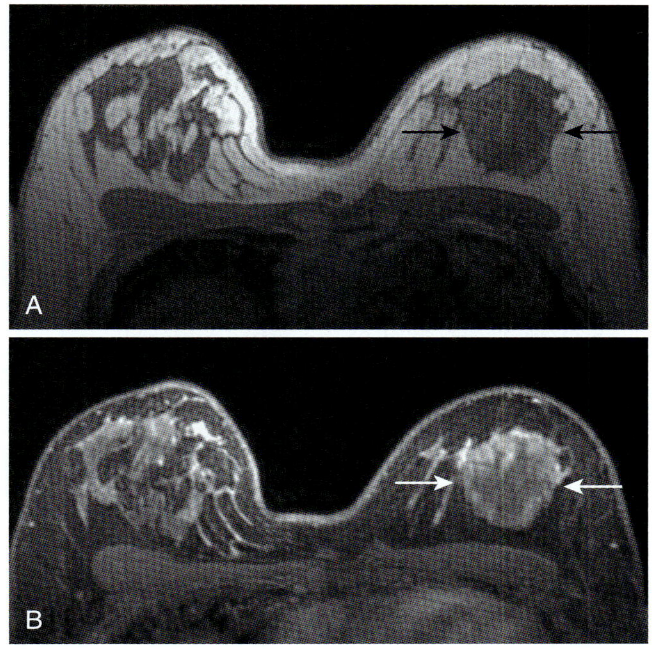

FIGURE 7.22 Diabetic mastopathy is shown. **A,** T1-weighted non–fat-suppressed MRI scan shows an isointense round mass (*between arrows*) with slightly irregular margins in the left breast. **B,** T1-weighted contrast-enhanced MRI scan shows minimal contrast enhancement of the left fibrous mass (*between arrows*). *(From Apple SK, Dascalos JM, Bassett L: Solid benign lesions of the breast. In Bassett L, Mahoney MC, Apple SK, D'Orsi CJ, editors:* Breast imaging, *Philadelphia, 2011, Elsevier Saunders, pp 278-279.)*

Lipoma

Lipoma is a benign fatty tumor that may occur anywhere in the breast. Most lipomas are located in the subcutaneous fat. They may manifest as soft, mobile palpable masses or incidental findings on screening mammography. The cause of lipomas is unknown.

Lipomas have a classic appearance on mammography, presenting as a completely radiolucent mass with a thin radiopaque capsule. On ultrasound, they may be isoechoic to adjacent fat lobules or mildly hyperechoic. Occasionally, lipomas may contain multiple echogenic septa that course parallel to the skin.[1]

On MRI, lipomas present as oval masses with smooth margins. Their signal intensity follows that of normal fatty tissue in the breast on all sequences. They have high signal intensity identical to the adjacent normal fatty tissue on T1-weighted non–fat-suppressed sequences. On T1-weighted fat-suppressed sequences, their signals are suppressed to the same degree as the adjacent normal fat (Figure 7.23).

Hamartoma

Hamartomas are benign breast lesions composed of a variety of normal breast constituents, including fat, glandular tissue, and fibrous connective tissue. Other names, such as *fibroadenolipoma* or *lipofibroadenoma* have been used to reflect the dominant tissue types within the mass. The lesion may be a result of dysgenesis rather than a true tumor. Most of hamartomas are detected in pre- and perimenopausal women. They are variable in size but usually measure several centimeters in diameter. Clinically, hamartomas are found either incidentally on screening mammograms or in patients presenting with painless palpable masses.

On mammograms, hamartomas may have a classic appearance of a circumscribed mass containing both fat and soft tissue density surrounded by a thin radiopaque capsule. When a hamartoma contains a very small amount of fat, it may mimic a fibroadenoma or circumscribed carcinoma. Its sonographic appearance is also variable. It often appears as a mass with smooth margins, containing areas of low-level internal echogenicity interspersed with irregular areas of hyperechogenicity.[1]

On MRI, a hamartoma appears as an encapsulated mass with a heterogeneous appearance. Some contrast enhancement can be seen in the glandular elements on T1-weighted postcontrast images (Figure 7.24).

Hemangioma

Hemangiomas are benign vascular tumors that may occur in males or females with a wide reported age range (18 months

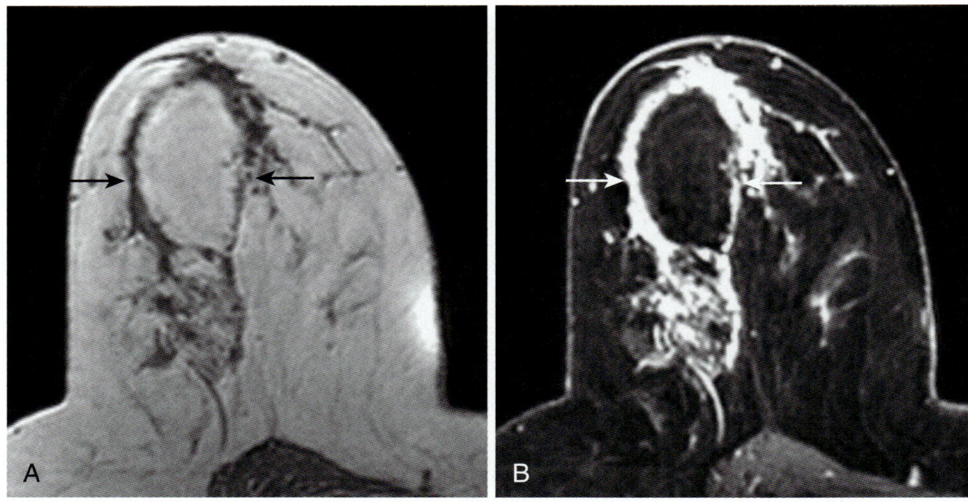

FIGURE 7.23 Lipoma is shown in MRI scans of a 34-year-old woman with a strong family history of premenopausal breast cancer who presented for high-risk screening, with incidental finding of lipoma in the right breast. **A,** Axial T1-weighted non–fat-suppressed noncontrast image shows an oval, circumscribed high signal intensity mass *(between arrows)*. **B,** Axial T1-weighted fat-suppressed postcontrast image shows suppressed signals in the mass *(between arrows)* identical to the adjacent normal fatty tissue.

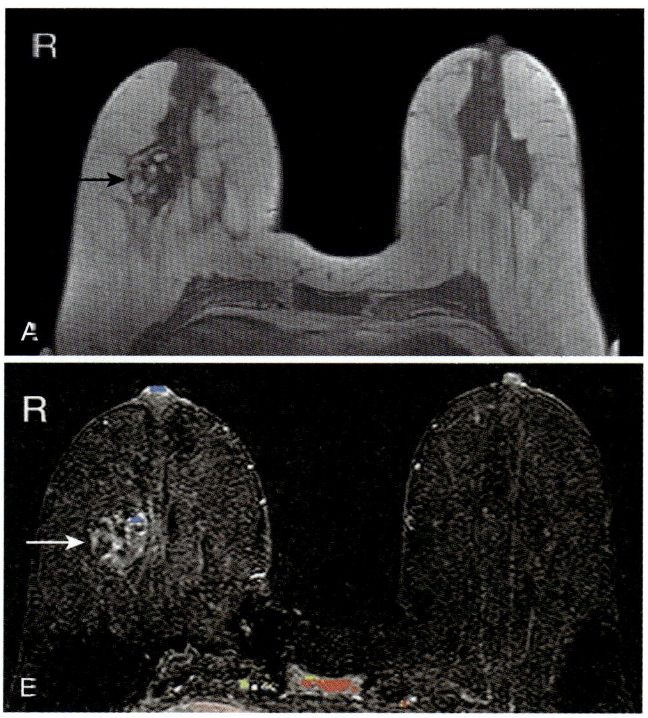

FIGURE 7.24 Hamartoma is shown. **A,** Axial T1-weighted non–fat-suppressed breast MRI scan demonstrates an oval mass with smooth margins *(arrow)* in the right breast with both fat and soft tissue signal intensity. **B,** Axial T1-weighted subtraction fat-suppressed postcontrast image shows prominent glandular elements in the mass with some contrast enhancement. *(From Apple SK, Dascalos JM, Bassett L: Solid benign lesions of the breast. In Bassett L, Mahoney MC, Apple SK, D'Orsi CJ, editors:* Breast imaging, *Philadelphia, 2011, Elsevier Saunders, p 267.)*

to 32 years). They have been found in 1.3% of mastectomy specimens and 11% of postmortem specimens of the female breast.[37,38] Perilobular hemangiomas refer to hemangiomas that are microscopic lesions (2-4 mm in size), found incidentally in breast biopsy specimens. Larger hemangiomas may be a clinically palpable mass or may be detected by breast imaging. These lesions are classified as capillary or cavernous hemangiomas, depending on the size of their vascular channels. Considerable emphasis is placed on the distinction between subcutaneous and intraparenchymal vascular lesions of the breast. The former virtually all prove to be benign, whereas the majority of the latter were found to be angiosarcomas.[8]

Most hemangiomas are small and asymptomatic, found incidentally on mammography. Mammographically, most hemangiomas are oval or lobular isodense masses with circumscribed or microlobulated margins. Rarely, punctate microcalcifications are seen, representing phleboliths.[39-41] Sonographically, hemangiomas usually appear as superficial oval solid masses with circumscribed lobular margins and a parallel orientation. Their echo textures are variable, ranging from hypoechoic, isoechoic, to hyperechoic, or complex (heterogeneous). Indistinct margins are less often seen and are associated with hyperechoic lesions. Hemangiomas are less conspicuous sonographically when the lesions are hypoechoic or isoechoic.[39,40] The vascularity on color Doppler study is variable, with both hypo- and hypervascularity being described.[39,42] Large cavernous hemangiomas may present as a mass containing multiple cystic spaces.[42]

The MRI appearance of hemangiomas is variable, depending on the size and subtype of the lesions. Small incidental hemangiomas show focal area of rapid intense enhancement mimicking malignancy[1] (Figure 7.25).

Four reports on MRI of cavernous hemangiomas of the breast are found in the literature.[41-44] On T1-weighted precontrast sequences, most lesions are isointense to the glandular tissue. On T2-weighted images, they appear as well-defined lobular masses with high signal intensity and septations. Stagnant, slowly flowing blood and thrombosis are presumably responsible for the high T2 signal intensity.[43] Large cavernous hemangiomas can be very heterogeneous in appearance, with low signal intensities on both T1- and T2-weighted sequences, owing to different stages of thrombosis.[42] Two reports describe slow, gradual, filling-in of injected contrast from the periphery, with incomplete enhancement up to 30 minutes after contrast injection.[41,42] Yet two other reports describe a rapid central nodular enhancement in the early phase, with these areas showing plateau kinetics during the delayed phase. The remaining

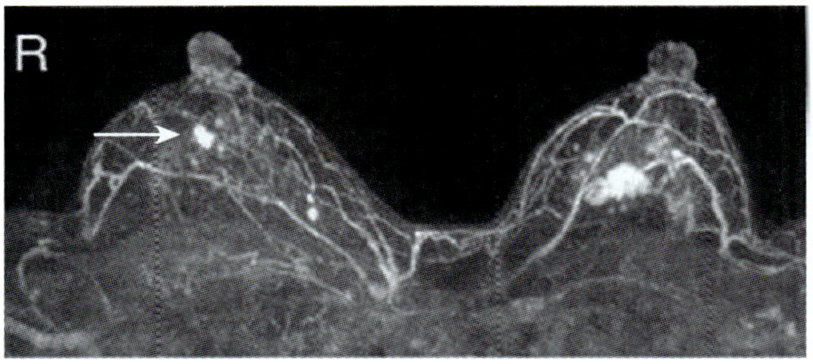

FIGURE 7.25 Hemangioma is shown. A 50-year-old female patient presented with a biopsy-proved left breast invasive ductal carcinoma for breast MRI to evaluate extent of disease. Three-dimensional MIP image shows an incidental 8 × 4 mm homogeneously enhancing oval, irregularly marginated mass present in the anterior right breast at the 6 o'clock position (*arrow*). Histology after MRI-guided biopsy showed a capillary hemangioma *(From Apple SK, Dascalos JM, Bassett L: Solid benign lesions of the breast. In Bassett L, Mahoney MC, Apple SK, D'Orsi CJ, editors:* Breast imaging, *Philadelphia, 2011, Elsevier Saunders, p 267.)*

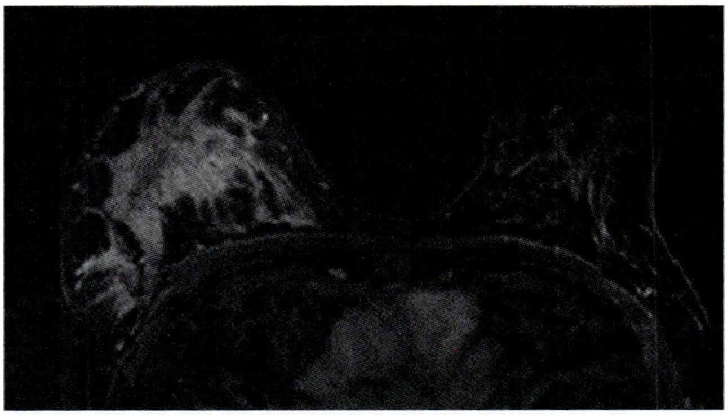

FIGURE 7.26 Mastitis is shown. Subtraction MRI scan showing multiple, adjacent, poorly defined areas of intensely enhancing inflammatory tissue in the right breast. *(From Iglesias A, Arias M, Santiago P, et al.: Benign breast lesions that simulate malignancy: Magnetic resonance imaging with radiologic-pathologic correlation,* Curr Probl Diagn Radiol *36:66-82, 2007.)*

areas exhibited patchy, slow, and gradual enhancement.[43,44] The mixed pattern of enhancement may be explained by the coexistence of rapidly enhancing capillary hemangiomas and slowly enhancing cavernous hemangiomas. This was confirmed by histopathologic findings in one report.[44] MRI is useful in assessing the extent of the hemangioma and possible chest wall involvement before surgery. In pediatric cases, MRI is also valuable in assessing the relationship of the hemangioma to the breast bud of immature breasts.[45]

The main differential diagnosis for a hemangioma is an angiosarcoma. Complete excision of a hemangioma is necessary for accurate diagnosis because the majority of vascular tumors arising from the breast parenchyma are malignant. It is prudent to perform an excisional biopsy after a core needle biopsy reveals a vascular tumor. In cases in which postbiopsy imaging indicates that the core biopsy procedure removed most or all of a histologically benign lesion and a tissue marker has been left at the biopsy site, imaging follow-up can be an alternative to excisional biopsy.[8,40]

Inflammatory Lesions

Mastitis

Mastitis is a condition of inflammation of the breast parenchyma that can be infectious or noninfectious in cause. Infections may be caused by bacteria, fungi, or parasites. Alternatively, a noninfectious local inflammatory reaction or immune response may occur, causing accumulation and infiltration of lymphocytes (lymphocytic mastitis), plasma cells (plasma cell mastitis), or granuloma formation (granulomatous mastitis).[1]

Acute pyogenic bacterial mastitis during lactation is common, most often caused by staphylococcal or streptococcal infection. Stasis of milk or cracks in the skin of the nipple may allow retrograde dissemination of bacteria, which may progress to abscess formation. Nonpuerperal mastitis is frequently associated with subareolar abscess and duct ectasia. *Staphylococcus aureus* or anaerobic organisms are commonly grown.[1,3]

Clinically, acute infectious mastitis presents as a breast induration with tenderness, swelling, skin erythema, and cellulitis. The induration may progress to a fluctuant abscess. Systemic symptoms of fever and chills may be present. Nonpyogenic or noninfectious mastitis may have more subtle presentations, such as pain and a lump. Mammography shows skin and trabecular thickening from breast edema. An abscess, if present, appears as an oval mass with indistinct margins. On ultrasound, skin thickening and parenchymal edema are visible. The abscess appears as an irregular hypoechoic or anechoic mass with indistinct margins, sometimes with fluid-debris levels and usually with posterior acoustic enhancement.[1]

Liu and Peng[46] studied 27 cases of nonpuerperal mastitis with MRI and found 22 cases presented as nonmasslike enhancement and 5 cases as masses. The majority (21 of 22) of the nonmasslike enhancement showed heterogeneous parenchymal enhancement (Figure 7.26). There were signs of rim or rimlike enhancement in 59% (16 of 27) of all cases, with the central contents showing fluid signal (hyperintensity on T2-weighted sequence), presumably because of abscess formation.

On MRI, an abscess appears as a high signal collection on T2-weighted image, with signal intensity corresponding to the water content of the abscess. The surrounding tissue and skin may also demonstrate high T2 signal intensity depicting varying degrees of edema. The abscess mass shows intermediate signal on T1-weighted images, with the surrounding capsule showing lower signal intensity compared with the signal intensity of the contents of abscess. Postcontrast T1-weighted images show no enhancement of the contents of the abscess but show peripheral enhancement of the capsule and surrounding tissue (Figure 7.27).

The most important differential diagnosis for mastitis is inflammatory breast carcinoma. Differentiation of these two conditions with contrast-enhanced MRI remains challenging because of a significant overlap of morphology and enhancement kinetics.[47-49] According to Renz and colleagues,[48] breast MRI may be able to detect and differentiate between underlying abscess and breast carcinoma in

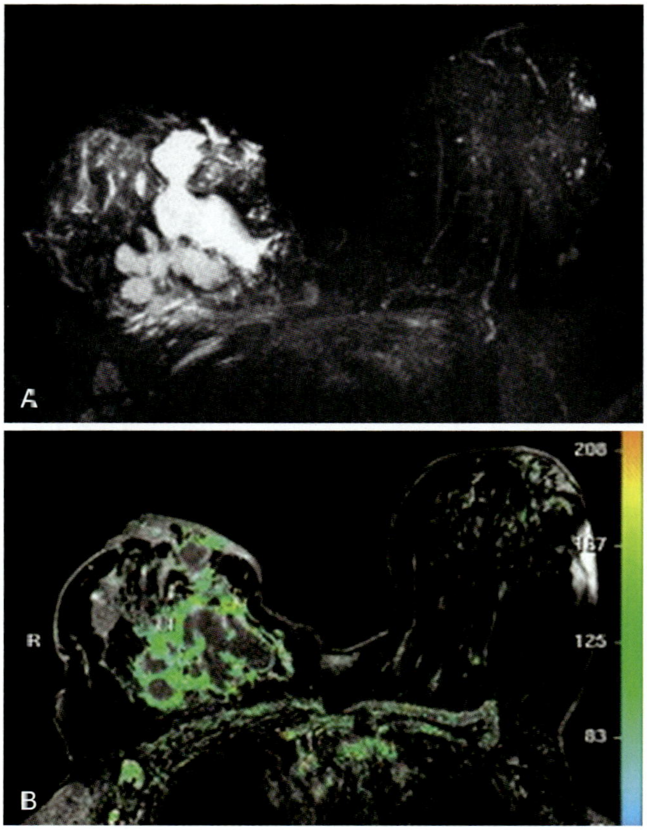

FIGURE 7.27 Tuberculous abscess is seen in a 3-D MIP reconstructed T2 STIR image of right breast (**A**), which shows a thick-walled multilocular cystic lesion of intermediate-high signal intensity attributed to its turbid inspissated content. The entire extent of the right breast abscess, as well as the ipsilateral enlarged axillary node, can be easily seen. **B,** Axial T1-weighted high-resolution isotropic volume excitation (THRIVE) image taken 3.3 minutes after contrast administration with color overlay shows intense marginal enhancement of the abscess cavity. The time/intensity curve showed a medium rate of initial uptake with delayed persistent kinetics *(From Mansour SM, Abolfotooh A: Does MRI help in the assessment of inflammatory breast disorders?* Egypt J Radiol Nucl Med *43:487-497, 2012.)*

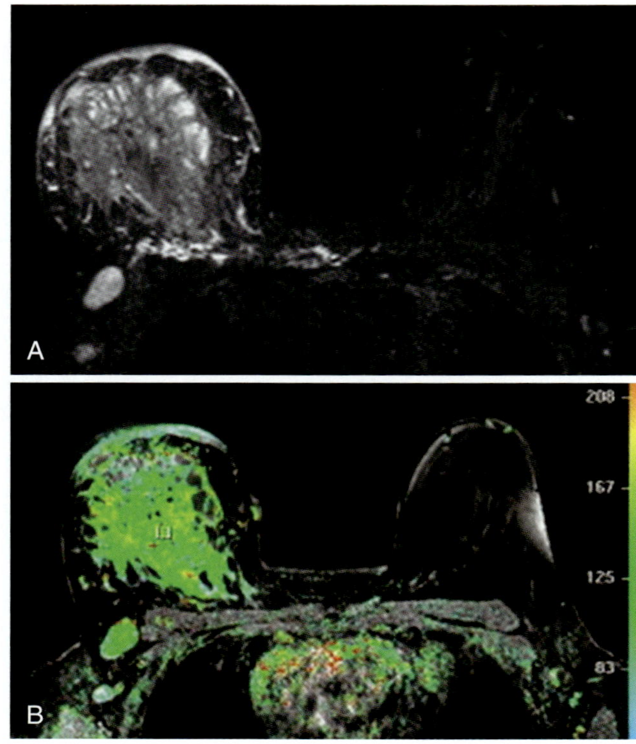

FIGURE 7.28 Nonspecific granulomatous mastitis is shown. **A,** T2 STIR axial image of the right breast shows the breast to be studded with multiple, variable-sized, complicated cystic spaces mingled with diffuse tissue infiltration of intermediate-high signal intensity. Note right diffuse skin thickening, peripectoral edema, and an ipsilateral axillary enlarged node. **B,** Axial THRIVE image taken 3.3 minutes after contrast administration with color overlay shows intense enhancement of the breast infiltration and marginal enhancement of the associated cystic spaces. Note skin enhancement. The time/intensity analysis showed early rapid and delayed washout kinetics. *(From Mansour SM, Abolfotooh A: Does MRI help in the assessment of inflammatory breast disorders?* Egypt J Radiol Nucl Med *43:487-497, 2012.)*

some cases by considering multiple dynamic and morphologic criteria.[48] However, because inflammatory carcinoma is an aggressive form of invasive breast cancer, a histological diagnosis by punch skin biopsy is still needed if any diagnostic doubt exists, especially in cases in which the clinical symptoms do not decrease after a trial of antibiotic therapy.

Idiopathic granulomatous mastitis occurs in young women between the ages of 20 and 40 years and is frequently associated with a recent pregnancy. Histologically, it shows lobulocentric granulomatous inflammation. The usual clinical patient presents with a palpable, extra-areolar or retroareolar mass that is often tender. Axillary lymphadenopathy may be present. The condition may recur in 38% of cases, if not excised completely. Patients do not have granulomatous disease at extra-mammary sites, which differentiates it from other granulomatous disorders. It often mimics infection or malignancy and remains a diagnosis of exclusion. Biopsy is often necessary to establish the diagnosis. Complete resection, corticosteroid therapy, or both are recommended.[1,50]

Mammography may show an ill-defined mass or a focal asymmetry. Ultrasound typically shows multiple clustered hypoechoic masses. There are very few published MRI scans of granulomatous mastitis. Figure 7.28 illustrates a case of idiopathic granulomatous mastitis characterized by multiple complicated cystic spaces intermingled with tissue of intermediate to high T2 signal intensity that enhances intensely with early rapid and delayed washout kinetics.[47]

Periductal Mastitis

Periductal mastitis is a condition seen in young women, usually in their early 30s. It is strongly associated with cigarette smoking. It may present with recurrent episodes of periareolar sepsis and thickening. Other symptoms include noncyclical central breast pain, nipple retraction, nipple discharge, and mammary fistula. The acute form is treated with antibiotics. Surgery with total duct excision may be needed for chronic infections or mammary fistula.[3]

There is no systemic review of the MRI features of acute or chronic periductal mastitis in the literature. Figure 7.29 illustrates an example of biopsy-proved chronic periductal

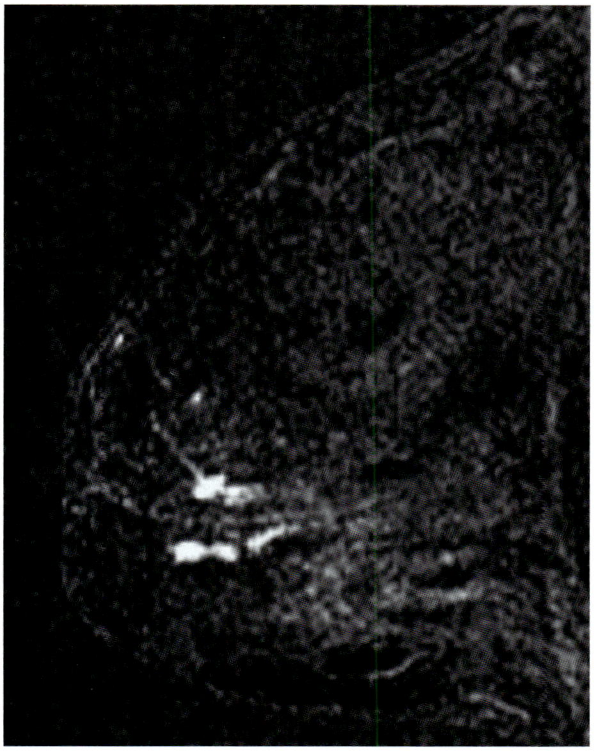

FIGURE 7.29 Chronic periductal mastitis is shown in a 32-year-old woman who was a heavy smoker with a strong family history of breast cancer undergoing screening breast MRI. Sagittal subtraction T1-weighted postcontrast image demonstrates clumped nonmass-like enhancement in a ductal distribution in the retroareolar region. The enhancement pattern was rapid initial uptake and delayed plateau kinetics. Biopsy revealed chronic periductal mastitis.

mastitis. It demonstrates clumped nonmasslike enhancement in a ductal distribution, a pattern indistinguishable from that of DCIS.

Inflammatory Granuloma

Granulomas may be found adjacent to silicone implants (silicone granulomas) or within surgical scars (foreign body giant cell granuloma). They may appear as a mass with circumscribed or ill-defined margins on mammography[51] and as a hypoechoic lesion with acoustic shadowing on ultrasound.[52] The MRI appearance of inflammatory granuloma is variable, depending on the degree of active inflammation or fibrosis. A fibrosed granuloma will be low in signal intensity on both T1- and T2-weighted sequences with minimal to no enhancement after contrast injection. Inflammatory granulomas with high water contents will show low signal intensity on T1-weighted images and high signal intensity on T2-weighted images. They may show rapid and avid initial enhancement with delayed washout kinetics, mimicking malignancy (Figure 7.30). The enhancement may persist for up to 3 years.[21] If the lesion is small, well defined, near a breast implant, or in a patient with recent surgery, inflammatory granuloma may be a consideration, and short interval follow-up MRI rather than biopsy may be considered.

Trauma- and Therapy-Related Conditions

Fat Necrosis

Fat necrosis is a common benign condition resulting from breast trauma. It may result from blunt trauma to the breast but more often occurs after surgery or radiation therapy.

The initial event in fat necrosis is disruption of fat cells accompanied by hemorrhage and an influx of histiocytes. This is followed by progressive infiltration by multinucleated histiocytes, hemosiderin deposition, and calcification. Fibrosis

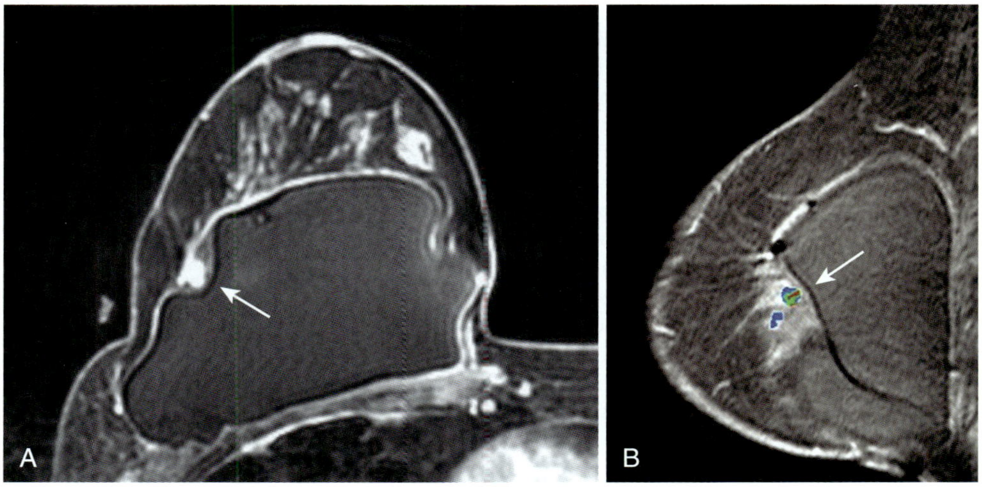

FIGURE 7.30 Inflammatory granuloma is shown in a 71-year-old woman with a history of right breast cancer treated with lumpectomy and bilateral silicone implants 9 years ago. The silicone implants were later revised to saline implants. **A,** Axial T1-weighted fat-suppressed postcontrast image of the right breast shows a small lobular enhancing mass (*arrow*) just deep to the capsule, indenting the shell of the saline implant. **B,** Corresponding sagittal image with color overlay shows the mass to have mixed enhancement kinetics, predominantly delayed plateau (*green*). Biopsy revealed inflammatory granuloma.

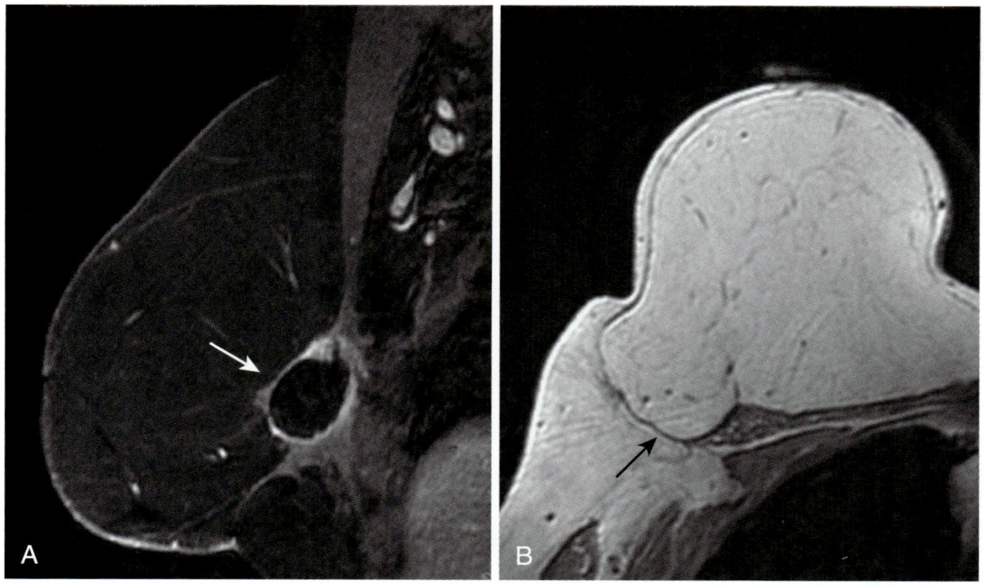

FIGURE 7.31 Fat necrosis is shown in a 50-year-old woman with a history of right breast cancer after mastectomy and transverse rectus abdominis myocutaneous (TRAM) flap reconstruction, with a new palpable mass in the reconstructed breast. **A,** Sagittal T1-weighted fat-suppressed contrast-enhanced image of the reconstructed breast shows central nonenhancing fat with a thin, slightly irregular enhancing rim (*white arrow*). **B,** Axial T1-weighted noncontrast image without fat suppression shows high-intensity fat signal identical to the adjacent normal fat (*black arrow*). Note the typical peripheral location of fat necrosis in a flap.

develops peripherally, enclosing an area of necrotic fat and cellular debris that may become cystic. In the later stages, reactive inflammatory components are replaced by fibrosis, which contracts into a scar. Loculated degenerated fat or oil can persist for months or years within a cyst surrounded by such a scar.[8] The imaging features of fat necrosis are variable, depending on its histologic stage and degree of fibrosis.

Clinically, fat necrosis may mimic carcinoma by presenting as a palpable mass or associated findings such as pain, skin dimpling, and nipple retraction. Some patients may not recall trauma to the breast and may be asymptomatic, with fat necrosis detected incidentally on mammography.

Mammographically, its most classic appearance is an oil cyst without or with rim calcification. When the central fat component is not visible, fat necrosis may mimic carcinoma by appearing as a focal asymmetry, an ill-defined or spiculated mass, architectural distortion with skin retraction, or as indeterminate microcalcifications. With time, the microcalcifications eventually evolve into typically benign coarse dystrophic calcifications. On ultrasound, fat necrosis may appear as an ill-defined echogenic area; a hypoechoic or isoechoic solid mass; or as a complex cystic mass with internal echoes, bands, or mural nodules. Its margins range from well circumscribed to indistinct to spiculated. Depending on the stage of fat liquefaction or fibrosis, it may show posterior acoustic enhancement or shadowing.[53,54] On MRI, fat necrosis often appears as a rim-enhancing mass with irregular margins and central nonenhancing fat (Figure 7.31). Its appearance varies widely with the amount of fat and the extent of inflammation and fibrosis. Fibrosis causes mass effect and architectural distortion, and the degree of inflammation dictates the degree of enhancement. Although a thin rim of enhancement is a common feature, the rim may also be thick, irregular, or spiculated (Figure 7.32). The degree and pattern of

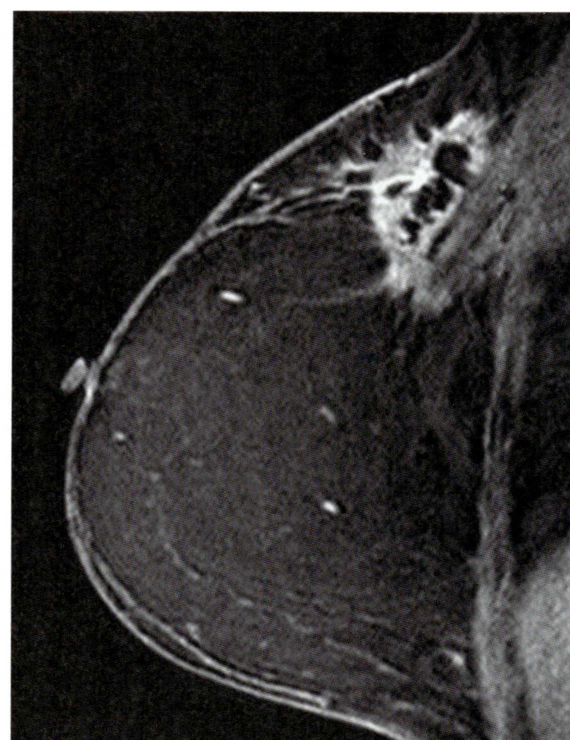

FIGURE 7.32 Fat necrosis is seen in a 66-year-old woman with a history of right breast cancer, treated with mastectomy and reconstruction. MRI is performed for follow-up of an enhancing mass in the right breast mound. Sagittal T1-weighted fat-suppressed contrast-enhanced image shows an irregular enhancing mass in the superior posterior breast mound, with multifocal central nonenhancing fat. Note the irregular thick enhancing wall with spiculated margins and typical peripheral location of fat necrosis in a flap.

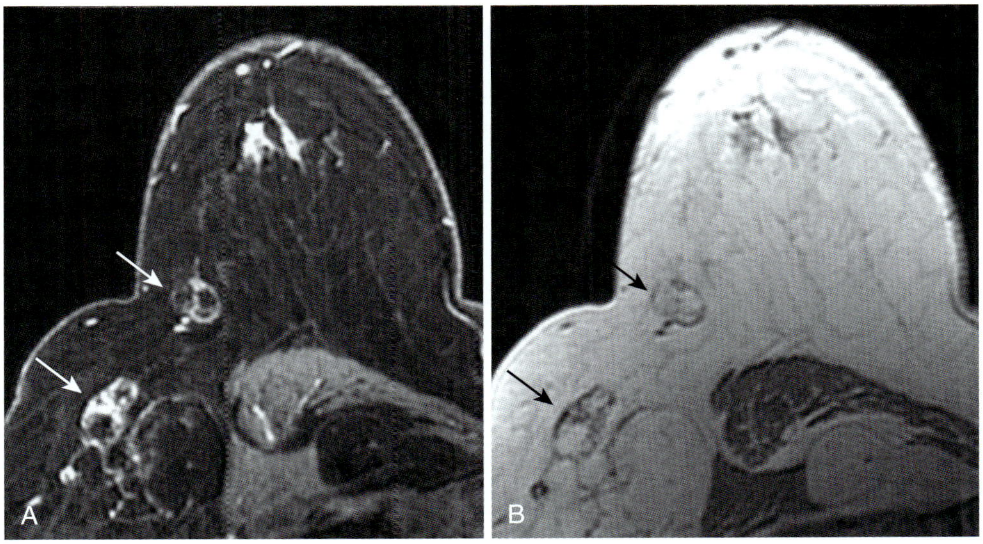

FIGURE 7.33 Fat necrosis is seen in a 36-year-old woman with a history of atypical ductal hyperplasia, undergoing high-risk screening MRI. **A,** Axial T1-weighted fat-suppressed postcontrast image shows two areas of fat necrosis (*white arrows*) with thin enhancing rims and enhancing internal septations in the upper outer quadrant of right breast. **B,** Axial T1-weighted noncontrast image without fat suppression depicts the fat contents with high signal intensity (*black arrows*) identical to the adjacent normal fat. The patient recalled a previous incident of a seat belt injury to the right breast during a motor vehicle accident.

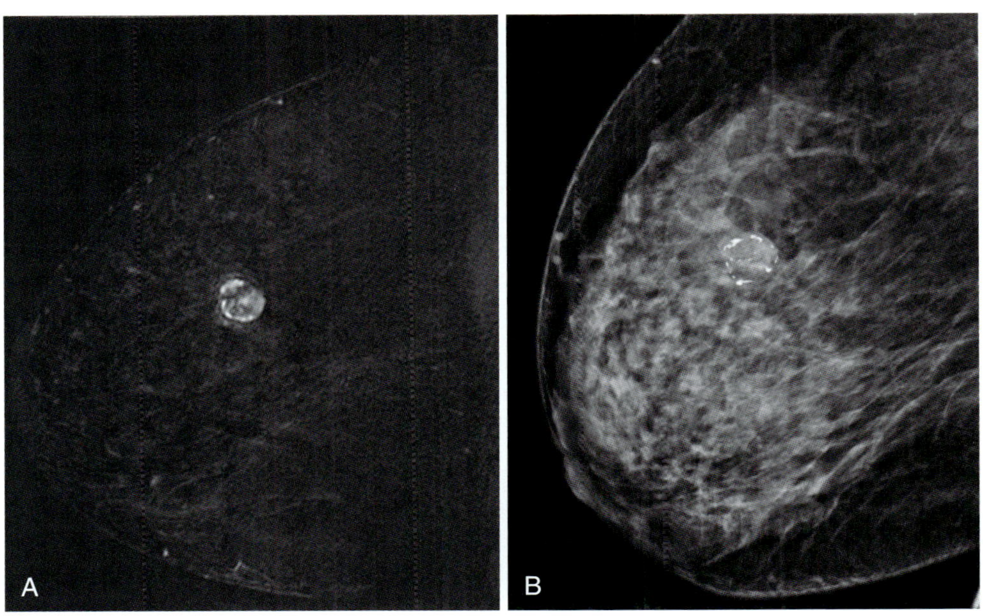

FIGURE 7.34 Fat necrosis is seen in MRI images of a 51-year-old woman with a suspicious mass in the left breast on mammography. **A,** Sagittal subtraction T1-weighted postcontrast image in the opposite breast shows a circumscribed oval mass with an enhancing thin rim and nonspecific heterogeneous internal enhancement. **B,** Digital mammogram of the same breast in mediolateral projection shows characteristic benign rim calcifications, highly suggestive of calcifying fat necrosis.

enhancement vary widely from slow to rapid initially, with persistent, plateau, or even washout delayed kinetics. A fat-fluid level or thin enhancing internal septations may be present within the central fat collection (Figure 7.33). Fat necrosis may also appear as an enhancing focus, or clumped nonmasslike enhancement when it contains a minimal amount of fat.[55]

The presence of nonenhancing loculated liquid fat is the key to diagnosing fat necrosis. The best sequence to detect the fat content is the precontrast, T1-weighted sequence without fat suppression. On these images, fat shows high signal intensity similar to fat elsewhere in the breast or slightly lower signal intensity because of hemorrhagic or inflammatory contents[54] (see Figures 7-31 and 7-33). On fat-suppressed T1-weighted images, the loculated fat will show suppression of signals similar to the adjacent fat as well as a lack of contrast enhancement.[55]

The specificity of MRI for fat necrosis can be further improved by correlation with mammography to detect oil cyst or coarse microcalcifications (Figure 7.34) and by its typical location. Fat necrosis due to blunt trauma is usually superficial in location (see Figure 7.33). It is commonly seen in the inferior central breast after reduction mammoplasty or in the periphery of reconstruction flap (see

Figures 7-31 and 7-32) where the blood supply is more tenuous.[55] These considerations may allow differentiation of fat necrosis from recurrent carcinoma, avoiding unnecessary biopsy. However, fat necrosis may be indistinguishable from cancer on MRI because of the absence of gross lipid and the prominence of fibrosis, and biopsy will be necessary for histologic confirmation.

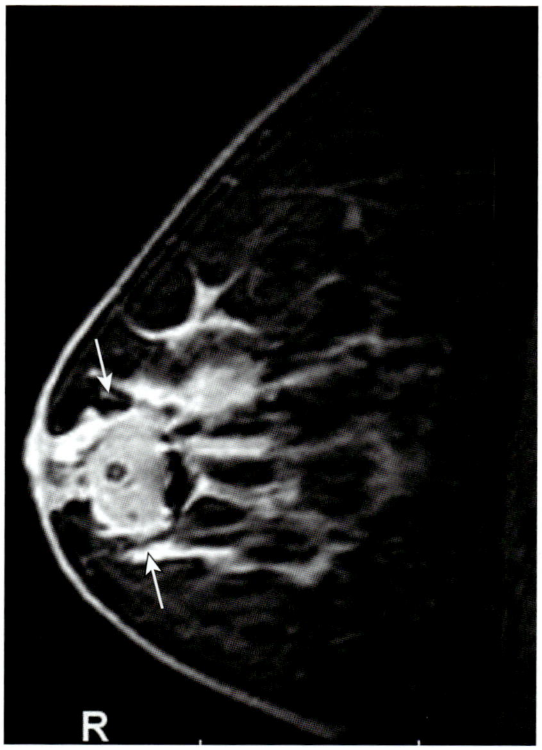

FIGURE 7.35 Hyperacute hematoma is seen in a 46-year-old woman undergoing MRI-guided biopsy of a right retroareolar mass. Sagittal T1-weighted fat-suppressed postcontrast image shows an acute hematoma (*between arrows*) after insertion of the biopsy trocar (*small black circle* in the center of hematoma). Note the mildly hyperintense signal of the hematoma, identical to the enhancing parenchyma.

Hematoma

Hematomas are commonly encountered on breast MRI in patients who have undergone recent core-needle biopsy or surgical excision. Although the temporal evolution of the MRI appearance of intracranial and musculoskeletal hematomas has been well documented in the literature, the same is not true for breast hematomas. It has been proposed that the evolution of an intramuscular hematoma differs from an intracranial hematoma because of the rich blood supply and rapid healing of the intramuscular entity.[56] It is reasonable to expect the MRI appearance of an intramammary hematoma to parallel that of the intramuscular hematoma because of a similar physiologic environment.

The MRI signal patterns commonly encountered in a hematoma at different stages are strongly influenced by the oxidation state of hemoglobin and its breakdown products (oxyhemoglobin, deoxyhemoglobin, methemoglobin, ferritin, and hemosiderin).[57]

A hyperacute intramuscular hematoma is of intermediate signal intensity on T1-weighted and high signal intensity on T2-weighted sequences.[56] However, a hyperacute hematoma is encountered only on breast MRI during MRI-guided biopsy. It typically shows signal hyperintensity on T1-weighted images owing to enhancement by gadolinium contrast agent (Figure 7.35). Acute hematoma shows intermediate signal intensity on T1-weighted and low signal on T2-weighted sequences because of intracellular deoxyhemoglobin. The postbiopsy or postsurgical hematomas seen on breast MRI are usually in the subacute stage. These are high in signal intensity on T1-weighted sequences because of methemoglobin. On T2-weighted sequences, they may be signal hypointense during the early subacute stage (intracellular methemoglobin) or signal hyperintense during the late subacute stage (extracellular methemoglobin). With further aging, a peripheral dark rim caused by hemosiderin within macrophages may appear (Figure 7.36). Marked signal heterogeneity in a hematoma caused by blood in varying stages of evolution is not uncommon. A chronic hematoma is usually of low signal intensity on both T1- and T2- weighted sequences owing to hemosiderin deposition.[56,57]

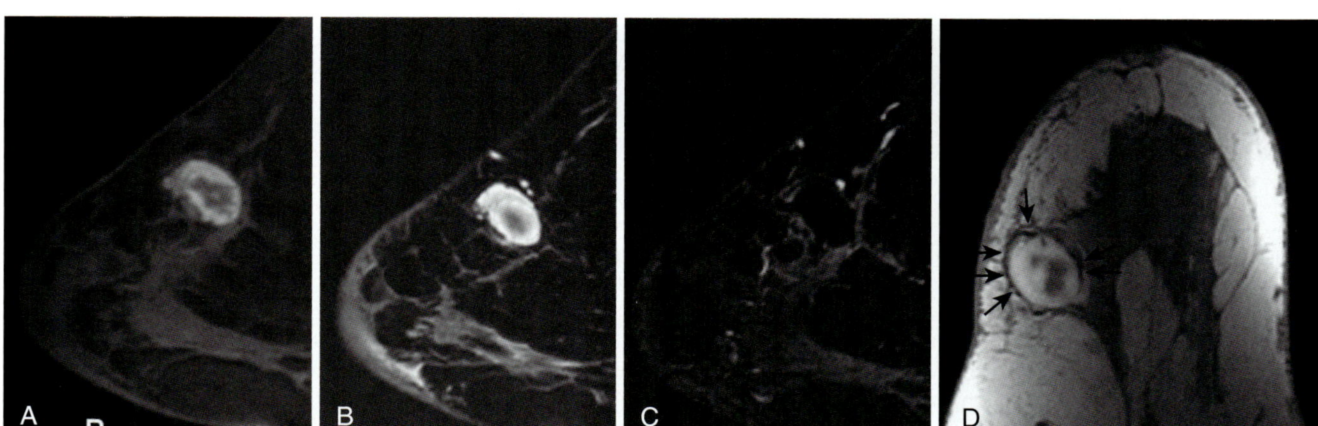

FIGURE 7.36 Subacute hematoma is seen in a 55-year-old woman, 3 weeks after large core biopsy of an invasive lobular carcinoma of the right breast, undergoing MRI to assess extent of disease. **A,** Sagittal T1-weighted fat-suppressed precontrast image shows an oval mass of predominantly high signal intensity. **B,** Sagittal T2-weighted fat-suppressed image shows even higher signal intensity of the hematoma. **C,** Sagittal T1-weighted postcontrast subtraction image confirms the absence of contrast enhancement. **D,** Axial T1-weighted precontrast image without fat suppression depicts the thin dark peripheral rim of hemosiderin deposition (*small arrows*).

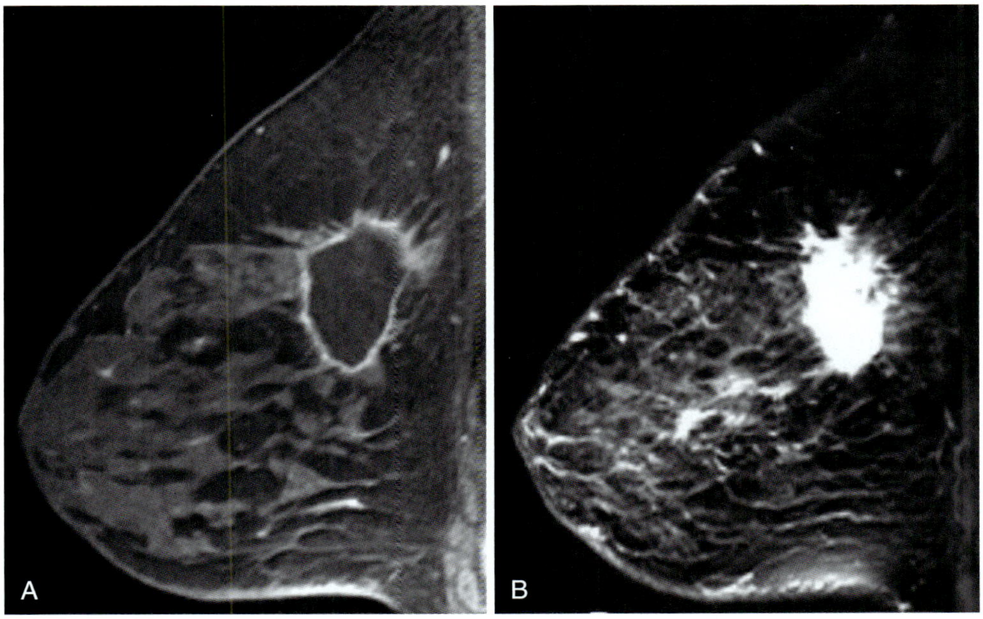

FIGURE 7.37 Seroma in a 48-year-old woman with a history of recent lumpectomy for a phyllodes tumor in the upper outer quadrant of the right breast. The tumor contains a 1-mm focus of high-grade DCIS. MRI was performed to assess residual disease. **A,** Sagittal T1-weighted fat-suppressed postcontrast image reveals a low signal intensity fluid-filled cavity surrounded by a thin enhancing rim that is associated with mild surrounding architectural distortion. **B,** Sagittal fat-suppressed T2-weighted image depicts the homogeneous high signal intensity of the seroma fluid.

Seroma

Seroma is a common finding on breast MRI after lumpectomy. It appears as a circumscribed fluid-filled cavity with a thin, mildly enhancing rim. The nonenhancing seroma cavity usually contains simple fluid that shows low signal intensity on T1-weighted sequences and homogeneously high signal intensity on T2-weighted images (Figure 7.37). However, it may contain blood or fat or a mixture of them. It is important to inspect the rim of seroma for focal thickening and enhancement that may suggest residual or recurrent tumor. Li and associates[58] studied the MR images of 248 women before and after breast conservation therapy. They reported persistence of seroma in 3.7% of patients at 6 or more years after treatment. Postsurgical seromas usually diminish in size over time and are often replaced by architectural distortion and scar formation.[58]

Lumpectomy Site Enhancement

During the immediate postoperative period, enhancement at the lumpectomy site is a normal finding.[59] Although rim enhancement is seen in the presence of a seroma, a focal enhancement pattern is noted in the absence of a seroma.[58] Some earlier reports suggested that enhancement at the surgical site is abnormal after 18 to 24 months.[60,61] However, Li and colleagues[58] found continued enhancement at the seroma or scar in 15% of 60 women in their study with MRI performed 5 or more years after treatment. In women showing enhancement early after treatment, it persisted in 43% of 37 cases with follow-up of 5 or more years. Such enhancement is most persistent in women with fat necrosis.[58] Their study also found that stability and gradual regression of these findings are the typical pattern, usually achieving stability by 3 years after therapy. Increasing enhancement, especially masslike enhancement, is not a usual pattern and should raise concern about recurrent tumor and prompt biopsy.[58]

Parenchymal Scar

Postsurgical scar is the most common benign cause of architectural distortion on breast imaging. It has a variable appearance on mammograms, often being denser and more distorted on one of the two views and barely perceptible on the orthogonal projection. Ultrasound usually reveals an irregular hypoechoic mass with posterior acoustic shadowing, mimicking carcinoma.[62]

On MRI, a postsurgical scar appears as architectural distortion with long spicules radiating from surgical bed. A central seroma, or lipid collection in association with fat necrosis, may be seen (Figure 7.38). Signal voids often reflect surgical clips, dystrophic calcification, or hemosiderin deposition (Figure 7.39). Surgical scars tend to enhance within the first 6 months, but generally do not enhance more than 18 months after treatment. However, persistent enhancement beyond 5 years[58] or delayed appearance of enhancement in the presence of fat necrosis up to 32 months after surgery, has been reported.[63] Although rare, such delayed enhancement will necessitate biopsy to exclude recurrent malignancy.

Post-Radiation Changes

Post-radiation changes of the breast, including edema and enhancement of the skin and parenchyma are visible on MRI and diminish over time.[58,60] According to Heywang-Köbrunner and associates,[60] the irradiated breast tissue

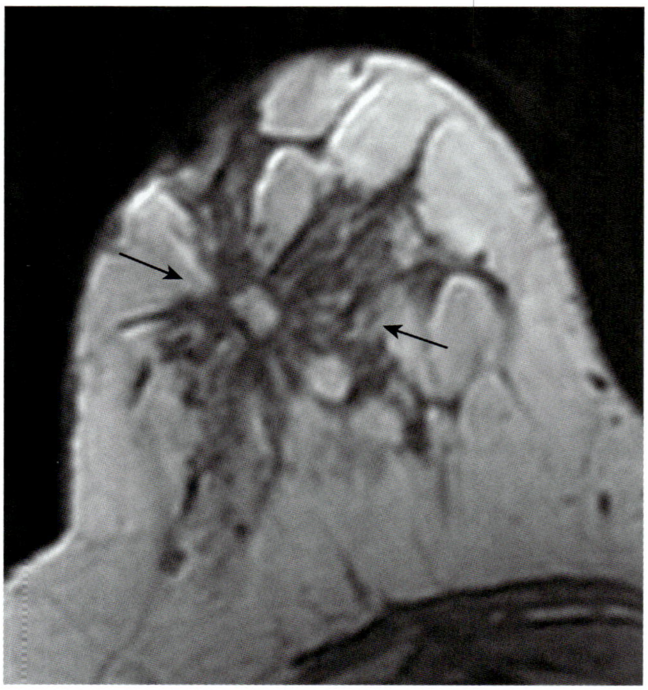

FIGURE 7.38 Postsurgical scar is seen in MRI scan of a 34-year-old woman with a history of surgical resection of atypical ductal hyperplasia in the right breast. Follow-up axial T1-weighted noncontrast image without fat suppression shows a postsurgical scar containing central high signal intensity fat (*between arrows*). Note overlying postsurgical skin thickening.

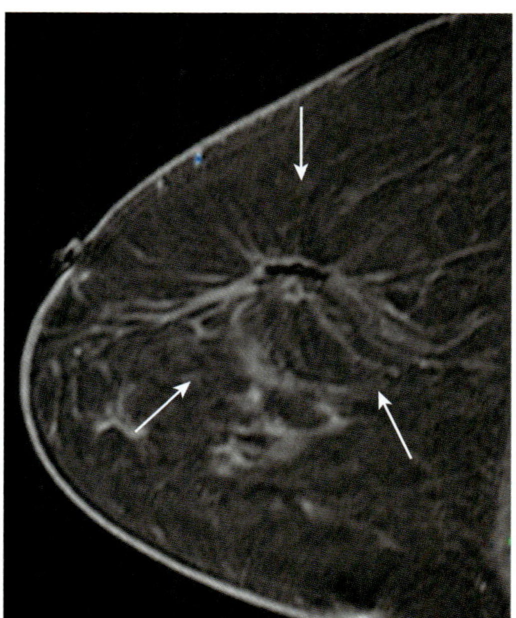

FIGURE 7.39 Postsurgical scar is seen in MRI scan of a 68-year-old woman with a remote history of lumpectomy in the right breast, recently diagnosed with left breast carcinoma. Sagittal T1-weighted fat-suppressed postcontrast image depicts architectural distortion (*between arrows*) from the surgical scar. Note minimal contrast enhancement of the scar and signal void in the center caused by surgical staples.

shows strong and significant patchy or diffuse enhancement during the first 9 months after radiation. Between 10 and 18 months, the amount and rate of enhancement decreased with individual variations. More than 18 months after therapy, enhancement was insignificant in 93% of cases. Based on this and other reports, the use of breast MRI in differentiation of scar versus tumor recurrence is well accepted, if performed later than 12 to 18 months after completion of radiation therapy but is discouraged before this time point. Such recommendation was based on the assumption or experience that postradiation enhancement of breast parenchyma may obscure recurrent tumor and radiation may suppress enhancement of the tumors, making them less detectable.[59-61] However, according to a report by Morakkabati and colleagues,[64] the radiation-induced changes were much less severe and subsided faster than expected, peaking at 3 months after therapy and decreasing by 6 months (Figure 7.40). This allowed detection and characterization of recurrent tumor or benign lesions with diagnostic accuracies similar to nonirradiated breasts during the early postradiation time frame.[64] Li and associates[58] also found that parenchymal enhancement and cystic changes showed a rapid decrease in both treated and untreated breasts by 6 months after treatment and continued to decrease more slowly over time. Although these changes were more pronounced in the treated breast, such bilateral decrease in enhancement appears to be due to the influence of systemic changes affecting both breasts, such as chemotherapy, hormonal therapy, and natural aging processes.[58]

Figure 7.41 illustrates the chronic effect of radiation, with striking decrease in size and parenchymal enhancement in the irradiated breast, compared with those characteristics in the untreated breast. The normal hormonal enhancement in the untreated breast should not be mistaken for an abnormal finding.

Li and coworkers[58] reported that the MRI pattern of edema as seen on T2 imaging and skin thickening may persist for years, with 20% of patients showing T2 edema at 4 years and 25% of patients showing skin thickening at 5 years after completion of therapy.[58] The skin changes may have a linear border with a nonanatomic configuration that corresponds to the radiation portal.[65]

Lymphedema

Because the arm, breast and adjacent trunk quadrant share lymphatic drainage via the axilla, it is expected that lymphedema can also occur in the breast and ipsilateral trunk quadrant, with or without arm swelling after breast cancer therapy.[66] Both surgery and radiation therapy involving routes of lymphatic drainage of the breast and axilla are implicated in the development of trunk, extremity, and breast edema. The frequency of breast lymphedema appears to depend on the extent of axillary surgery and breast radiation. Fibrosis that develops after radiation, affecting lymphatic drainage, may be a contributing factor. Other risk factors include large and/or pendulous breasts, acute postoperative breast edema, seroma, wound infection, and obesity.[66,67] Clinically, breast lymphedema occurs 6 to 12 months after radiation therapy, with gradual resolution within 1 to 3 years.[67] Patients report swelling and heaviness

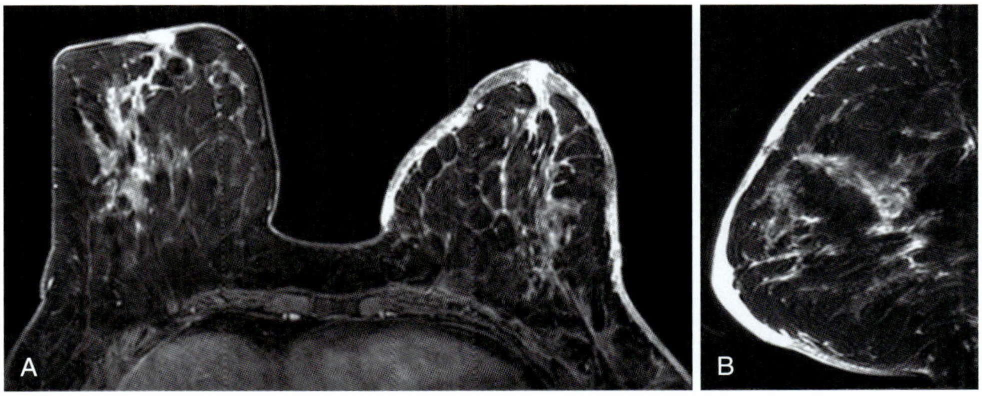

FIGURE 7.40 Postradiation changes are seen in MRI scans of a 72-year-old woman 6 months after lumpectomy and whole breast radiation to the left breast for treatment of carcinoma. **A,** Bilateral axial T1-weighted fat-suppressed contrast-enhanced MRI shows diffuse thickening and enhancement of skin. Note mild trabecular thickening in the breast. **B,** Sagittal T2-weighted fat-suppressed image of left breast demonstrates skin thickening, coarsened stromal pattern, and high T2 signal because of postradiation edema.

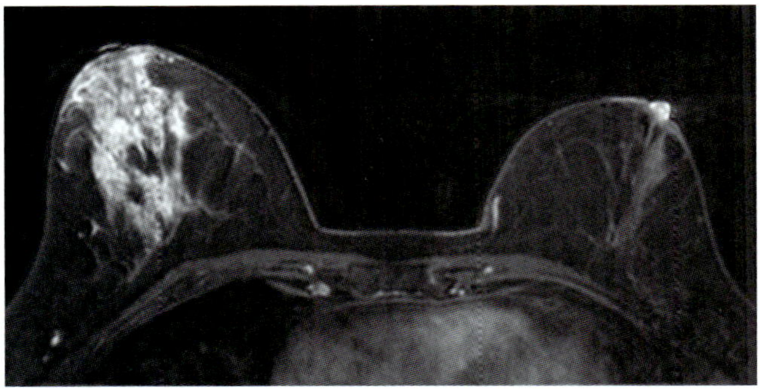

FIGURE 7.41 Postradiation changes are seen in a 40-year-old woman 2 years after lumpectomy and radiation of the left breast undergoing surveillance MRI. Bilateral axial T1-weighted fat-suppressed contrast-enhanced MRI scan shows significantly decreased size and parenchymal enhancement in the treated left breast. The marked hormonal enhancement of the right breast is normal and should not be mistaken as abnormal.

of the affected breast with heat and tender erythema, leading to significant functional impairment. Peau d'orange effects resulting from edema and fibrosis may also be seen.[66]

Although clinical examination remains the most practical means of assessment for breast edema, ultrasonography is found to be a more reliable assessment method.[68] Sonographically, lymphedema appears as skin thickening and parenchymal edema that is more pronounced in the dependent portion of the breast. Important differential diagnoses in cases of chronic breast lymphedema include subacute cellulitis; seroma, hematoma, and abscess; inflammatory breast cancer; recurrent or new primary breast cancer; and cutaneous angiosarcoma.[66] MRI is useful in assessing the extent of edema and fibrosis as well as excluding underlying abscess or tumor.

There are few reports in the literature on the MRI appearance of breast lymphedema.[65] Figure 7.42 illustrates such a case seen at our institution. On T1-weighted fat-suppressed images, there is marked thickening of skin and connective tissue septae separating fat lobules. On T2-weighted fat-suppressed images, these thickened structures show diffuse signal hyperintensity consistent with edema. After injection of gadolinium-based IV contrast, there is mild enhancement of the thickened dermis, whereas the parenchymal enhancement is similar to or minimally greater than the untreated contralateral breast. The enhancement pattern is slow and persistent. This MRI scan appearance is similar to the MRI findings reported by Khanna and coworkers[69] in massive localized lymphedema of lower extremity in morbidly obese patients. The MRI features reflect the histopathologic findings of lymphedema, including dermal fibrosis, lymphangiectasia, and fat partitioned by fibrous septae composed of abundant fibrillary collagen fibers separated by edema.[69]

Normal and Physiologic Findings

Lymph Nodes

An intramammary lymph node is a lymph node found within the breast parenchyma. The majority of lymph nodes seen on mammography are in the upper outer quadrant, but they may be found anywhere in the breast. On mammography, they appear as oval or reniform circumscribed noncalcified masses containing a radiolucent central or eccentric fatty hilus. On ultrasound, they appear as oval, well-circumscribed mass with a hypoechoic cortex of uniform thickness and a hyperechoic fatty hilum that exhibits color flow signals on Doppler study.[1,21]

On MRI, a normal intramammary lymph node is a kidney-shaped structure with a high signal intensity, fatty hilum on T1-weighted non–fat-suppressed images. Its cortex is of intermediate signal intensity on T1-weighted images and high signal intensity on T2-weighted images. Lymph nodes enhance rapidly and homogeneously, most commonly with initial rapid and delayed washout kinetics. The combination of an oval mass with smooth margins, fat signal intensity of the fatty hilum, and high signal on T2-weighted images is virtually diagnostic of an intramammary lymph node.[1,21] They are frequently related to a coursing vessel that can sometimes be seen entering its hilum (Figure 7.43). Occasionally, the fatty hilum is inconspicuous and biopsy may be needed to differentiate from malignancy because of its prominent washout kinetics (Figure 7.44).

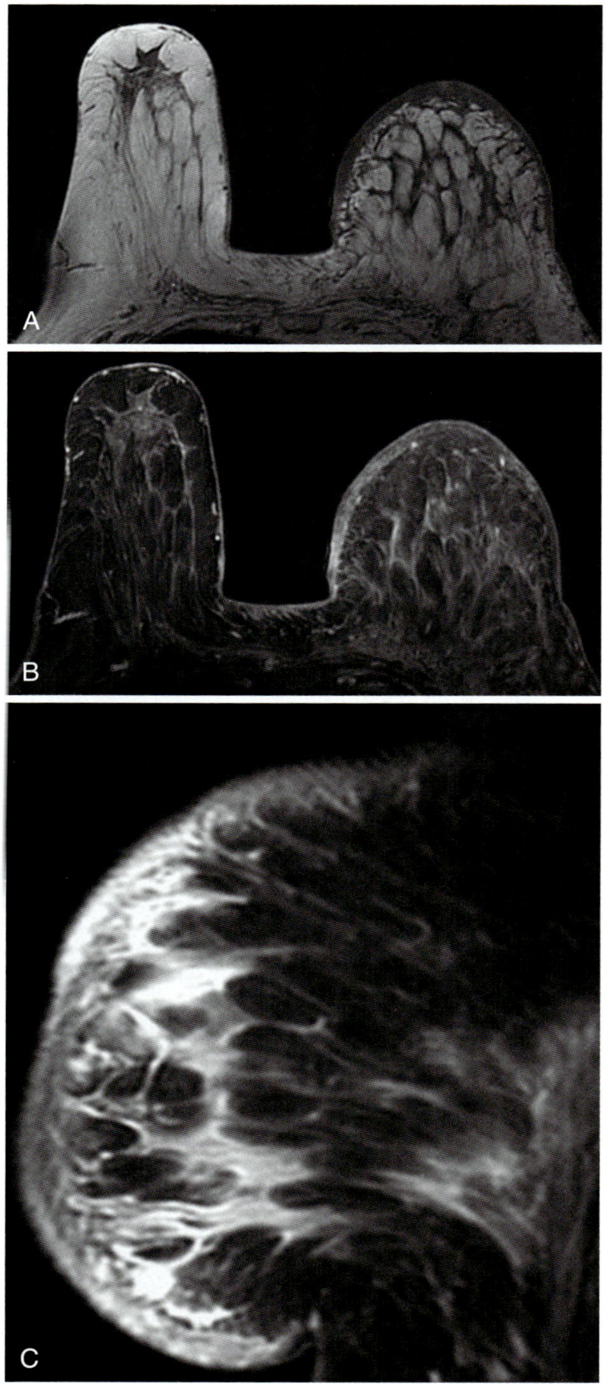

FIGURE 7.42 Breast lymphedema is seen in a 72-year-old woman with a history of left breast cancer treated with lumpectomy and whole breast radiation 2 years earlier, presenting with complaints of increasing swelling, firmness, and heaviness of left breast. Clinical examination shows pitting edema and warmth to touch without erythema. Breast MRI was performed to rule out tumor recurrence. **A,** Bilateral axial T1-weighted precontrast image without fat suppression shows diffuse skin thickening and thickened connective tissue septae separating fat lobules in left breast. **B,** Bilateral axial T1-weighted fat-suppressed postcontrast image shows mild diffuse enhancement of the dermis. The enhancement of underlying parenchyma is slightly greater than the right breast. **C,** Sagittal T2-weighted fat-suppressed image of the left breast shows diffuse signal hyperintensity of the dermis and connective tissue septae consistent with edema. Clinical examination was consistent with lymphedema.

Background Parenchymal Enhancement

Background parenchymal enhancement refers to the enhancement of normal fibroglandular tissue after intravenous contrast injection at breast MRI.[70] It is thought that such enhancement is related to the endogenous hormone status and fluctuates with the menstrual cycle, being highest during weeks 1 and 4 and lowest during week 2.[71,72] More than 50% of enhancing "lesions" encountered when scans are performed outside of week 2 of the menstrual cycle will resolve when rescanning during midcycle.[71] Noncyclic intrinsic variability of parenchymal enhancement within an individual over time has also been observed.[71] The underlying cause of such enhancement is not fully understood, but may be related to elevated metabolic activity associated with progesterone and mediated by a histamine-like effect of estrogen that causes hyperemia, vasodilatation, and capillary leakiness, which are the same factors underlying contrast enhancement of breast lesions on MRI.[2,73]

Background parenchymal enhancement on MRI may be focal or diffuse. The focal enhancement may be masslike, with well-circumscribed or irregular margins, hence mimicking malignancy.[71,72] Nonmasslike enhancement may be stippled, in a diffuse or patchy distribution, commonly in the peripheral part of the breast (Figures 7-45 and 7-46). The enhancement is usually bilaterally symmetric, unless affected by previous unilateral radiation or surgery (see Figure 7.41). Although the velocity of enhancement initially varies from slow to rapid, it usually has a benign delayed time-intensity curve. Kuhl and colleagues[71] reported that 75% to 89% of normal parenchymal enhancement have type I (persistent) kinetics, with the remaining cases exhibiting type II (plateau) curves. None had a malignant type III (washout) curve.[71]

Because of the potential for background parenchymal enhancement to interfere with interpretation of breast MRI in a fashion similar to breast density with mammography, it is anticipated that the upcoming new American College of Radiology Breast Imaging Reporting and Data System (BI-RADS) MRI lexicon will contain classification of such enhancement: minimal (≤25% enhancement of glandular tissue), mild (25%-50% enhancement of glandular tissue), moderate (50%-75% enhancement of glandular tissue), or marked (>75% enhancement of glandular tissue).[74] T1-weighted postcontrast three-dimensional (3-D) maximum-intensity projection (MIP) images are the most suitable for assessment of the degree of background enhancement because they display the enhancing parenchyma of the entire breast. Figure 7.47 illustrates the BI-RADS classification.

Figure 7.47 also serves to demonstrate the dramatic cyclical change in parenchymal enhancement in a 36-year-old patient scanned during week 2 (Figure 7.47, *A*) and week 4 (Figure 7.47, *D*) of her menstrual cycle. Background parenchymal enhancement has been found to increase in postmenopausal women undergoing hormone replacement therapy.[75,76] Conversely, there is report of significant reduction of the breast background enhancement after treatment with aromatase inhibitors compared with baseline MRI.[77] Figure 7.47 also illustrates the effect of hormonal replacement therapy on a 55-year-old postmenopausal woman, with moderate background enhancement while on hormone

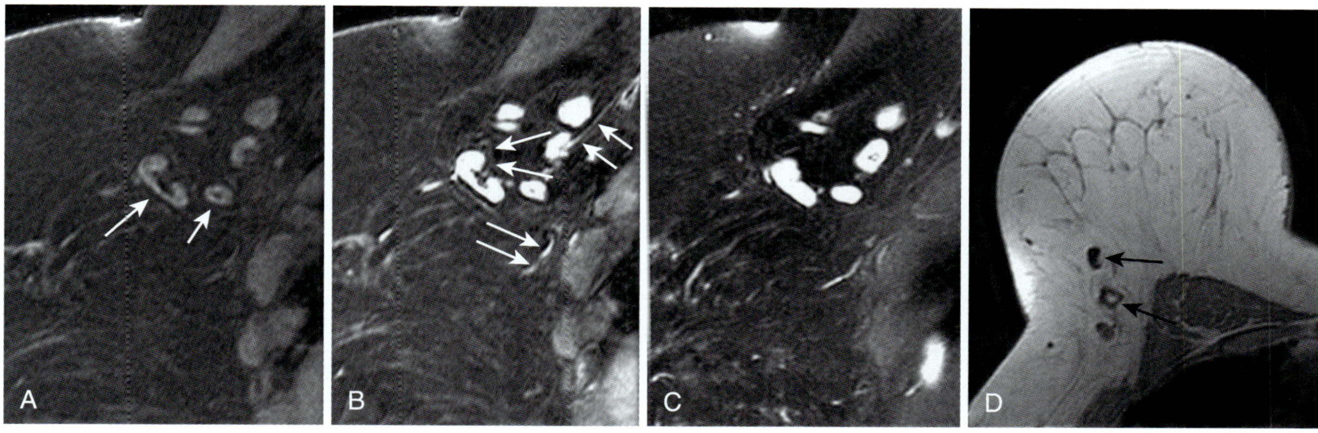

FIGURE 7.43 Intramammary lymph nodes are shown in a 52-year-old woman with a history of left breast cancer after left mastectomy and right reduction mammoplasty, undergoing high-risk screening MRI. **A,** Sagittal T1-weighted fat-suppressed precontrast image shows multiple circumscribed masses including a reniform mass with eccentric areas of fat suppression (*long arrow*) and an oval mass with a central focus of fat suppression (*short arrow*). **B,** On corresponding T1-weighted fat-suppressed postcontrast image, the lymph nodes enhance rapidly and homogeneously. Note vessels coursing into the hilum (*paired arrows*). **C,** Lymph nodes are signal hyperintense on the T2-weighted fat-suppressed image. **D,** Axial T1-weighted noncontrast image without fat suppression illustrates the hilar and central high signal intensity fat (*arrows*) identical to the normal fat in the breast.

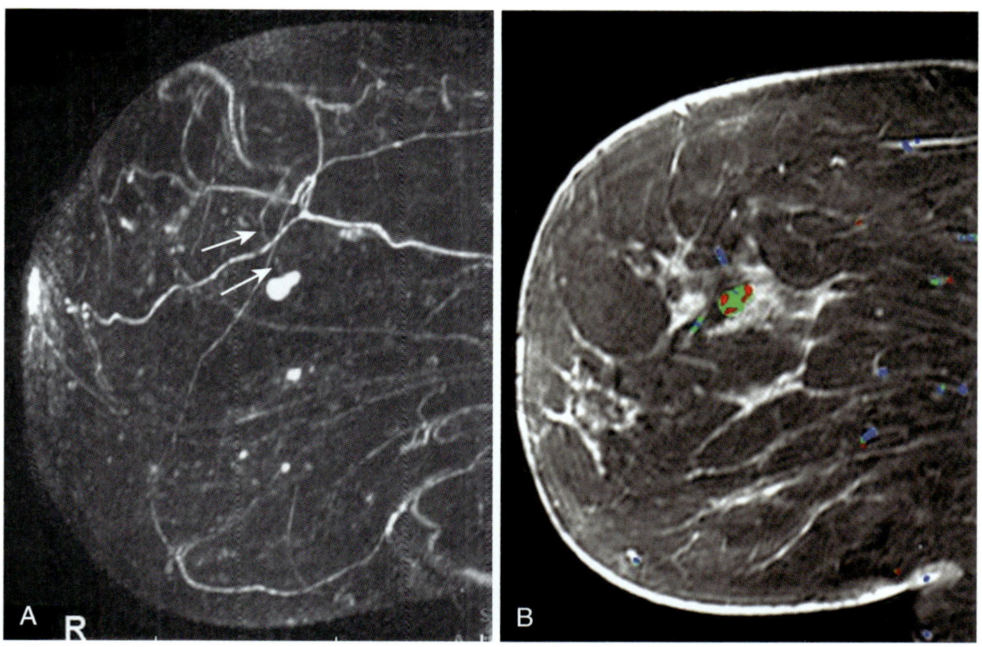

FIGURE 7.44 Intramammary lymph node is seen in a 57-year-old woman with a strong family history of breast cancer undergoing high-risk screening MRI. **A,** Sagittal T1-weighted fat-suppressed postcontrast 3-D MIP image of the right breast depicts a 1.1-cm brightly enhancing mass with smooth lobular margins in the upper outer quadrant. The mass is near a blood vessel (*paired arrows*) but does not show visible fat content. Evaluation of an axial T1-weighted non–fat-saturated image (not shown) also did not reveal obvious fat content. **B,** Color map of enhancement kinetics shows rapid enhancement with delayed plateau (*green*) and washout (*red*) kinetics. The lesion is signal hyperintense on a T2-weighted fat-suppressed image (not shown).

replacement therapy (Figure 7.47, C) and only mild enhancement after the therapy is discontinued for 2 months (Figure 7.47, B). These examples underscore the importance of scheduling nonemergent breast MRI during week 2 (day 7 to 14) of the menstrual cycle for premenopausal patients. When possible, hormone replacement therapy should be discontinued 6 to 8 weeks before breast MRI is performed. However, most centers do not insist on such timing or discontinuation in cases in which an important clinical problem exists, such as staging for newly diagnosed breast cancer. At our institution, we encountered a case of DCIS obscured by parenchymal enhancement (Figure 7.48).

It has been postulated that normal parenchymal enhancement may increase false-positive biopsy rates by presenting as focally enhancing masses and may also cause false-negative studies by obscuring small cancers. Baltzer and associates[78] found the relative number of false positive findings to be highest (5 of 10, 50%) in the group with multiregional,

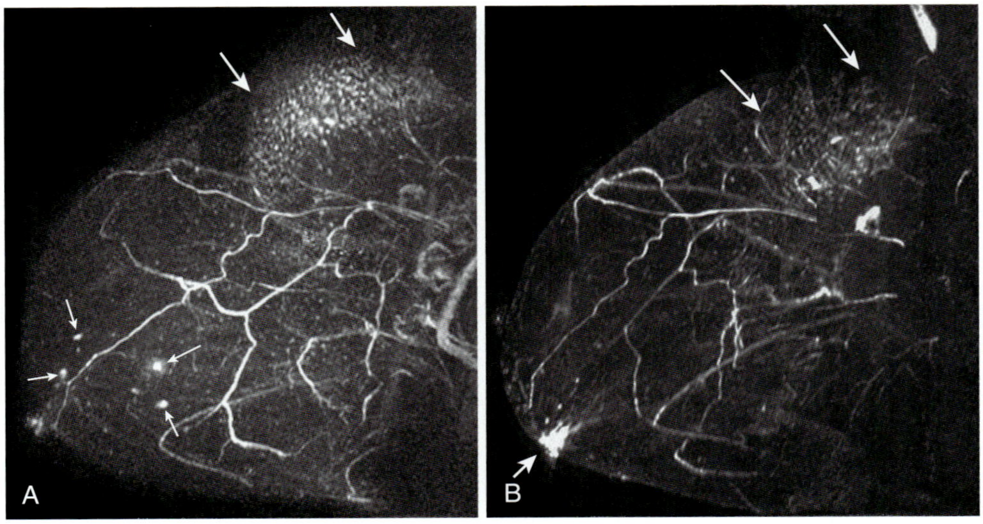

FIGURE 7.45 Background parenchymal enhancement is seen in a 42-year-old woman with a history of right nipple inversion and negative mammogram undergoing MRI for problem solving. **A,** T1-weighted fat-suppressed postcontrast subtraction MIP image of the right breast shows four small enhancing foci (*small arrows*) in the anterior breast and regional stippled enhancement (*double arrows*) with persistent kinetics in the posterior upper breast. **B,** Follow-up MRI 6 months later shows resolution of the four enhancing foci and diminished regional stippled enhancement (*double arrows*) on a scan with overall better vascular enhancement, confirming the physiologic natures of these enhancement. Note normal strong enhancement in an inverted nipple (*single arrow*).

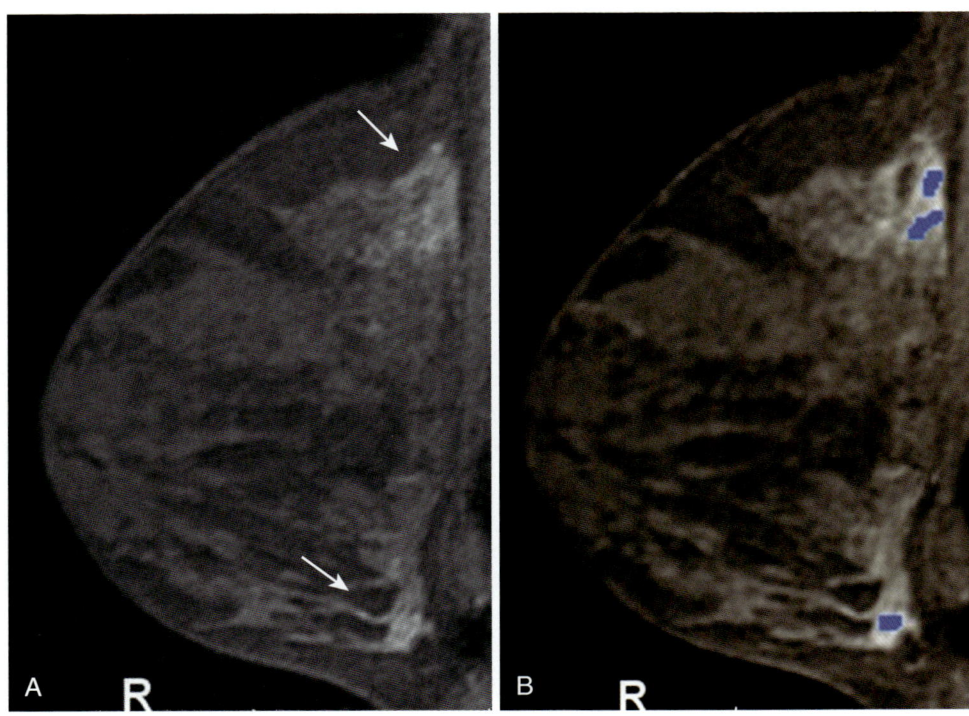

FIGURE 7.46 Background parenchymal enhancement is shown in a 38-year-old *BRCA*-positive woman undergoing high-risk screening breast MRI. **A,** Sagittal T1-weighted fat-suppressed postcontrast image depicts two patchy areas of low-level nonmasslike enhancement (*arrows*) in the peripheral aspects of the dense breast parenchyma. **B,** Color map of enhancement kinetics shows delayed persistent curves (*blue*).

intermediate to strong background enhancement. Hambly and colleagues[70] found mild, moderate, and marked background enhancement to be associated with a significantly lower rate of BI-RADS category 1 and 2 assessments and a significantly higher rate of BI-RADS category 3 assessments. However, there was no significant difference in the biopsy rate or cancer detection rate among the different enhancement categories.[70] A recent study by DeMartini and coworkers[74] also showed that increased background parenchymal enhancement is associated with a higher abnormal interpretation rate but not related to significant differences in positive biopsy rate, cancer yield, and sensitivity or specificity of breast MRI.[74]

It is important to note that background parenchymal enhancement is not necessarily associated with the amount of fibroglandular tissue or mammographic density.[74] King and associates[79] found increased background parenchymal enhancement to be strongly predictive of breast cancer odds,

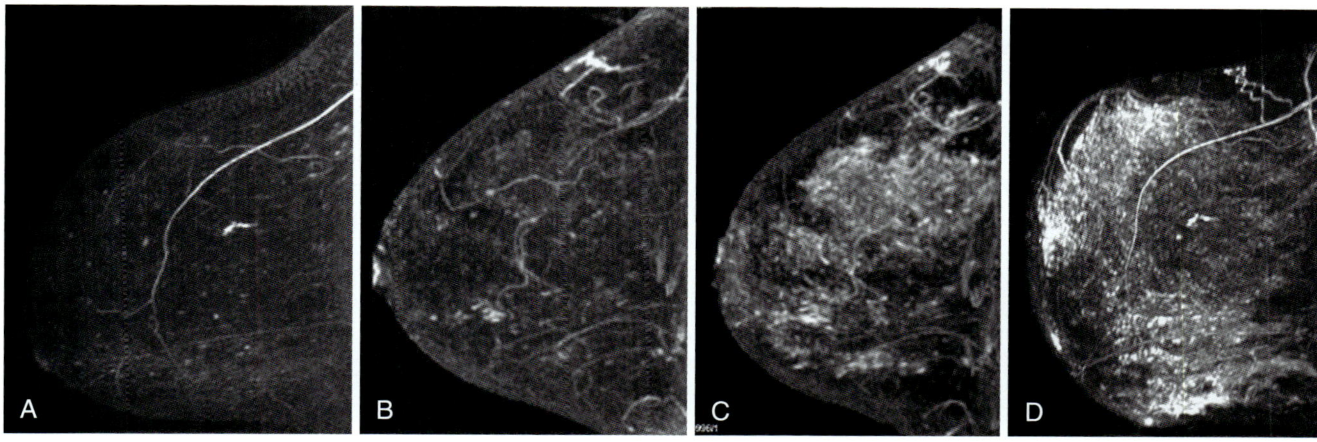

FIGURE 7.47 Classification of background parenchymal enhancement and the effect of hormonal status is shown. **A,** Minimal (≤25% enhancement of glandular tissue). **B,** Mild (25%-50% enhancement of glandular tissue). **C,** Moderate (50%-75% enhancement of glandular tissue). **D,** Marked (>75% enhancement of glandular tissue). A and D are images of a 36-year-old premenopausal woman during week 2 and week 4 of her menstrual cycle, respectively. The linear enhancement in the upper breast was stable and considered benign. B and C are images of a 55-year-old postmenopausal woman without and with hormone replacement therapy, respectively.

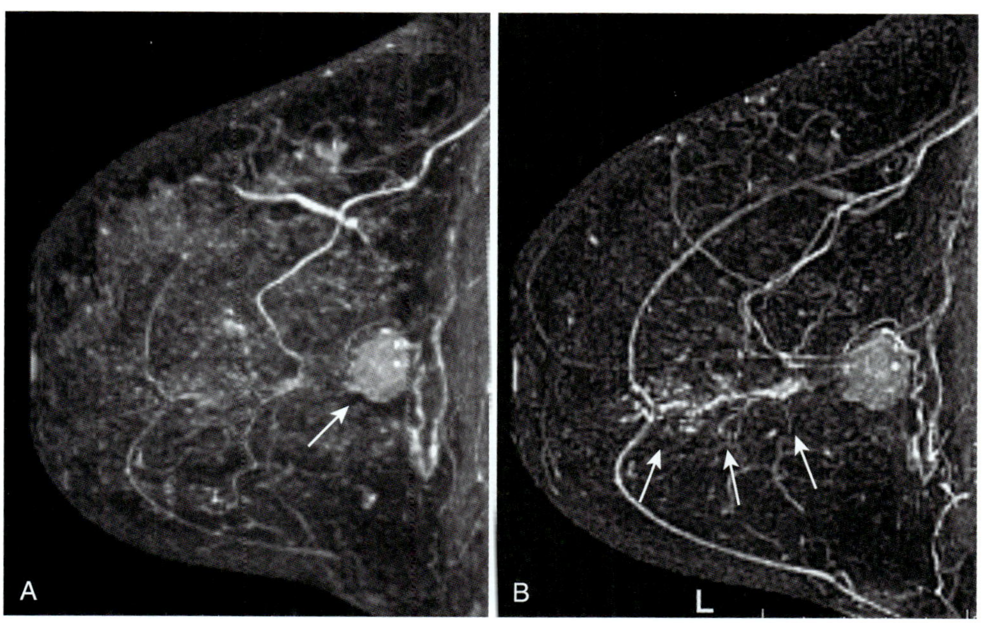

FIGURE 7.48 DCIS obscured by parenchymal enhancement is seen in a 42-year-old woman with newly diagnosed breast cancer undergoing staging breast MRI. **A,** T1-weighted postcontrast subtraction 3-D MIP image shows the known carcinoma in the central posterior aspect of the left breast (*arrow*) and moderate background parenchymal enhancement. No other suspicious mass or nonmasslike enhancement is seen. **B,** Repeat scan during week 2 of her menstrual cycle shows reduced background enhancement, which allows visualization of clumped nonmass-like enhancement in a ductal distribution (*arrows*) that proved to represent DCIS by biopsy.

whereas the association between the amount of fibroglandular tissue and breast cancer odds was weak. Figures 7-49 and 7-50 illustrate the lack of correlation between mammographic density and background parenchymal enhancement.

Normal Nipple

It is essential to be familiar with the normal MRI appearance of the nipple-areolar complex to avoid false-positive and false-negative interpretations. Assurance of a normal nipple would also allow a more cosmetically appealing nipple-conserving breast surgery in treating breast cancer.

The characteristic two-layer appearance of the nipple-areolar complex is seen on MRI as a 1- to 2-mm-thick linear area of dermal enhancement with a nonenhancing central zone (Figure 7.51, *A*). Occasionally there is also a linear band of enhancement passing through the nonenhancing region (Figure 7.51, *B*).[80] Although Friedman and colleagues originally described this single linear enhancement, we have frequently observed multiple parallel linear enhancing bands at our institution (Figure 7.51, C). Normal nipple may enhance mildly (Figure 7.51, *D*), moderately, intensely (Figure 7.51, *E*), or not at all, depending on the blood supply. Intense enhancement is due to a rich blood supply.[2] There should not be any nodular or irregular enhancement along the posterior border of a normal nipple.[80]

Benign Nipple Inversion

The terms *retraction* and *inversion* of the nipple are often used interchangeably, but such usage is inexact. Retraction is applied when only a slitlike area is pulled inward, and inversion is used when the entire nipple is pulled inward, sometimes far enough to lie below the surface of the breast.[81] Both conditions may be congenital or acquired and unilateral or bilateral.[81] Because the nipple normally enhances, an inverted nipple may mimic a subareolar mass,[65,81] especially if only the MIP image is analyzed (see Figures 7-45 and 7-52). However, care must be taken to identify a subtle true subareolar mass responsible for the nipple inversion, as in this situation.

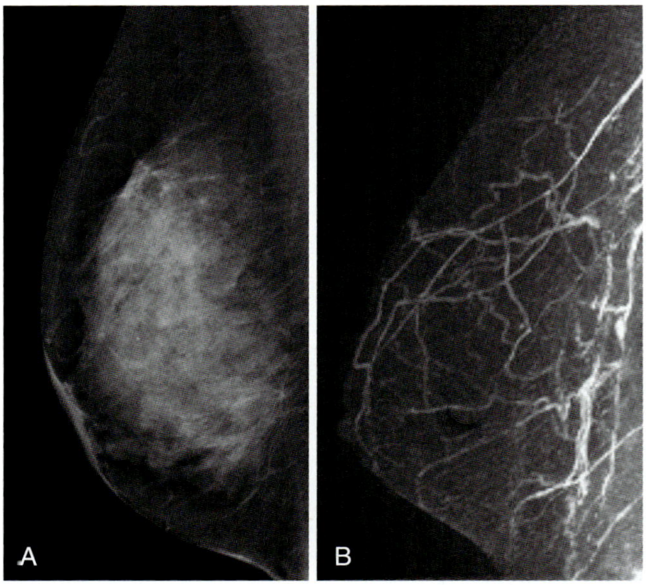

FIGURE 7.49 A dense breast with minimal background parenchymal enhancement is shown on mammogram and MRI. **A,** A 43-year-old woman with very dense mammogram. **B,** T1-weighted postcontrast subtraction 3-D MIP MRI scan on the same date shows minimal background parenchymal enhancement in the same breast.

Skin Lesions

Epidermal Inclusion Cyst and Sebaceous Cyst

Epidermal inclusion cysts and sebaceous cysts are regularly encountered at breast MRI. When occurring in the breast skin, these epithelial cysts are usually in the inframammary, axillary, and parasternal regions and at the nipple-areolar complex.[65] Although these two terms are often used interchangeably, they are actually different conditions by etiology and histopathology. Epidermal inclusion cysts usually arise from obstruction of the infundibular portion of the hair follicle or can be caused by traumatic or surgical implantation or squamous metaplasia of a sweat duct. Microscopically, they are lined by keratinizing squamous epithelium. Sebaceous cysts are retention cysts, arising from the acral surface of the skin by implantation of the epidermis into the dermis. Histologically, they are lined by three to four layers of keratinocytes, without the intercellular bridges seen in epidermal inclusion cysts.[1] *Steatocystoma multiplex* is a rare autosomal dominant disorder in which numerous steatocystomas, pathologically resembling sebaceous cysts, develop in the skin of the anterior chest and axilla.[65]

Both cysts have similar contents of keratin debris.[1] They are similar in clinical presentation and imaging

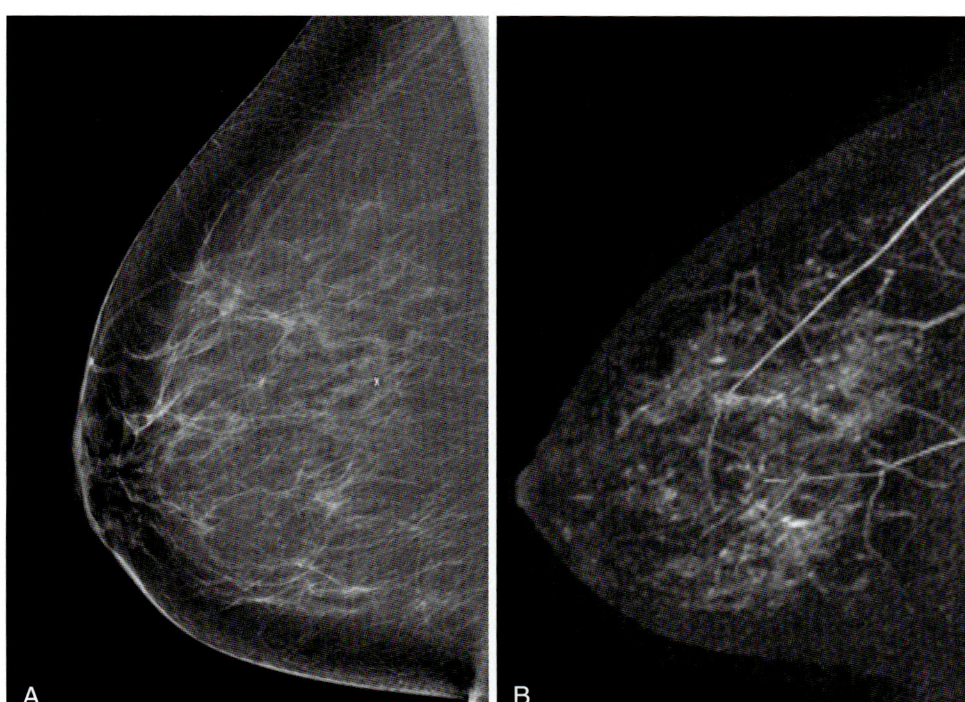

FIGURE 7.50 A relatively fatty breast with moderate background parenchymal enhancement is shown on mammogram and MRI. **A,** A 41-year-old woman with mediolateral mammogram that shows scattered fibroglandular density. **B,** T1-weighted postcontrast subtraction 3-D MIP MRI scan on the same date shows moderate background parenchymal enhancement.

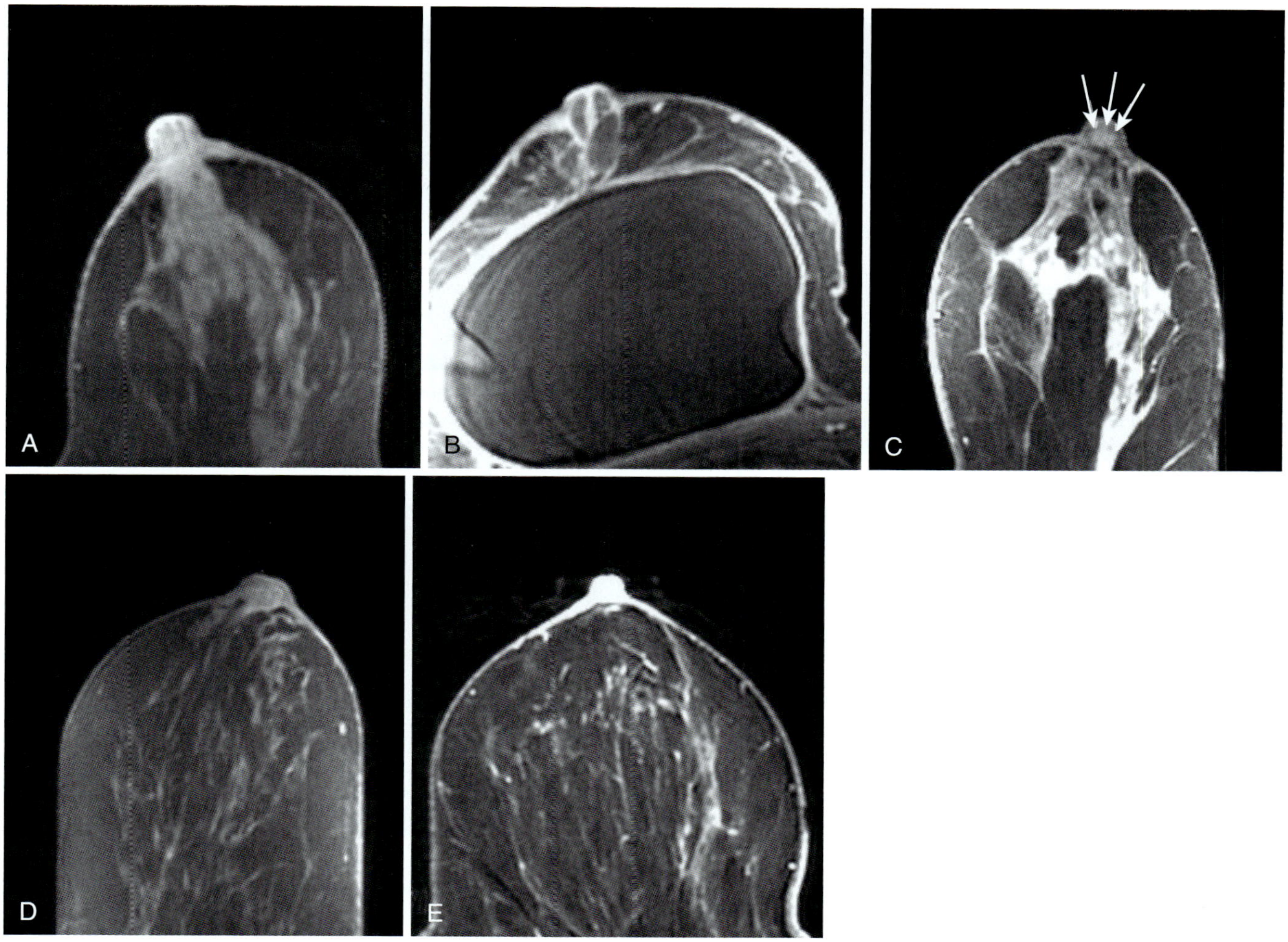

FIGURE 7.51 Patterns of normal nipple enhancement are illustrated. Multiple axial T1-weighted fat-suppressed postcontrast images show patterns and degrees of enhancement in a normal nipple. **A**, Normal skin enhancement. **B**, Single linear enhancement in the center of the nipple. **C**, Multiple parallel linear enhancements (*arrows*). **D**, Mild enhancement. **E**, Intense enhancement.

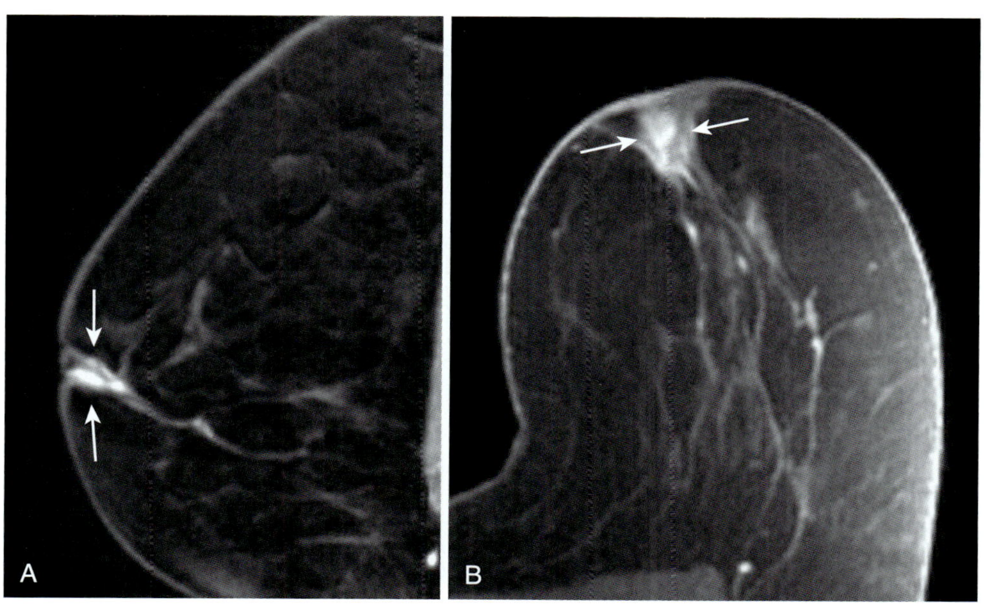

FIGURE 7.52 Benign nipple inversion is shown in a 65-year-old woman with a 3-year history of nipple inversion undergoing follow-up breast MRI. Sagittal (**A**) and axial (**B**) T1-weighted fat-suppressed postcontrast images illustrate an enhancing inverted nipple (*between arrows*) without a retroareolar mass.

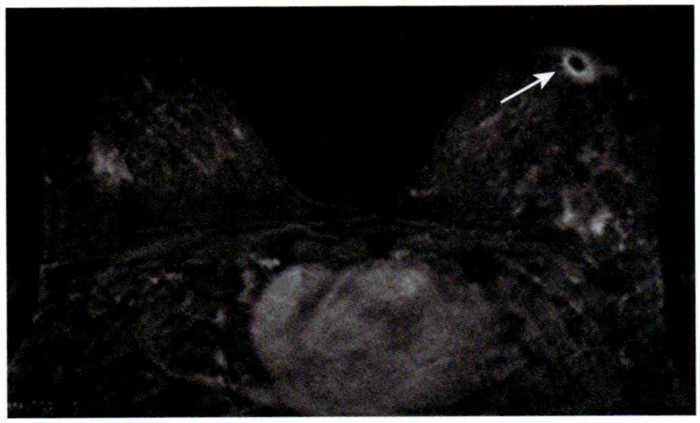

FIGURE 7.53 An epidermal inclusion cyst is shown on MRI. Axial postcontrast subtraction image shows retroareolar enhancing tissue surrounding a small nodule with rim enhancement (*arrow*) in the left breast. *(From Iglesias A, Arias M, Santiago P, et al.: Benign breast lesions that simulate malignancy: magnetic resonance imaging with radiologic-pathologic correlation,* Curr Probl Diagn Radiol *36:66-82, 2007.)*

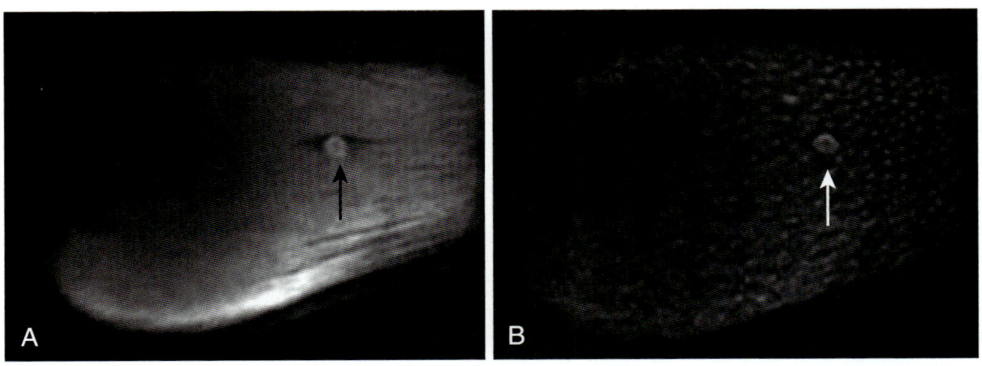

FIGURE 7.54 A sebaceous cyst is shown in a 52-year-old woman with a strong family history of breast cancer undergoing screening MRI. **A,** Sagittal T1-weighted fat-suppressed postcontrast image, in the most medial slice of left breast shows a small, circumscribed lesion of the skin with rim enhancement (*black arrow*). Note suboptimal fat suppression. **B,** Corresponding sagittal T2-weighted fat-suppressed image shows its low-signal fat content due to fat suppression (*white arrow*).

features. Clinically, they appear as asymptomatic, palpable masses in the superficial skin or subcutaneous tissue. A small, blackened pore may be seen at the dome of the lesions. They are frequently associated with pain and drainage when inflamed or ruptured. Mammographically, they appear as circumscribed, round, or oval masses that may project over the breast parenchyma. Heterogeneous microcalcifications, when present, are found in the keratin debris.[82] Sonographically, they arise from the skin or immediate subcutaneous tissue, with skin surrounding the mass occasionally showing the *claw sign* or a connecting tail from the mass to the skin surface. They are circumscribed and contain low-level internal echoes owing to the thick keratin debris.[1] They may be seen rising into the dermis on sonography.[82] It has been reported that epidermal cysts associated with reduction mammoplasty may be located less superficially, and biopsy is sometimes necessary for diagnosis.[82]

The literature concerning the MRI appearance of these cysts is limited.[2,21,65] On MRI, the lesions appear as well-defined subcutaneous masses of intermediate signal intensity on T1-weighted images and heterogeneously high signal intensity on T2-weighted images.[21] These cysts may have peripheral rim enhancement (Figure 7.53) or even appear to exhibit solid internal progressive enhancement on postcontrast T1-weighted images, a finding that may be secondary to volume averaging. Occasionally, the lesion may appear signal hypointense on fat-suppressed T2-weighted images because of its fat contents (Figure 7.54). It may appear as a retroareolar or superficial mass with peripheral enhancement, making it difficult to differentiate from a malignant lesion and necessitating biopsy (see Figure 7.53). Biopsy may be avoided if characteristic clinical and imaging findings, including extension into dermis on sonogram, are present.[21,82]

References

1. Bassett L, Mahoney MC, Apple SK, D'Orsi CJ, editors: *Breast imaging*, Philadelphia, PA, 2011, Elsevier Saunders, pp 239–388.
2. Morris EA, Liberman L: *Breast MRI: diagnosis and intervention*, New York, NY, 2005, Springer-Verlag Science+Business Media.
3. O'Malley FP, Pinder SE, editors: *Breast pathology*, Philadelphia, PA, 2006, Elsevier Churchill Livingston.
4. van den Bosch MA, et al: Magnetic resonance imaging characteristics of fibrocystic change of the breast, *Invest Radiol* 40:436–441, 2005.
5. Chen JH, Nalcioglu O, Su MY: Fibrocystic change of the breast presenting as a focal lesion mimicking breast cancer in MR imaging, *J Magn Reson Imaging* 28:1499–1505, 2008.
6. Liberman L, Morris EA, Dershaw DD, Abramson AF, Tan LK: Ductal enhancement on MR imaging of the breast, *AJR Am J Roentgenol* 181:519–525, 2003.
7. Oztekin PS, Tuncbilek I, Kosar P, Gultekin S, Ozturk FK: Nodular sclerosing adenosis mimicking malignancy in the breast: magnetic resonance imaging findings, *Breast J* 17:95–97, 2011.
8. Rosen PP: *Rosen's breast pathology*, ed 3, Philadelphia, PA, 2009, Lippincott Williams and Wilkins.

9. Hochman MG, Orel SG, Powell CM, Schnall MD, Reynolds CA, White LN: Fibroadenomas: MR appearances with radiologic-histopathologic correlation, *Radiology* 204:123–129, 1997.
10. Nunes LW, Schnall MD, Siegelman ES, et al: Diagnostic performance characteristics of architectural features revealed by high spatial-resolution MR imaging of the breast, *AJR Am J Roentgenol* 169:409–415, 1997.
11. Wurdinger S, Herzog AB, Fischer DR, et al: Differentiation of phyllodes breast tumors from fibroadenoma on MRI, *AJR Am J Roentgenol* 185:1317–1321, 2005.
12. Tan H, Zhang S, Liu H, et al: Imaging findings in phyllodes tumors of the breast, *Eur J Radiol* 81:e62–e69, 2012. Epub 2011 Feb 25.
13. Monzawa S, Yokokawa M, Sakuma T, et al: Mucinous carcinoma of the breast: MRI features of pure and mixed forms with histopathologic correlation, *AJR Am J Roentgenol* 192:W125–W131, 2009.
14. Eiada R, Chong J, Kulkarni S, Goldberg F, Muradali D: Papillary lesions of the breast: MRI, ultrasound, and mammographic appearances, *AJR Am J Roentgenol* 198:264–271, 2012.
15. Jones KN, Glazebrook KN, Reynolds C: Pseudoangiomatous stromal hyperplasia: imaging findings with pathologic and clinical correlation, *AJR Am J Roentgenol* 195:1036–1042, 2010.
16. Polger MR, Denison CM, Lester S, Meyer JE: Pseudoangiomatous stromal hyperplasia: mammographic and sonographic appearances, *AJR Am J Roentgenol* 166:349–352, 1996.
17. Cohen MA, Morris EA, Rosen PP, Dershaw DD, Liberman L, Abramson AF: Pseudoangiomatous stromal hyperplasia: mammographic, sonographic and clinical patterns, *Radiology* 198:117–120, 1996.
18. Teh HS, Chiang SH, Leung JWT, Tan SM, Kent Mancer JF Rapidly enlarging tumoral pseudoangiomatous stromal hyperplasia in a 15-year-old patient. Distinguishing sonographic and magnetic resonance imaging findings and correlation with histologic findings, *J Ultrasound Med* 26:1101–1106, 2007.
19. Masannat YA, Whitehead S, Hawley I, Apthorp L, Shah EF: Pseudoangiomatous stromal hyperplasia: a case report, *Case Report Med* 2010:549–643, 2010.
20. Ryu EM, Whang IY, Chang ED: Rapidly growing bilateral pseudoangiomatous stromal hyperplasia of the breast, *Korean J Radiol* 11:355–358, 2010.
21. Iglesias A, Arias M, Santiago P, Rodriguez M, Mafias J, Saborido C: Benign breast lesions that simulate malignancy: magnetic resonance imaging with radiologic-pathologic correlation, *Curr Probl Diagn Radiol* 36:66–82, 2007.
22. Baskin H, Layfield L, Morrell G: MRI appearance of pseudoangiomatous stromal hyperplasia causing asymmetric breast enlargement, *Breast J* 13:203–210, 2007.
23. Powell CM, Cranor ML, Rosen PP: Pseudoangiomatous stromal hyperplasia (PASH): a mammary stromal tumor with myofibroblastic differentiation, *Am J Surg Pathol* 19:270–277, 1995.
24. Drinka EK, Bargaje A, Ersahin CH, et al: Pseudoangiomatous stromal hyperplasia (PASH) of the breast: a clinicopathological study of 79 cases, *Int J Surg Pathol* 20:54–58, 2012.
25. Sklair-Levy M, Samuels TH, Catzavelos C, Hamilton P, Shumak R: Stromal fibrosis of the breast, *AJR Am J Roentgenol* 177:573–577, 2001.
26. Lee SJ, Mahoney MC, Khan S: MRI features of stromal fibrosis of the breast with histopathologic correlation, *AJR Am J Roentgenol* 197:755–762, 2011.
27. Glazebrook KN, Renolds CA: Mammary Fibromatosis, *AJR Am J Roentgenol* 193:856–860, 2009.
28. Lee SJ, Mahoney MC: The protean manifestations of granular cell tumor of the breast, *Breast J* 17:201–203, 2011.
29. Scaranelo AM, Bukhanov K, Crystal P, Mulligan AM, O'Malley FP: Granular cell tumour of the breast: MRI findings and review of the literature, *Br J Radiol* 80:970–974, 2007.
30. Maki DD, Horne D, Damore LJ II, Jones C: Magnetic resonance appearance of granular cell tumor of the breast, *Clinical imaging* 33:395–397, 2009.
31. Kohashi T, Kataoka T, Haruta R, et al: Granular cell tumor of the breast: report of a case, *Hiroshima J Med Sci* 48:31–33, 1999.
32. Okada K, Ozeki K, Ishida T, Isomoto I, Matsuo T, Mochinago N: Granular cell tumor of the breast: a case report describing dynamic MR mammography, *Breast Cancer* 5:179–182, 1998.
33. Haj M, Weiss M, Herskovits T: Diabetic sclerosing lymphocytic lobulitis of the breast, *J Diabetes Complications* 18:187–191, 2004.
34. Baratelli GM, Riva C: Diabetic fibrous mastopathy: sonographic-pathologic correlation, *J Clin Ultrasound* 33:34–37, 2005.
35. Wong KT, Tse GM, Yang WT: Ultrasound and MR imaging of diabetic mastopathy, *Clin Radiol* 57:730–735, 2002.
36. Tuncbilek N, Karakas HM, Okten O: Diabetic fibrous mastopathy: dynamic contrast-enhanced magnetic resonance imaging findings, *Breast J* 10:359–362, 2004.
37. Rosen PP, Ridolfi RL: The perilobular hemangioma, a benign vascular lesion of the breast, *Am J Clin Pathol* 68:21–23, 1977.
38. Lesueur GC, Brown RW, Bhathal PS: Incidence of perilobular hemangioma in the female breast, *Arch Pathol Lab Med* 107:308–310, 1983.
39. Glazebrook KN, Morton MJ, Reynolds C: Vascular tumors of the breast: mammographic, sonographic, and MRI appearances, *AJR Am J Roentgenol* 184:331–338, 2005.
40. Mesurolle B, Sygal V, Lalonde L, et al: Sonographic and mammographic appearances of breast hemangioma, *AJR Am J Roentgenol* 191: W17–W22, 2008.
41. Courcoutsakis NA, Hill SC, Chow CK, Gralnick H: Breast hemangiomas in a patient with Kasaback-Merritt syndrome: imaging findings, *AJR Am J Roentgenol* 169:1397–1399, 1997.
42. Kim SM, Kim HH, Gong G, Ahn SH: Cavernous haemangioma of the breast, *Br J Radiol* 79:e177–e180, 2006.
43. Vuorela AL: MRI of breast hemangioma, *J Comput Assist Tomogr* 22:1009–1010, 1998.
44. Hayasaka K, Tanaka Y, Saitoh T, Takahashi M: Gadolinium-enhanced dynamic MRI of breast hemangioma, *Comput Med Imaging Graph* 27:493–495, 2003.
45. Miaux Y, Lemarchand-Venencie F, Cyna-Gorse F, et al: MR imaging of breast hemangioma in female infants, *Pediatr Radiol* 22:463–464, 1992.
46. Liu H, Peng W: Morphological manifestations of nonpuerperal mastitis on magnetic resonance imaging, *J Magn Reson Imaging* 33:1369–1374, 2011.
47. Mansour SM, Abolfotooh A: Does MRI help in the assessment of inflammatory breast disorders? *Egypt J Radiol Nucl Med* 43:487–497, 2012.
48. Renz DM, Baltzer PA, Bottcher J, et al: Magnetic resonance imaging of inflammatory breast carcinoma and acute mastitis. A comparative study, *Eur Radiol* 18:2370–2380, 2008.
49. Rieber A, Tomczak RJ, Mergo PJ, Wenzel V, Zeitler H, Brambs HJ: MRI of the breast in the differential diagnosis of mastitis versus inflammatory carcinoma and follow-up, *J Comput Assist Tomogr* 21:128–132, 1997.
50. Tuli R, O'Hara BJ, Hines J, Rosenberg AL: Idiopathic granulomatous mastitis masquerading as carcinoma of the breast: a case report and review of the literature, *Int Semin Surg Oncol* 4:21, 2007.
51. Sabate JM, Clotet M, Gomez A, et al: Radiologic evaluation of uncommon inflammatory and reactive breast disorders, *Radiographics* 25:411–414, 2005.
52. Mesuroll B, Ariche-Cohen M, Mignon F, et al: Small focal area of acoustic shadowing in the breast, *J Ultrasound Med* 30:88–97, 2002.
53. Taboada JL, Stephens TW, Krishnamurthy S, Brandt KR, Whitman GJ: The many faces of fat necrosis in the breast, *AJR Am J Roentgenol* 192:815–825, 2009.
54. Chala LF, de Barros N, de Camargo Moraes P, et al: Fat necrosis of the breast: mammographic, sonographic, computed tomography, and magnetic resonance imaging findings, *Curr Probl Diagn Radiol* 33:106–126, 2004.
55. Daly CP, Jaeger B, Sill DS: Variable appearances of fat necrosis on breast MRI, *AJR Am J Roentgenol* 191:1374–1380, 2008.
56. Lee YS, Kwon ST, Kim JO, Choi ES: Serial MR imaging of intramuscular hematoma: experimental study in a rat model with the pathologic correlation, *Korean J Radiol* 12:66–77, 2011.
57. Bush CH: The magnetic resonance imaging of musculoskeletal hemorrhage, *Skeletal Radiol* 29:1–9, 2000.
58. Li J, Dershaw DD, Lee CF, Joo S, Morris EA: Breast MRI after conservation therapy: usual findings in routine follow-up examinations, *AJR Am J Roentgenol* 195:799–807, 2010.
59. Lewis-Jones HG, Whitehouse GH, Leinster SJ: The role of magnetic resonance imaging in the assessment of local recurrent breast carcinoma, *Clin Radiol* 43:197–204, 1991.
60. Heywang-Köbrunner S, Schlegel A, Beck R, et al: Contrast-enhanced MRI of the breast after limited surgery and radiation therapy, *J Comput Assist Tomogr* 17:891–900, 1993.
61. Dao TH, Rahmouni A, Campana F, Laurent M, Asselain B, Fourquet A: Tumor recurrence versus fibrosis in the irradiated breast: differentiation

with dynamic gadolinium-enhanced MR imaging, *Radiology* 187: 751–755, 1993.
62. Shaheen R, Schimmelpenninck CA, Stoddart L, Raymond H, Slanetz PJ: Spectrum of diseases presenting as architectural distortion on mammography: multimodality radiologic imaging with pathologic correlation, *Semin Ultrasound CT MRI* 32:351–362, 2011.
63. Solomon B, Orel S, Reynolds C, Schnall MD: Delayed development of enhancement in fat necrosis after breast conservation therapy: a potential pitfall of MR imaging of the breast, *AJR Am J Roentgenol* 170: 966–968, 1998.
64. Morakkabati N, Leutner CC, Schmiedel A, Schild HH, Kuhl CK: Breast MR imaging during or soon after radiation therapy, *Radiology* 229:893–906, 2003.
65. Kalli S, Freer PE, Rafferty EA: Lesions of the skin and superficial tissue at breast MR imaging, *RadioGraphics* 30:1891–1913, 2010.
66. Williams A: Breast and trunk oedema after treatment for breast cancer, *J Lymphoedema* 1:32–39, 2006.
67. Mondry TE, Johnstone PAS: Manual lymphatic drainage for lymphedema limited to the breast, *J Surg Oncol* 81:101–104, 2002.
68. Ronka RH, Pamilo MS, von Smitten KA, Leidenius MH: Breast lymphedema after breast conserving treatment, *Acta Oncol* 43:551–557, 2004.
69. Khanna M, Naraghi AM, Salonen D, et al: Massive localised lymphoedema: clinical presentation and MR imaging characteristics, *Skeletal Radiol* 40:647–652, 2011.
70. Hambly NM, Liberman L, Dershaw DD, Brennan S, Morris EA: Background parenchymal enhancement on baseline screening breast MRI: impact on biopsy rate and short-interval follow-up, *AJR Am J Roentgenol* 196:218–224, 2011.
71. Kuhl CK, Bieling HB, Gieseke J, et al: Healthy premenopausal breast parenchyma in dynamic contrast-enhanced MR imaging of the breast: normal contrast medium enhancement and cyclical-phase dependency, *Radiology* 203:137–144, 1997.
72. Müller-Schimpfle M, Ohmenhäuser K, Stoll P, Dietz K, Claussen CD: Menstrual cycle and age: influence on parenchymal contrast medium enhancement in MR imaging of the breast, *Radiology* 203:145–149, 1997.
73. Vogel PM, Geariade NG, Fetter BF, et al: The correlation of histologic changes in the human breast with the menstrual cycle, *Am J Pathol* 104:23–24, 1981.
74. DeMartini WB, Liu F, Peacock S, Eby PR, Gutierrez RL, Lehman CD: Background parenchymal enhancement on breast MRI: impact on diagnostic performance, *AJR Am J Roentgenol* 198:W373–W380, 2012.
75. Delille JP, Slanetz PJ, Yeh ED, Kopans DB, Halpern EF, Garrido L: Hormone replacement therapy in postmenopausal women: breast tissue perfusion determined with MR imaging—initial observations, *Radiology* 235:36–41, 2005.
76. Reichenbach JR, Przetak C, Klinger G, Kaiser WA: Assessment of breast tissue changes on hormonal replacement therapy using MRI: a pilot study, *J Comput Assist Tomogr* 23:407–413, 1999.
77. Mousa NA, Eiada R, Crystal P, Nayot D, Casper RF: The effect of acute aromatase inhibition on breast parenchymal enhancement in magnetic resonance imaging: a prospective pilot clinical trial, *Menopause* 19: 420–425, 2012.
78. Baltzer PA, Dietzel M, Vag T, et al: Clinical MR mammography: impact of hormonal status on background enhancement and diagnostic accuracy, *Rofo* 183:441–447, 2011.
79. King V, Brooks JD, Bernstein JL, Reiner AS, Pike MC, Morris EA: Background parenchymal enhancement at breast MR imaging and breast cancer risk, *Radiology* 260:50–60, 2011.
80. Friedman EP, Hall-Craggs MA, Mumtaz H, Schneidau A: Breast MR and the appearance of the normal and abnormal nipple, *Clin Radiol* 52:854–861, 1997.
81. Nicholson BT, Harvey JA, Cohen MA: Nipple-areolar complex: normal anatomy and benign and malignant processes, *Radiohics* 29: 509–523, 2009.
82. Denison CM, Ward VL, Lester SC, et al: Epidermal inclusion cysts of the breast: Three lesions with calcifications, *Radiology* 204:493–496, 1997.

CHAPTER 8

MRI of High-Risk Breast Lesions

Su-Ju Lee
Mary C. Mahoney

Some benign pathologic entities of the breast, when diagnosed at image-guided core needle biopsies, have the potential to be upgraded to invasive carcinoma or ductal carcinoma in situ (DCIS) upon complete excision by surgery. These entities are collectively categorized as *high-risk lesions* and include atypical ductal hyperplasia (ADH), flat epithelial atypia (FEA), atypical lobular hyperplasia (ALH), lobular carcinoma in situ (LCIS), papillary lesions, radial scar, phyllodes tumor, and mucocele-like lesions.[1] This chapter describes magnetic resonance imaging (MRI) features of these lesions.

Atypical Ductal Hyperplasia

ADH defines a group of epithelial proliferative lesions that have some, but not all, of the features of DCIS, either by lack of a major defining cytologic feature of carcinoma or by having the features to a lesser extent than true DCIS (i.e., involvement of a single duct and size of less than 2 mm in diameter)[2,3] The most common types of ADH architecture are the cribriform and micropapillary patterns. The average age of women with ADH is late 40s. ADH is associated with a 4 to 5 times relative risk of development of breast cancer within 10 to 15 years after breast biopsy. The absolute risk of developing cancer in women with ADH after age 40 to 45 years is about 10% in the ensuing 15 years. The risk of cancer is at any site and in either breast.[3]

ADH is clinically occult, usually detected on screening mammograms as suspicious microcalcifications. With the extensive use of screening mammography, there has been a significant increase in the diagnosis of ADH. It is found in approximately 10% of screen-directed biopsies.[3] There are no reported characteristic features of ADH on sonography.

No studies to date show definitive and specific characteristics of ADH on MRI. According to published data by Liberman and colleagues,[4] ADH may appear as masses or areas of nonmasslike enhancement. Figure 8.1 illustrates ADH presenting as a mass, and Figure 8.2 shows ADH, coexisting with flat epithelial atypia (FEA), as extensive nonmasslike enhancement in ductal and segmental distributions.

Distinction between ADH and DCIS on histopathology can be difficult. It is even more challenging on core needle biopsy samples because of fragmentation and the limited quantity of tissue.[2,3] A study of the published data by Heller and Moy[5] showed ADH to be the most common high-risk lesion detected on MRI and to have the highest upgrade rate to carcinoma on subsequent excision among all high-risk lesions. The reported rates of underestimation of malignancy of ADH (upgrade rates) are highly variable, ranging from 16% to 50%.[4–8] Given the high upgrade rate, it has long been established that a diagnosis of ADH on core needle biopsy warrants surgical excision.

Flat Epithelial Atypia (Columnar Cell Changes/Hyperplasia with Atypia)

Columnar cell changes refer to a condition in which the normal epithelial cell layer of the terminal ductal tubular unit (TDLU) is replaced by one or two layers of taller columnar epithelial cells that have basal nuclei and apical cytoplasmic snouts. When these columnar cells show cellular stratification with more than two cell layers, the entity is described as columnar cell hyperplasia. Columnar cell change with atypia and columnar cell hyperplasia with atypia are collectively referred to as flat epithelial atypia (FEA).[3] The number of FEA cases diagnosed is increasing because of advances in breast imaging and increasing use of core needle biopsy. FEA is usually diagnosed in premenopausal women between the ages of 35 and 50 years. However, the incidence of FEA is not well established.

FEA is a clinically silent entity that often appears as suspicious microcalcifications on mammography. When visible on sonography, FEA lesions appear most often as masses with irregular shapes, microlobulated margins, and hypoechoic or complex echotexture.[9] No MRI features specific to FEA have been reported. Figure 8.3 illustrates a case of biopsy-proved FEA appearing as a small mass. Figure 8.4 is a case of FEA associated with ADH presenting as clumped nonmass-like enhancement in a segmental distribution on a background of fibrocystic changes.

FEA is frequently associated with low-grade DCIS, invasive tubular carcinoma, lobular neoplasia (i.e., ALH, LCIS), and invasive lobular carcinoma.[10] The "Rosen triad" describes the association of columnar cell lesion, tubular carcinoma, and lobular neoplasia.[11] FEA shows some genetic similarities to low-grade DCIS and invasive carcinoma.[12] It appears likely that FEA may represent a precursor lesion of, or risk

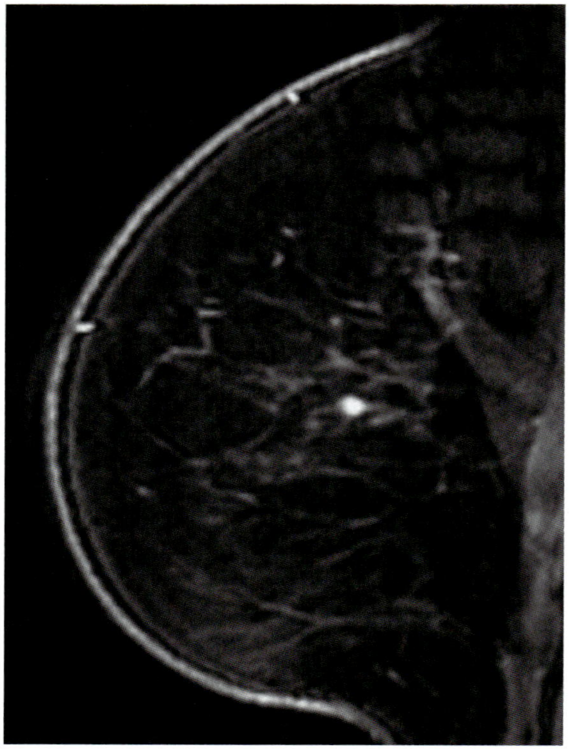

FIGURE 8.1 ADH is seen in a 58-year-old woman with a history of a small enhancing mass seen on MRI at another institution, undergoing follow-up breast MRI. Sagittal T1-weighted fat-suppressed postcontrast image of the left breast shows a small, circumscribed, 6 × 5 mm mass with homogeneous rapid enhancement and washout kinetics. MRI-guided core needle biopsy revealed ADH.

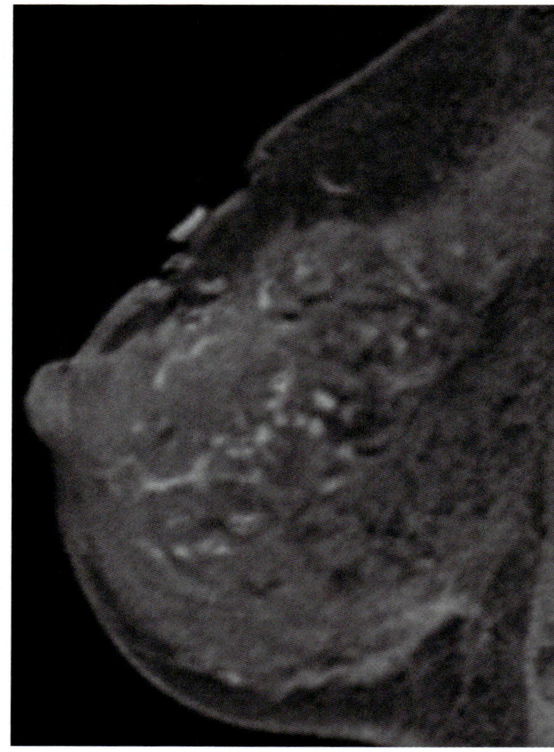

FIGURE 8.2 ADH and FEA are seen in a 65-year-old woman with suspicious amorphous microcalcifications in ductal and segmental distributions on mammography, extensively involving the upper inner quadrant and central zone of the right breast. Core needle biopsies at two separate sites showed ADH and FEA. Surgical excisions at both sites showed no carcinoma. The patient underwent MRI for high-risk screening. Sagittal T1-weighted fat-suppressed postcontrast MR image of the right breast shows a large area of clumped nonmasslike enhancement in ductal and segmental distributions, matching the distribution of microcalcifications. It showed a slow to medium rate of initial enhancement with delayed persistent kinetics. This is consistent with the prior diagnosis of FEA and ADH, although low-grade DCIS cannot be excluded based on these imaging features. Note surgical scar in the skin and an overlying fiducial.

factor for low-grade DCIS or invasive carcinoma.[3] Several studies showed that FEA diagnosed by core needle biopsy was upgraded to DCIS or invasive carcinoma on subsequent surgical excision in 14% to 21% of cases.[7,9,13-15] However, Piubello and associates[16] reported 0% upgrade rate in 20 cases of pure FEA on surgical excision in their series and suggested that FEA diagnosed by 11 gauge vacuum-assisted core needle biopsy may be managed with close imaging follow-up without surgery. Although more research is needed to determine the optimal clinical management of FEA, it is prudent to consider surgical excision when imaging-guided needle biopsy yields pure FEA, given the reported upgrade rates.

Lobular Neoplasia

ALH and LCIS are relatively uncommon lesions, collectively identified as lobular neoplasia. Both entities have identical cytologic features, consisting of round, small cells with increased nuclear-to-cytoplasmic ratios, and are defined histologically by differing degrees of involvement and distention of acini in the terminal ductal lobular unit (TDLU). The true incidence of lobular neoplasia is unknown but estimated to be 1% to 3.6%. It is most commonly found in premenopausal women, with a mean age of 44 to 46 years. Lobular neoplasia is often multicentric (approximately 50% of cases) and bilateral in up to 30% of cases. These lesions are considered to be generalized risk factors for subsequent breast cancer, with a relative risk of 4 to 5 times for ALH and 8 to 10 times for LCIS. Current and ongoing epidemiologic and molecular studies support the notion that lobular neoplasias may also be precursor lesions.[3]

Lobular neoplasia is clinically silent. Although it was previously regarded as an incidental finding on a biopsy performed for other reasons, recent reports show most of these lesions to be visible on imaging, albeit with nonspecific features.[17,18] Destounis and coworkers[17] reported that 54 of 64 biopsy-proven cases of LCIS were visible mammographically, appearing as microcalcifications, focal asymmetries, architectural distortions with or without calcifications, or masses with or without calcifications. Microcalcifications have been observed near or within involved TDLUs.[3] There is no report of specific ultrasonographic features of lobular neoplasia.

To date, there are no reports that describe specific characteristics of lobular neoplasia on breast MRI. Experience at our institution shows that they may appear as nonmasslike enhancement (Figure 8.5), a focus (Figure 8.6), or a mass (Figure 8.7). When appearing as a mass, the enhancement kinetics are medium or rapid in the early phase, and mixed persistent, plateau, and washout kinetics in late phase.

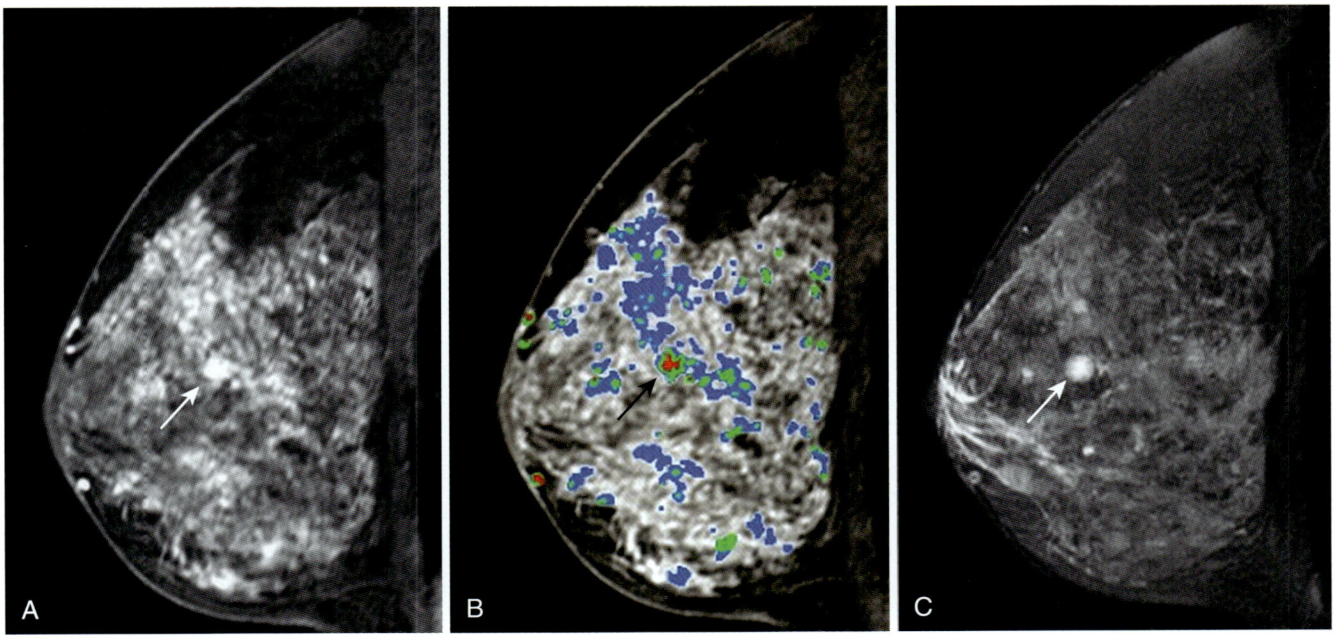

FIGURE 8.3 FEA in a 54-year-old woman with a history of a large carcinoma of the left breast undergoing staging breast MRI. **A,** Sagittal T1-weighted fat-suppressed postcontrast image of the right breast reveals a small mass (*arrow*) on a background of moderate physiologic enhancement. The lesion is signal isointense and invisible before contrast injection. **B,** A color map of enhancement kinetics shows predominantly worrisome washout (*red*) and plateau (*green*) kinetics in the lesion (*black arrow*). Note the persistent (blue) kinetics in the background physiologic enhancement. **C,** It is signal hyperintense on the T2-weighted fat-suppressed image (*white arrow*). Biopsy showed FEA.

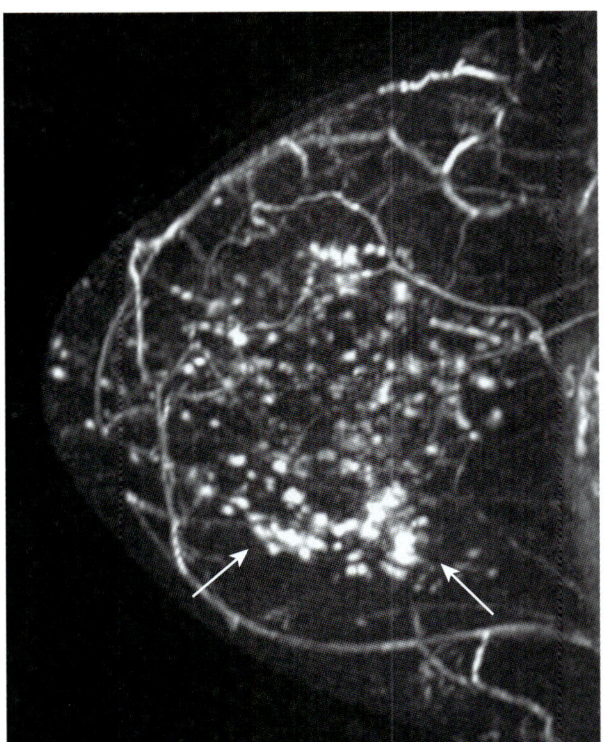

FIGURE 8.4 FEA and ADH are seen an a 64-year-old woman with a history of right breast cancer treated with mastectomy. Subtraction maximum-intensity projection (MIP) image of left breast shows clumped nonmasslike enhancement in a segmental distribution in the inferior breast (*between arrows*) and prominent background enhancement. Biopsy revealed FEA and ADH on a background of fibrocystic changes.

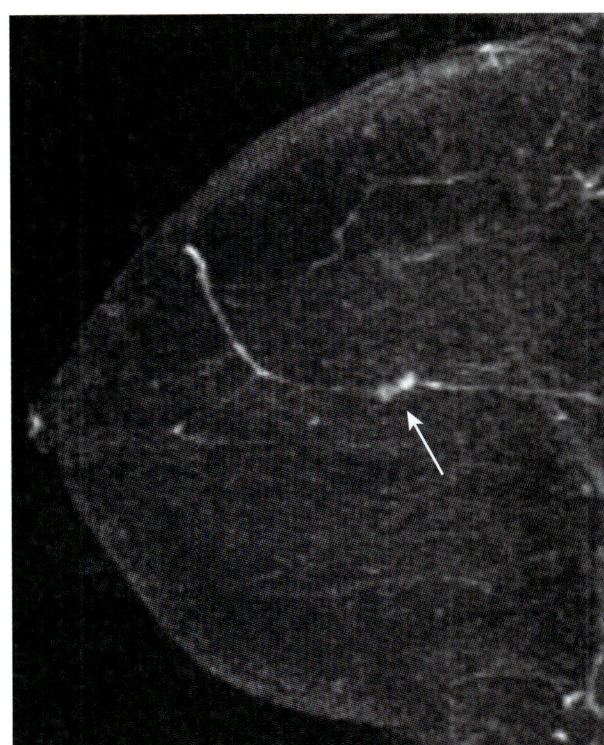

FIGURE 8.5 ALH is seen in a 59-year-old woman undergoing screening breast MRI. Subtraction T1-weighted postcontrast image shows a small linear area of clumped nonmasslike enhancement (*arrow*). Biopsy revealed ALH. There was no upgrade to carcinoma at surgical excision.

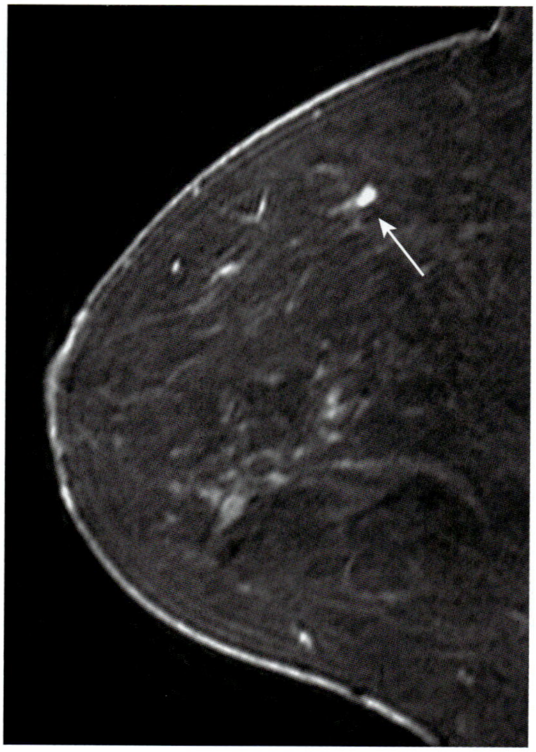

FIGURE 8.6 LCIS is seen in a 66-year-old woman with a history of ALH found at reduction mammoplasty, undergoing annual surveillance screening breast MRI. Sagittal T1-weighted fat-suppressed postcontrast image of left breast reveals a new dominant focus at 12 o'clock (*arrow*). It showed medium to rapid initial enhancement and mixed persistent and plateau kinetics. Biopsy showed LCIS.

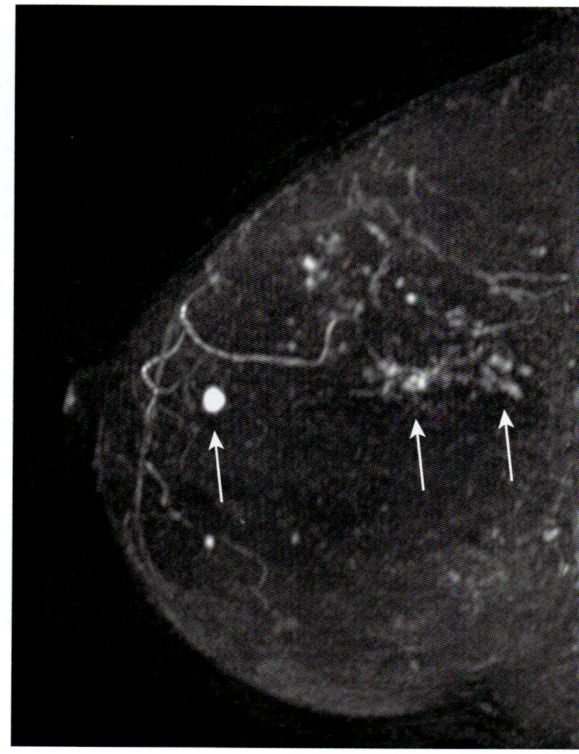

FIGURE 8.7 LCIS is seen in a 55-year-old woman with a highly suspicious mass in the left breast and suspicious microcalcifications in the upper central right breast on mammography. Subtraction T1-weighted postcontrast thin MIP image of the right breast shows two lesions along 9 o'clock: a small round enhancing mass (*single arrow*) in the anterior breast and clumped nonmasslike enhancement in a ductal distribution (*double arrows*) in the posterior breast, matching the suspicious microcalcifications. The mass showed rapid and medium rate of enhancement with mixed persistent, plateau, and washout kinetics. On core needle biopsy, the anterior mass revealed LCIS and the posterior nonmasslike enhancement showed widespread LCIS and DCIS. No tumor upgrade was found on mastectomy.

Lobular neoplasia is second to ADH in terms of incidence among high-risk lesions.[5] In a large series, Brem and colleagues[19] reported upgrade rates to malignancy of 23% for lobular neoplasia diagnosed on core needle biopsy (25% for LCIS and 22% for ALH). Four other smaller series reported upgrade rates for lobular neoplasia ranging from 19% (Mahoney et al.) to 50% (Crystal et al.).[17,18,20,21] Although there is some controversy,[22,23] surgical excision is usually recommended after a diagnosis of lobular neoplasia on core needle biopsies. This is especially true in the cases of mammographically detected lesions or variants of LCIS such as pleomorphic LCIS and LCIS with central necrosis, both of which have more aggressive behaviors than usual LCIS. There are divergent views regarding the appropriate treatment of patients in whom lobular neoplasia has been diagnosed. Management options include increased surveillance with physical examination, mammography, and MRI, as well as chemoprevention with female hormone antagonists such as Tamoxifen and Raloxifene. Bilateral mastectomy may be considered for women with a very strong family history of breast cancer or a breast and ovarian cancer susceptibility (*BRCA*) gene mutation.[24]

Papillary Lesions

Papillary lesions of the breast may be classified as solitary intraductal papillomas, multiple intraductal (peripheral) papillomas, atypia-DCIS within a papilloma, micropapillary DCIS, and papillary carcinoma.[3,25] Benign papillary lesions include solitary and multiple intraductal papillomas and papillomas with atypia. A distinction must be made between multiple intraductal papillomas and intraductal papillomatosis. *Intraductal papillomatosis* is used to describe microscopic ductal hyperplasia.[26]

Papillomas are benign ductal neoplastic lesions composed of arborizing fronds of fibrovascular stroma with a stalk, covered with proliferative ductal epithelium and myoepithelial cells. They may be solitary or multiple and are usually found in perimenopausal women, although they have been increasingly diagnosed in younger asymptomatic patients because of the widespread use of screening mammography and breast ultrasound.[3,25]

Solitary Intraductal Papilloma

Solitary papillomas are usually found centrally in the subareolar major lactiferous duct and cause bloody or serous nipple discharge when symptomatic. They are often nonpalpable but may appear as a palpable mass when large. They range from 3 to 5 mm to several centimeters in size.[3]

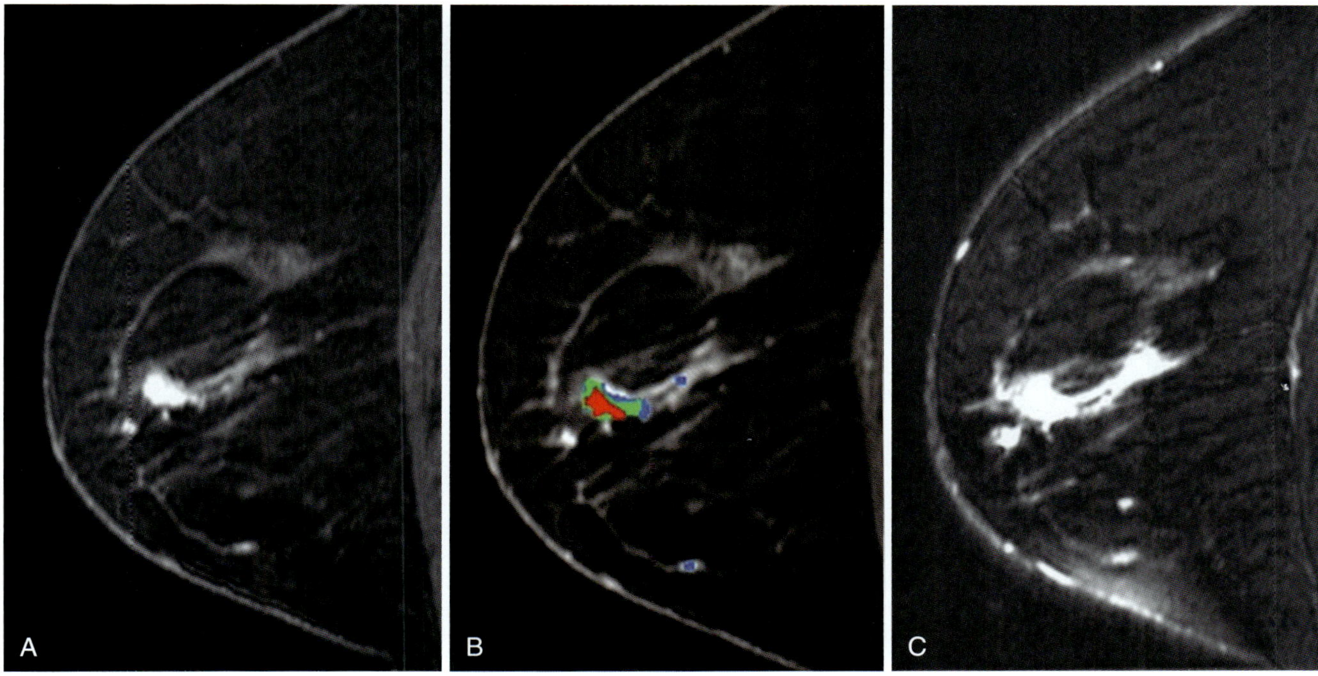

FIGURE 8.8 Solitary intraductal papilloma is seen in MRI images of a 51-year-old woman with bloody left nipple discharge. Ultrasound showed a retroareolar intraductal mass at 12 o'clock. **A,** Sagittal T1-weighted fat-suppressed postcontrast image shows a 1.5-cm ill-defined irregular mass with homogeneous enhancement. Note a small protein-rich cyst anterior to it. **B,** Color overlay shows rapid early enhancement with delayed washout (*red*) and plateau (*green*) kinetics. **C,** Sagittal T2-weighted fat-suppressed image shows the mass associated with ductal dilatation and obscured by ductal content. Biopsy demonstrated a solitary intraductal papilloma.

Papillomas may be so small as to be mammographically occult. They may also be seen as a circumscribed mass or dilated duct or as microcalcifications.[27] Sonographically, they may appear as a smooth hypoechoic mass within an ectatic duct or as a complex mass with a solid component.[24] Color Doppler imaging may show the mass arising from a vascular feeding pedicle.[27]

There are a few reports on the MRI appearance of papilloma.[25,27-31] On MRI, papillomas may appear as a mass with smooth or irregular margins, often associated with a dilated duct, or they may appear as a complex cystic and solid mass. Summarized from the reports of Tominaga,[29] Bhattarai,[30] and Kurz and colleagues,[31] the three most common features suggestive of papillomas are retroareolar location, homogeneous enhancement, and a dilated duct. Bhattarai and coworkers found the associated dilated ducts to show T1 and T2 signal hyperintensity, likely owing to hemorrhage and mixed-age blood products.[30] Tominaga and colleagues observed that irregular papillomas completely filled the ductal lumen and were surrounded by fibrosis of the periductal fibroglandular tissue.[29]

Papillomas are isointense in signal to fibroglandular tissue on T1-weighted precontrast images. They are iso- to slightly hyperintense on fat-suppressed T2-weighted images. The intraductal mass may be obscured by ductal contents on T2-weighted images (Figure 8.8). Papillomas enhance avidly and rapidly, with variable persistent, plateau, or washout kinetics in the delayed phase. Washout kinetics are less common, but not rare, making differentiation from malignancy impossible without biopsy. There are no reported definitive MRI morphologic or kinetic features that predict upgrade of papillomas to malignancy.[5]

Multiple Intraductal Papillomas

Multiple intraductal papillomas arise from the TDLU and are usually peripherally located. Therefore the condition is also named *multiple peripheral papillomatosis*. Except for their multiplicity and origination from TDLU, they have the same features as solitary papillomas on breast MRI (Figure 8.9).

The diagnosis of intraductal papilloma is associated with an increased risk of developing breast carcinoma relative to the general population. The risk is higher (up to threefold) with multiple peripheral papillomas and extends equally to both breasts.[32]

Juvenile Papillomatosis

Juvenile papillomatosis is an entity first described by Rosen and colleagues in 1980 in a group of adolescents and young women with a constellation of changes usually described as components of fibrocystic disease.[33] This hereditary condition carries a slightly increased risk for malignancy. It may be a marker for families at risk for breast cancer, because 28% to 33% of affected women have a family history of breast carcinoma. With further follow-up, the frequency of positive family history exceeds 50%. "The female relatives of patients most likely to be affected by breast carcinoma are their mothers and maternal aunts."[26]

Summary

The presence of atypia in a papilloma confers a relative breast cancer risk 7.5 times that of a papilloma without atypia.[3] A papilloma with atypia is associated with malignancy in as

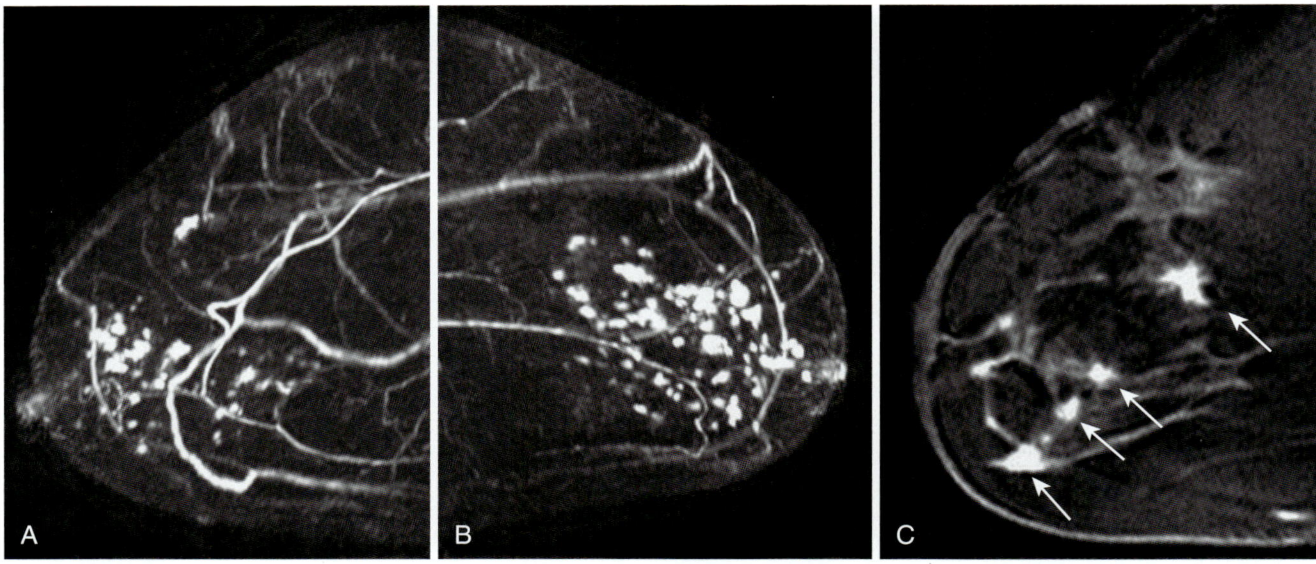

FIGURE 8.9 Multiple peripheral papillomas are seen in MRI images of a 49-year-old woman with a history of surgical excision of an atypical papilloma. Follow-up mammogram showed an area of architectural distortion away from the surgical site. Problem-solving breast MRI was performed after unsuccessful biopsy. **A,** Sagittal postcontrast subtraction MIP image of the right breast shows numerous enhancing masses with smooth, lobulated, or spiculated margins in a retroareolar, ductal distribution. **B,** Sagittal postcontrast subtraction MIP image of the left breast shows similar findings of numerous small enhancing masses. **C,** Sagittal T1-weighted fat-suppressed postcontrast image of right breast shows multiple irregular masses with ill-defined or spiculated margins distributed in the ductal system (*arrows*). MRI-guided biopsies of the two most suspicious masses were reported as peripheral papillomas with fibrocystic changes.

many as 67% of cases.[34] There is consensus that papillomas with atypia diagnosed on core needle biopsy should be surgically excised. The need for surgical excision of papillomas without atypia is controversial. There are reported upgrade rates of papilloma as low as 3%, which some authors have used to support mammographic follow-up over surgical excision.[34] However, because of the focal nature of atypia in papillary lesions and the frequent fragmentation on tissue samples, some recent studies recommend surgical excision, showing upgrade rates of up to 29% for papillary lesions thought to be benign at initial core biopsy.[28,35,36]

Radial Scar and Complex Sclerosing Lesion

Radial scar is a benign sclerosing breast lesion of unknown cause, characterized by a central fibroelastotic core with radiating ducts and lobules exhibiting various proliferative changes. The term *complex sclerosing lesion* is used if the lesion is larger than 1 cm or composed of several closely contiguous fibroelastotic areas.[3] Rosen prefers the term *radial sclerosing lesions* for both entities.[26] Both lesions are not truly scars and are unrelated to trauma or surgery.

Because radial scars are clinically silent, they are usually incidental findings on screening mammography or breast biopsies performed for other indications. Mammographically, they appear as a spiculated mass or an area of architectural distortion, often with radiating, long thin spicules and central lucency (Figure 8.10, *A*). They may have central density and microcalcifications in up to 37% of cases, making differentiation from invasive carcinoma even more difficult.[24] Sonographically, a radial scar most commonly appears as an irregular hypoechoic mass without or with posterior shadowing.[24,37] Microscopically, a radial sclerosing lesion may mimic a tubular carcinoma or a low-grade invasive ductal carcinoma.[3]

There are conflicting reports on the MRI appearance of radial scars in the literature. Earlier images published by Nunes and colleagues[38] showed them as nonenhancing areas of architectural distortion. Pediconi and coworkers[39] and Baum and associates[40] reported that 100% (12/12) and 80% (12/15), respectively, of mammographic architectural distortions proved to be radial scars were nonenhancing on MRI. Linda and associates[41] reported variable MR appearances of 29 biopsy-proven radial sclerosing lesions (31% MR-occult, 69% masses, 25% architectural distortions, 20% nonmass lesions, and 5% foci). In their series, a mass lesion with irregular morphology suspicious for invasive carcinoma was the most frequent appearance of radial scar. When visible as architectural distortion, it was better appreciated on precontrast images, with absent or mild contrast uptake and benign kinetics. There was also high variability of delayed enhancement kinetics, ranging from persistent to washout.[41] Figure 8.10, *B*, and Figure 8.11 illustrate an enhancing complex sclerosing lesion and a radial scar associated with sclerosing adenosis.[42] The relative risk for carcinoma after diagnosis of radial scar in women is 1.8, and it increases to 5.8 when concurrent atypical hyperplasia is present.[24]

Because of its association with tubular carcinomas, invasive and in situ ductal carcinomas, LCIS and ADH, radial scar is considered a high-risk lesion and when it is diagnosed on core needle biopsy, excisional biopsy is usually recommended by most radiologists and pathologists to exclude sampling error.[42] Brenner and colleagues[43] suggested that the diagnosis of radial scar based on core needle biopsy is reliable in cases in which there is no associated atypical hyperplasia, particularly when large amounts of tissue

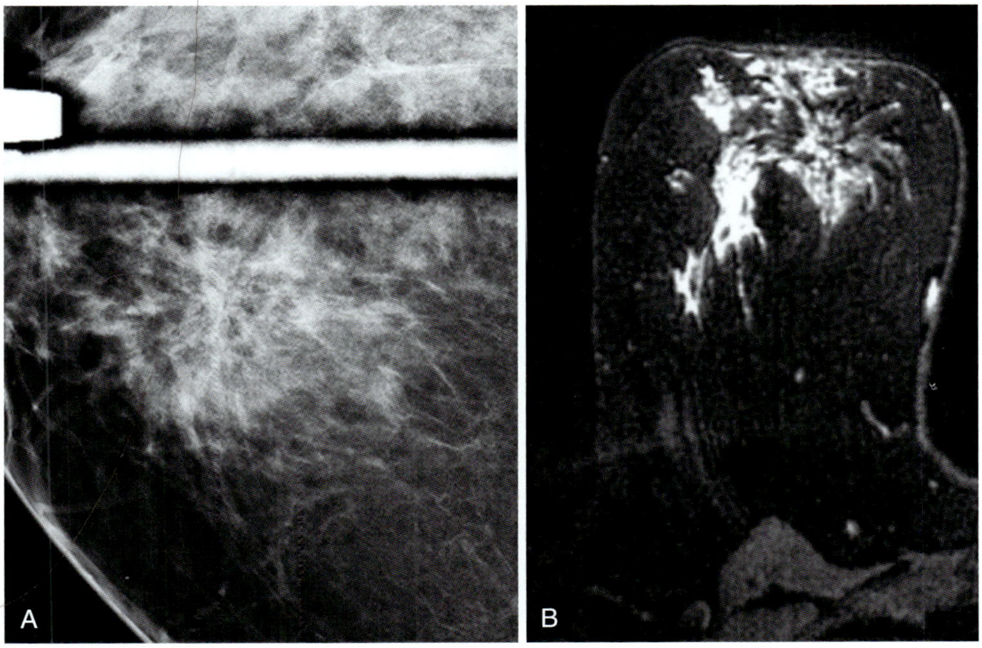

FIGURE 8.10 A complex sclerosing lesion is seen in a 41-year-old woman with architectural distortion on screening mammogram. **A,** Spot-compression view mammogram confirms architectural distortion. **B,** Axial contrast-enhanced MRI of the right breast shows spiculated architectural distortion with enhancement similar to adjacent parenchyma in the upper inner breast. Biopsy showed a complex sclerosing lesion. *(From Shaheen R, Schimmelpenninck CA, Stoddart L, et al: Spectrum of diseases presenting as architectural distortion on mammography: multimodality radiologic imaging with pathologic correlation,* Semin Ultrasound CT MRI *32:351-362, 2011.)*

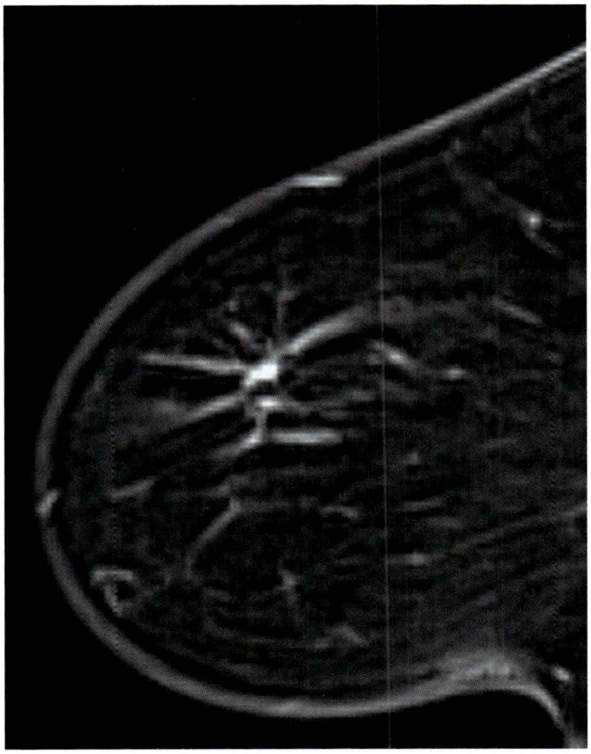

FIGURE 8.11 Radial scar with sclerosing adenosis is seen in a woman with architectural distortion on mammography. Sagittal contrast-enhanced MRI scan of the left breast shows a contrast enhancing focal area of architectural distortion. The enhancement pattern is progressive (persistent). Stereotactic biopsy showed sclerosing adenosis. However, surgical excision revealed radial scar with sclerosing adenosis. *(From Shaheen R, Schimmelpenninck CA, Stoddart L, et al: Spectrum of diseases presenting as architectural distortion on mammography: Multimodality radiologic imaging with pathologic correlation,* Semin Ultrasound CT MRI *32:351-362, 2011.)*

are removed with large core (11 gauge or larger) vacuum-assisted biopsy devices, and the mammographic findings are reconciled with the histologic findings.

Phyllodes Tumor

Phyllodes tumor is a rare neoplasm composed of epithelial and stromal components, with a reported incidence of less than 1% of all female breast tumors. It was previously known as cystosarcoma phyllodes to reflect its cystic and leaflike appearance. The World Health Organization renamed it as phyllodes tumor in 1982. Phyllodes tumor is similar to fibroadenoma in that it is a fibroepithelial lesion with both epithelial and stromal proliferations. However, phyllodes tumor has a much greater stromal cellularity than a fibroadenoma. The average age of presentation, between 40 and 52 years, is a decade to two later than the typical presenting age for a fibroadenoma.[3,24] Histologically, phyllodes tumors are classified as benign, borderline, and malignant, based on stromal cellularity, the number of mitotic figures per high-power field, margin characteristics, stromal overgrowth, and the presence of heterologous components and necrosis.[3]

The biologic behavior of phyllodes tumors is difficult to predict. The classification reflects an estimate of probable clinical course based on histologic grade. A benign phyllodes tumor will not metastasize and has a lower probability (20%) for local recurrence after excision. A borderline phyllodes tumor has a slight probability of metastasis (<5%) and is more likely to recur locally than the benign variety. A malignant phyllodes tumor will metastasize 22% of the time and is very prone to local recurrence (27%).[24,26]

Phyllodes tumors of all histologic grades have a propensity for local recurrence and should undergo wide local resection with 1- to 2-cm clear margins when diagnosed on core needle biopsy. Simple mastectomy should be considered for large, high-grade tumors.[44,45]

The classic clinical presentation of a phyllodes tumor is a rapidly enlarging, painless mass. Mammographically, it appears as a large circumscribed, noncalcified mass that is round, oval, or lobulated. When small, it has the same appearance as a fibroadenoma.[24] Calcifications are rare, seen in 4 of 51 (8%) benign and malignant phyllodes tumors studied by Liberman and colleagues.[46] An unusual form of phyllodes tumor that contains mature fat has been termed *lipophyllodes tumor.* Adipose differentiation in phyllodes tumors may range between mature fat and liposarcoma. Hence the presence of fat in these tumors on mammography does not exclude the possibility of a malignant phyllodes tumor. Sonographically, phyllodes tumors appear as a solid mass with inhomogeneous internal echoes and posterior acoustic enhancement. They sometimes contain small cystic spaces and have multilobulations.[24,46] According to Liberman and coworkers, a tumor diameter of 3 cm or more is associated with a higher likelihood of malignancy.[46] Tan and colleagues also found increased tumor size and irregular shape on sonography to correlate with increased malignancy rate in 24 phyllodes tumors.[47]

The number of reports on MRI of phyllodes tumors is limited. The reported MRI appearance of phyllodes tumors is variable. Farria and colleagues[48] and Kinoshita and coworkers[49] described MRI features of benign phyllodes tumors as oval or lobular masses with circumscribed margins, low signal intensity on T1-weighted images, high signal intensity on fat-suppressed T2-weighted sequences, and rapid initial enhancement on dynamic imaging. Farria and associates observed internal septations in one of four tumors, and Kinoshita and colleagues described gradual enhancement in some tumors. Wurdinger and coworkers[50] found phyllodes tumors to be well-defined, round or lobular masses containing internal septations, cystic spaces, and hemorrhage. Internal enhancement was usually heterogeneous, and contrast kinetic patterns varied between slow persistent, rapid plateau, and rapid washout. The authors concluded that phyllodes tumors and fibroadenomas cannot be precisely differentiated on breast MRI.[50] Yabuuchi and associates[51] identified several MRI findings that are suggestive of malignant phyllodes tumor on histopathology. These include tumor signal intensity higher than normal breast tissue on T1-weighted images (hemorrhage), cystic change with irregular wall (tumor necrosis), tumor signal intensity lower than or equal to normal breast tissue on T2-weighted images, and low apparent diffusion coefficient (ADC) on diffusion-weighted images (stromal hypercellularity).[51] Tan and colleagues[47] studied 24 phyllodes tumors on MRI and reported that all tumors showed signal hyperintensity on T2-weighted images and persistent enhancement kinetics during the delayed phases, irrespective of histologic grades. According to the authors, there tends to be a high frequency of benign tumors (3 of 4) among those with a slitlike pattern in enhanced images (Figure 8.12). However, six of nine malignant tumors in their series also exhibited slitlike changes according to the data presented.[47] In a single case report, Balaji and colleagues also described slitlike spaces in a benign phyllodes tumor.[52] This nonenhancing slitlike pattern likely correlates to the slitlike space between the leaflike pattern on histopathology.[47] All 11 borderline phyllodes tumors in Tan's series showed multilobular shape with low signal septations on T2-weighted images.[47] Figures 8.13 and 8.14 are examples of borderline and malignant phyllodes tumors, respectively, on MRI.

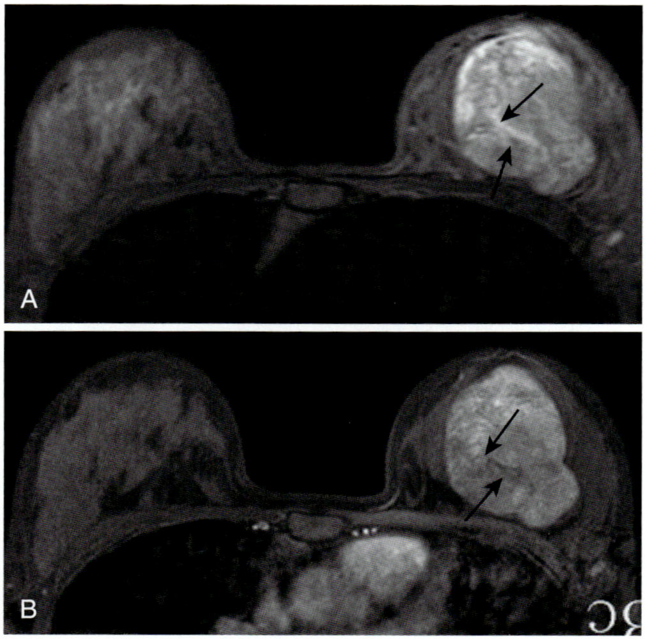

FIGURE 8.12 Benign phyllodes tumor of the left breast is seen in a 51-year-old woman. **A,** Axial T2-weighted MRI shows a slitlike high signal (between *arrows*) in the lobulated mass. **B,** Axial T1-weighted enhanced MRI shows nonenhancing slitlike signal (between *arrows*). Also note well-defined margins and heterogeneous high signals on the T2-weighted sequence that remain heterogeneous on the T1-weighted sequence. *(From Tan H, Zhang S, Liu H, et al: Imaging findings in phyllodes tumors of the breast,* Eur J Radiol *81:e62-e69 2012.)*

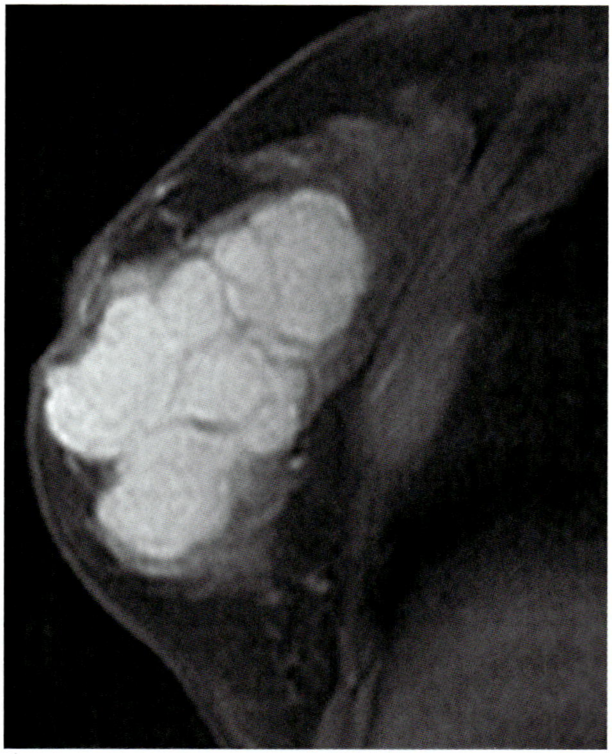

FIGURE 8.13 Borderline phyllodes tumor of the right breast is seen in a 44-year-old woman. Sagittal T1-weighted contrast-enhanced MRI image shows a brightly enhancing multinodular mass with nonenhancing internal septations. *(From Tan H, Zhang S, Liu H, et al: Imaging findings in phyllodes tumors of the breast,* Eur J Radiol *81:e62-e69 2012.)*

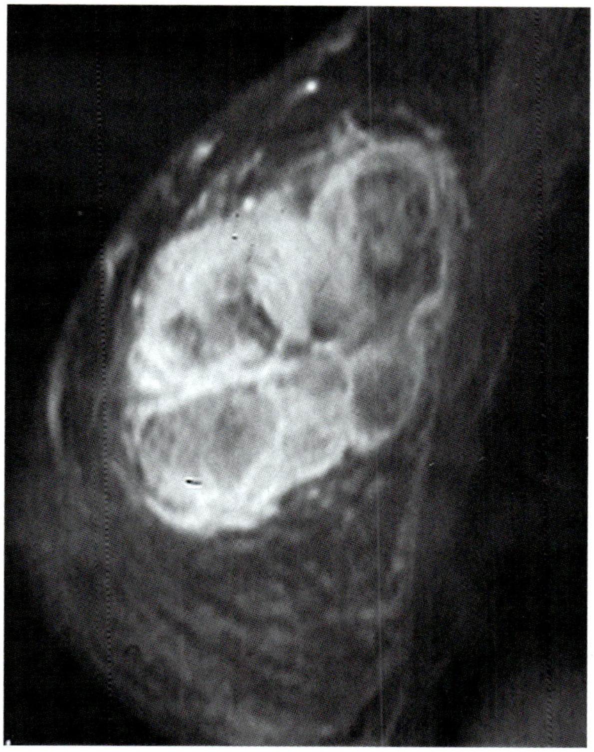

FIGURE 8.14 Malignant phyllodes tumor of the right breast is seen in a 33-year-old woman. Sagittal T1-weighted contrast enhanced MRI image shows a lobular, heterogeneously enhancing mass with enhancing septations. *(From Tan H, Zhang S, Liu H, et al: Imaging findings in phyllodes tumors of the breast.* Eur J Radiol *81:e62-e69 2012.)*

Mucocele-like Lesions

Mucocele-like lesions of the breast are uncommon lesions that were initially described by Rosen in 1986 as benign lesions consisting of multiple cysts with mucinous material that has ruptured and discharged the secretions and epithelium into the surrounding tissues.[53] The pathogenesis of these lesions is unknown, but excessive mucin secretions or ductal obstruction followed by incidental trauma may be responsible.[53] Subsequent studies in the pathology literature report its association with ADH, DCIS, and mucinous carcinoma.[54-58] These studies support the likelihood that mucocele-like lesions represent a continuum from benign mucin-containing lesions to mucinous DCIS to mucinous carcinoma, and these entities can coexist within one lesion. Because mucinous carcinoma can be diagnosed only when large numbers of discohesive atypical cells are present,[57] differentiation between a benign mucocele-like lesion and mucinous carcinoma on paucicellular fine needle aspirates or fragmented core biopsy specimens can be challenging. With a reported upgrade rate of benign mucocele-like lesions diagnosed on core biopsy between 0% and 43%, opinions vary regarding the management of these lesions.[59] In 2011, Jaffer and colleagues[59] reported an upgrade rate of 18% of these lesions diagnosed on core biopsy in their series, with the majority of cases upgraded to ADH, and only rarely to carcinoma. Because the upgrade to ADH carries significant clinical implications and changes the treatment of these patients, the authors maintained the previous pathologic recommendation of surgical excision for a benign mucocele-like lesion diagnosed at image-guided core biopsy on histology.[59-61]

The mucocele-like lesions are most often asymptomatic lesions detected on screening mammography as microcalcifications or as nodules that often contain calcifications.[62-64] Less frequently, they may present as a palpable mass. The most common mammographic presentation is the presence of microcalcifications.[63,64] Kim and colleagues[63] reported these microcalcifications as pleomorphic, often mixed with large coarse eggshell or fine linear calcifications. Leibman and associates[64] reported these as calcifications of intermediate concern. It was noted that microcalcifications in the malignant mucocele-like lesions extended over a wider area than those in the benign entity.[63]

On sonography, mucocele-like lesions may appear as multiple tubular or oval hypoechoic structures with low-level internal echoes resembling complex cysts, with no flow on color Doppler sonography.[62] They may also appear as single or multiple cysts, with calcified or noncalcified mural nodules.[63] The sonographic findings of benign mucocele-like lesions overlap with those of pure mucinous carcinoma.[62,63]

The reports on the MRI appearance of mucocele-like lesions in the literature are very limited. A case imaged with MRI showed a lesion containing multiple high signal intensity cystic spaces on T2-weighted images that do not enhance significantly after contrast injection. The lesion is associated with two small peripheral delayed enhancing masses, with the larger mass proved to be mucinous carcinoma on ultrasound-guided core biopsy. Upon surgical resection, histologic examination showed this to be a mucocele-like lesion associated with micropapillary type DCIS and mucinous carcinoma.[65]

Breast MRI and Management of High-Risk Lesions

Although the underestimation of ADH at percutaneous core biopsy has been well established and usually leads to recommendations for excision,[48] controversies exist in how to treat patients after core biopsy of other high-risk lesions, including benign papilloma, radial scar, lobular neoplasia, and flat epithelia atypia.[22,23] The management of papilloma and radial scar, in particular, is under scrutiny because of their low upgrade rates. The obstacles to achieving consensus in the management of these lesions include the lack of uniform standards for pathologic diagnosis and the wide variation of reported upgrade rates for each entity, in part because of small sample sizes.

With the exception of papillary lesions, which may have suggestive MRI imaging characteristics, review of the literature by Heller and Moy found no morphologic or kinetic MRI characteristics that were specific for other high-risk lesions. Furthermore, no imaging features were predictive of subsequent upgrade to malignancy.[5]

Some recent studies investigate the usefulness of breast MRI for treatment decisions, with promising results.[66-68] A prospective study of 32 cases by Pediconi and colleagues[66] suggests that MRI can improve the evaluation of lesions classified as borderline (lesions of uncertain malignant potential) at core needle biopsy, and follow-up rather than surgical biopsy might be performed in cases of nonsuspicious enhancement or no enhancement on breast MRI.[66] Another prospective study of 169 high-risk lesions by Linda and colleagues[67] showed negative predictive values of MRI as follows: for papilloma, 97.4%; for radial scar, 97.6%; for lobular neoplasia, 88.0%; and for ADH, 90.0%. They concluded that patients with papilloma and radial scar without suspicious MRI findings can safely undergo follow-up instead of surgery. With a retrospective study of 227 cases, Londero and associates[68] showed an 18% collective upgrade rate for all enhancing high-risk lesions, and only a 3% upgrade rate for the nonenhancing high-risk lesions on MRI. They concluded that dynamic MRI may allow reliable exclusion of invasive cancers among high-risk lesions diagnosed at needle biopsy.[68] However, future prospective multicenter studies are needed to confirm this new indication for breast MRI.

References

1. Javitt MC: Diagnosis and management of high-risk breast lesions: Aristotle's dilemma, *AJR Am J Roentgenol* 198:246–248, 2012.
2. Masood S, Rosa M: Borderline breast lesions: diagnostic challenges and clinical implications, *Adv Anat Pathol* 18:190–198, 2011.
3. O'Malley FP, Pinder SE, editors: *Breast pathology*, Philadelphia, PA, 2006, Churchill Livingston.
4. Liberman L, Holland AE, Marjan D, et al: Underestimation of atypical ductal hyperplasia at MRI-guided 9-gauge vacuum-assisted breast biopsy, *AJR Am J Roentgenol* 188:684–690, 2007.
5. Heller SL, Moy L: Imaging features and management of high-risk lesions on contrast-enhanced dynamic breast MRI, *AJR Am J Roentgenol* 198:249–255, 2012.
6. Eby PR, Ochsner JE, DeMartini WB, Allison KH, Peacock S, Lehman CD: Frequency and upgrade rates of atypical ductal hyperplasia diagnosed at stereotactic vacuum-assisted breast biopsy: 9- versus 11-gauge, *AJR Am J Roentgenol* 192:229–234, 2009.
7. Ingegnoli A, d'Aloia C, Frattaruolo A, et al: Flat epithelial atypia and atypical ductal hyperplasia: carcinoma underestimation rate, *Breast J* 16:55–59, 2010.
8. Strigel RM, Eby PR, DeMartini WB, et al: Frequency, upgrade rates, and characteristics of high-risk lesions initially identified with breast MRI, *AJR Am J Roentgenol* 195:792–798, 2010.
9. Solorzano S, Mesurolle B, Omeroglu A, El Khoury M, Kao E, Aldis A, et al: flat epithelial atypia of the breast: pathological-radiological correlation, *AJR Am J Roentgenol* 197:740–746, 2011.
10. Abdel-Fatah TM, Powe DG, Hodi Z, Lee AH, Reis-Filho JS, Ellis IO: High frequency of coexistence of columnar cell lesions, lobular neoplasia and low grade ductal carcinoma in situ with invasive tubular carcinoma and invasive lobular carcinoma, *Am J Surg Pathol* 31:417–426, 2007.
11. Brandt SM, Young GQ, Hoda SA: The "Rosen Triad": tubular carcinoma, lobular carcinoma in situ, and columnar cell lesions, *Adv Anat Pathol* 15:140–146, 2008.
12. Simpson PT, Gale T, Reis-Filho JS, et al: Columnar cell lesions of the breast: the missing link in breast cancer progression? A morphological and molecular analysis, *Am J Surg Pathol* 29:734–746, 2005.
13. Martel M, Barron-Rodriguez P, Ocal IT, Dotto J, Tavassoli FA: Flat DIN1 (flat epithelial atypia) on core biopsy: 63 cases identified retrospectively among 1,751 core biopsies performed over an 8-year period, *Virchows Arch* 2007(452):883–891, 1992-1999.
14. Kunju LP, Kleer CG: Significance of flat epithelial atypia on mammotome core needle biopsy: should it be excised? *Hum Pathol* 38:35–41, 2007.
15. Joseph Lee TY, MacIntosh RF, Rayson D, Barnes PJ: Flat epithelial atypia on breast needle core biopsy: a retrospective study with clinical-pathological correlation, *Breast J* 16:377–383, 2010.
16. Piubello Q, Parisi A, Eccher A, Barbazeni G, Franchini Z, Iannucci A: Flat epithelial atypia on core needle biopsy: which is the right management? *Am J Surg Pathol* 33:1078–1084, 2009.
17. Destounis SV, Murphy PF, Seifert PJ, et al: Management of patient diagnosed with lobular carcinoma in situ at needle core biopsy at a community-based outpatient facility, *AJR Am J Roentgenol* 198:281–287, 2012.
18. Linda A, Zuiani C, Furlan A, et al: Nonsurgical management of high risk lesions diagnosed at core needle biopsy: can malignancy be ruled out safely with breast MRI? *AJR Am J Roentgenol* 198:272–280, 2012.
19. Brem RF, Lechner MC, Jackman RJ, et al: Lobular neoplasia at percutaneous breast biopsy: variables associated with carcinoma at surgical excision, *AJR Am J Roentgenol* 190:637–641, 2008.
20. Crystal P, Sadaf A, Bukhanov K, McCready D, O'Malley F, Helbich TH: High-risk lesions diagnosed at MRI-guided vacuum-assisted breast biopsy: can underestimation be predicted? *Eur Radiol* 21:582–589, 2011.
21. Mahoney MC, Robinson-Smith TM, Shaughnessy EA: Lobular neoplasia at 11-gauge vacuum-assisted stereotactic biopsy: correlation with surgical excisional biopsy and mammographic follow-up, *AJR Am J Roentgenol* 187:949–954, 2006.
22. Georgian-Smith D, Lawton TJ: Controversies on the management of high-risk lesions at core needle biopsy from a radiology/pathology perspective, *Radiol Clin North Am* 48:999–1012, 2010.
23. Georgian-Smith D, Lawton TJ: Variations in physician recommendations for surgery after diagnosis of a high-risk lesion on breast core needle biopsy, *AJR Am J Roentgenol* 198:256–263, 2012.
24. Bassett L, Mahoney MC, Apple SK, D'Orsi CJ, editors: *Breast imaging*, ed 1, Philadelphia, PA, 2011, Saunders, pp 349–369.
25. Eiada R, Chong J, Kulkarni S, Goldberg F, Muradali D: Papillary lesions of the breast: MRI, ultrasound, and mammographic appearances, *AJR Am J Roentgenol* 198:264–271, 2012.
26. Rosen PP: *Rosen's breast pathology*, ed 3, Philadelphia, PA, 2009, Lippincott Williams and Wilkins.
27. Brookes MJ, Bourke AG: Radiological appearances of papillary breast lesions, *Clin Radiol* 63:1265–1273, 2008.
28. Daniel BL, Gardner RW, Birdwell RL, Nowels KW, Johnson D: Magnetic resonance imaging of intraductal papilloma of the breast, *Magn Reson Imaging* 21:887–892, 2003.
29. Tominaga J, Hama H, Kimura N, Takahashi S: Magnetic resonance imaging of intraductal papillomas of the breast, *J Comput Assist Tomogr* 35:153–157, 2011.
30. Bhattarai N, Kanemaki Y, Kurihara Y, Nakajima Y, Fukuda M, Maeda I: Intraductal papilloma: features on MR ductography using a microscopic coil, *AJR Am J Roentgenol* 186:44–47, 2006.
31. Kurz KD, Roy S, Saleh A, Diallo-Danebrock R, Skaane P: MRI features of intraductal papilloma of the breast: sheep in wolf's clothing? *Acta Radiol* 52:264–272, 2011.
32. Mulligan AM, O'Malley FP: Papillary lesions of the breast: a review, *Adv Anat Pathol* 14:108–119, 2007.
33. Rosen PP, Cantrell B, Mullen DL, DePalo A: Juvenile papillomatosis (Swiss cheese disease) of the breast, *Am J Surg Pathol* 4:3–12, 1980.
34. Sydnor MK, Wilson JD, Hijaz TA, Massey HD, Shaw de Paredes ES: Underestimation of the presence of breast carcinoma in papillary lesions initially diagnosed at core-needle biopsy, *Radiology* 242:58–62, 2007.
35. Liberman L, Tornos C, Huzjan R, Bartella L, Morris EA, Dershaw DD: Is surgical excision warranted after benign, concordant diagnosis of papilloma at percutaneous breast biopsy? *AJR Am J Roentgenol* 186:1328–1334, 2006.
36. Tseng HS, Chen YL, Chen ST, et al: The management of papillary lesion of the breast by core needle biopsy, *Eur J Surg Oncol* 35:21–24, 2009.
37. Cohen MA, Sferlazza SJ: Role of sonography in evaluation of radial scars of the breast, *AJR Am J Roentgenol* 174:1075–1078, 2000.
38. Nunes LW, Schnall MD, Orel SG, et al: Correlation of lesion appearance and histologic findings for the nodes of a breast MR imaging interpretation model, *RadioGraphics* 19:79–92, 1999.
39. Pediconi F, Occhiato R, Venditti F, et al: Radial scars of the breast: contrast-enhanced magnetic resonance mammography appearance, *Breast J* 11:23–28, 2005.
40. Baum F, Fischer U, Füzesi L, Obenauer S, Vosshenrich R, Grabbe E: The radial scar in contrast media-enhanced MR mammography, *Rofo* 172:817–823, 2000.
41. Linda A, Zuiani C, Londero V, Cedolini C, Girometti R, Bazzocchi M: Magnetic resonance imaging of radial sclerosing lesions (radial scars) of the breast, *Eur J Radiol* 81:3201–3207, 2012.
42. Shaheen R, Schimmelpenninck CA, Stoddart L, Raymond H, Slanetz PJ: Spectrum of diseases presenting as architectural distortion on mammography: multimodality radiologic imaging with pathologic correlation, *Semin Ultrasound CT MRI* 32:351–362, 2011.
43. Brenner RJ, Jackman RJ, Parker SH, Evans WP 3rd, Philpotts L, Deutch BM, et al: Percutaneous core needle biopsy of radial scars of the breast: when is excision necessary? *AJR Am J Roentgenol* 179:1179–1184, 2002.

44. Rowell MD, Perry RR, Hsiu JG, Barranco SC: Phyllodes tumors, *Am J Surg* 165:376–379, 1993.
45. Mangi AA, Smith BL, Gadd MA, Tanabe KK, Ott MJ, Souba WW: Surgical management of phyllodes tumors, *Arch Surg* 134:487–492, 1999.
46. Liberman L, Bonaccio E, Hamele-Bena D, Abramson AF, Cohen MA, Dershaw DD: Benign and malignant phyllodes tumors: mammographic and sonographic findings, *Radiology* 198:121–124, 1996.
47. Tan H, Zhang S, Liu H, et al: Imaging findings in phyllodes tumors of the breast, *Eur J Radiol* 81:e62–e69, 2012.
48. Farria DM, Gorczyca DP, Barsky SH, Sinha S, Bassett LW: Benign phyllodes tumor of the breast: MR imaging features, *AJR Am J Roentgenol* 167:187–189, 1996.
49. Kinoshita T, Fukutomi T, Kubochi K: Magnetic resonance imaging of benign phyllodes tumor of the breast, *Breast J* 10:232–236, 2004.
50. Wurdinger S, Herzog AB, Fischer DR, et al: Differentiation of phyllodes breast tumors from fibroadenoma on MRI, *AJR Am J Roentgenol* 185:1317–1321, 2005.
51. Yabuuchi H, Soeda H, Matsuo Y, et al: Phyllodes tumor of the breast: correlation between MR findings and histologic grade, *Radiology* 41:702–709, 2006.
52. Balaji R, Ramachandran KN: Magnetic resonance imaging of a benign phyllodes tumor of the breast, *Breast Care* 4:189–191, 2009.
53. Rosen PP: Mucocele-like tumors of the breast, *Am J Surg Pathol* 10:464–469, 1986.
54. Hamele-Bena D, Cranor ML, Rosen PP: Mammary mucocele-like lesions: benign and malignant, *Am J Surg Pathol* 20:1081–1085, 1996.
55. Chinyama CN, Davies JD: Mammary mucinous lesions: congeners, prevalence and important pathological associations, *Histopathology* 29:533–539, 1996.
56. Fisher CJ, Millis RR: A mucocele-like tumor of the breast associated with both atypical ductal hyperplasia and mucoid carcinoma, *Histopathology* 21 69–71, 1992.
57. Yeoh GPS, Cheung PSY, Chan KW: Fine-needle aspiration cytology of mucocele-like tumors of the breast, *Am J Surg Pathol* 23:552–559, 1999.
58. Weaver MG, Abdul-Karim FW, al-Kaisi N: Mucinous lesions of the breast: a pathological continuum, *Pathol Res Pract* 19:873–876, 1993.
59. Jaffer S, Bleiweiss IJ, Nagi CS: Benign mucocele-like lesions of the breast: revisited, *Mod Pathol* 24:683–687, 2011.
60. Jacobs TW, Connolly JL, Schnitt SJ: Nonmalignant lesions in breast core needle biopsies, *Am J Surg Pathol* 26:1095–1110, 2002.
61. Deschryver K, Radford DM, Schuh MR: Pathology of large caliber stereotactic biopsies in non-palpable breast lesions, *Semin Diagn Pathol* 16:224–234, 1999.
62. Glazebrook K, Reynolds C: Mucocele-like tumors of the breast: mammographic and sonographic appearances, *AJR Am J Roentgenol* 180:949–954, 2003.
63. Kim JY, Han BK, Choe YH, Ko YH: Benign and malignant mucocele-like tumors of the breast: mammographic and sonographic appearances, *AJR Am J Roentgenol* 185:1310–1316, 2005.
64. Leibman AJ, Staeger CN, Charney DA: Mucocelelike lesions of the breast: mammographic findings with pathologic correlation, *AJR Am J Roentgenol* 186:1356–1360, 2006.
65. Cho JS, Ryu HS, Ro HW, Lim HS, Park MH, Lee JS, et al: A mucocele-like tumor of the breast associated with ductal carcinoma in situ and mucinous carcinoma: a case report, *J Breast Cancer* 12:117–120, 2009.
66. Pediconi F, Padula S, Dominelli V, Luciani M, Telesca M, Casali V, et al: Role of breast MR imaging for predicting malignancy of histologically borderline lesions diagnosed at core needle biopsy: prospective evaluation, *Radiology* 257:653–661, 2010.
67. Linda A, Zuiani C, Furlan A, Lorenzon M, Londero V, Girometti R, et al: Nonsurgical management of high risk lesions diagnosed at core needle biopsy: can malignancy be ruled out safely with breast MRI? *AJR Am J Roentgenol* 198:272–280, 2012.
68. Londero V, Zuiani C, Linda A, Girometti R, Bazzocchi M, Sardanelli F: High-risk breast lesions at imaging-guided needle biopsy: usefulness of MRI for treatment decision, *AJR Am J Roentgenol* 199:W240–W250, 2012.

CHAPTER 9

MRI Evaluation of the Patient with Breast Cancer

Amy Argus
Mary C. Mahoney

In the absence of distant metastatic disease, breast cancer staging is based on the extent of local-regional disease in the breast and axilla. The American Joint Committee on Cancer TNM system is used to provide breast cancer patients and their clinicians criteria for determining prognosis and treatment options. The TNM system categorizes extent of disease using anatomic data from the primary tumor (T), regional lymph nodes (N), and distant metastases (M) (Tables 9-1 through 9-4).[1] Clinical staging is performed initially, then replaced by pathologic staging following complete resection of the primary tumor and lymph node sampling. The use of neoadjuvant treatments (medical treatment prior to surgery) requires accurate preoperative clinical staging. Additionally, although not always altering the TNM stage, the extent of in-breast disease is critical to surgical planning.

Before the modern era of breast magnetic resonance imaging (MRI), clinical staging and surgical treatments were based primarily on the clinical exam, mammography, and ultrasound. The ability of MRI to identify additional, otherwise occult disease in the breast has added increased sensitivity and complexity. Imaging findings supplemented with image-guided biopsy of the breast and suspicious lymph nodes are central to determining clinical stage. Imaging findings must be collected within 4 months of diagnosis and in the absence of disease progression in order to be considered for clinical staging.[1] Advances in breast cancer biologic markers (estrogen receptor [ER]/progesterone receptor [PR]/ human epidermal growth factor receptor 2[HER2]), multigene expression assays, and a better understanding of cancer biology may foretell prognosis and guide treatment more accurately than the solely anatomically-based TNM system. Today, treatment of newly diagnosed breast cancer incorporates both cancer biology and the TNM staging system.

Breast MRI is used to complement conventional mammographic and sonographic imaging for preoperative clinical staging and for surgical treatment planning based on the extent of disease in the ipsilateral breast. MRI provides a more accurate assessment of tumor size and distribution than physical exam, mammography, or ultrasound alone.[2] When MRI is combined with these, disease-extent sensitivity of 99% can be obtained.[2] A recent study found that 94% of radiology practices surveyed used MRI to evaluate the extent of known malignant disease before definitive treatment.[3] In this chapter, the assessment for extent of disease in patients with newly diagnosed breast cancer will be reviewed. This includes evaluation of the ipsilateral breast for the size and extent of the known (index) tumor; multifocal and multicentric malignancy; involvement of the skin, nipple, pectoralis muscle and chest wall; evaluation for regional metastatic lymph node involvement; and evaluation of the contralateral breast for occult synchronous malignancy. Additionally, breast cancer may also arise in unique forms when the primary breast lesion is unknown. This includes metastatic disease in the axilla with an unknown primary malignancy, Paget disease of the nipple, and inflammatory breast carcinoma. MRI is also used in evaluating breast cancer patients undergoing neoadjuvant treatment and in those whose tumors were found to have positive surgical margins after breast conserving surgery.

Evaluation of the Ipsilateral Breast

Index Tumor Size

Local tumor extent is classified into three types: unifocal, multifocal, and multicentric. Unifocal type is defined as only one malignant focus identified in the breast. Multifocal type is more than one malignant focus identified within the same quadrant of the breast. Multicentric type is greater than one malignant focus identified in multiple quadrants of the breast or separated by more than 4 cm. Multicentric disease is a contraindication to breast conservation therapy[4,5] (Figures 9.1 and 9.2).

The goal of breast MRI is to characterize the size of the known index malignancy and identify additional sites of occult malignancy to guide surgical planning. MRI demonstrates improved accuracy in determining pathologic tumor size over breast exam and conventional imaging.[6,7] However, both overestimation and underestimation of disease do occur, and it has not yet been defined in which cases this is most likely to happen. There is limited evidence suggesting that improved correlation between tumor size and pathologic measurement occurs with both high-grade invasive tumors and high-grade ductal carcinoma in situ (DCIS)

Table 9.1 The American Joint Committee on Cancer Staging System: Primary Tumor

Primary Tumor (T)	
The T classification of the primary tumor is the same regardless of whether it is based on clinical or pathologic criteria, or both. Size should be measured to the nearest millimeter. If the tumor size is slightly less or greater than a cutoff for a given T classification, it is recommended that the size be rounded to the millimeter reading that is closest to the cutoff. For example, a reported size of 1.1 mm is reported as 1 mm, or a size of 2.01 cm is reported as 2.0 cm. Designation should be made with the subscript "c" or "p" modifier to indicate whether the T classification was determined by clinical (physical examination or radiologic) or pathologic measurements, respectively. In general, pathologic determination should take precedence over clinical determination of T size.	
TX	Primary tumor cannot be assessed
T0	No evidence of primary tumor
Tis	Carcinoma in situ
Tis (DCIS)	Ductal carcinoma in situ
Tis (LCIS)	Lobular carcinoma in situ
Tis (Paget's)	Paget's disease of the nipple NOT associated with invasive carcinoma and/or carcinoma in situ (DCIS and/or LCIS) in the underlying breast parenchyma. Carcinomas in the breast parenchyma associated with Paget's disease are categorized based on the size and characteristics of the parenchymal disease, although the presence of Paget's disease should still be noted
T1	Tumor size ≤ 20 mm in greatest dimension
T1mi	Tumor ≤ 1 mm in greatest dimension
T1a	Tumor > 1 mm but ≤ 5 mm in greatest dimension
T1b	Tumor > 5 mm but ≤ 10 mm in greatest dimension
T1c	Tumor > 10 mm but ≤ 20 mm in greatest dimension
T2	Tumor > 20 mm but ≤ 50 mm in greatest dimension
T3	Tumor > 50 mm in greatest dimension
T4	Tumor of any size with direct extension to the chest wall and/or to the skin (ulceration or skin nodules).
Note: Invasion of the dermis alone does not qualify as T4	
T4a	Extension to the chest wall, not including only pectoralis muscle adherence/invasion
T4b	Ulceration and/or ipsilateral satellite nodules and/or edema (including peau d'orange) of the skin, which do not meet the criteria for inflammatory carcinoma
T4c	Both T4a and T4b
T4d	Inflammatory carcinoma (see "Rules for Classification")

Table 9.2 The American Joint Committee on Cancer Staging System: Lymph Nodes

Regional Lymph Nodes (N)	
Clinical	
NX	Regional lymph nodes cannot be assessed (e.g., previously removed)
N0	No regional lymph node metastases
N1	Metastases to movable ipsilateral level I, II axillary lymph node(s)
N2	Metastases in ipsilateral level I, II axillary lymph nodes that are clinically fixed or matted; or in clinically detected* ipsilateral internal mammary nodes in the *absence* of clinically evident axillary lymph node metastases
N2a	Metastases in ipsilateral level I, II axillary lymph nodes fixed to one another (matted) or to other structures
N2b	Metastases only in clinically detected * ipsilateral internal mammary nodes and in the *absence* of clinically evident level I, II axillary lymph node metastases
N3	Metastases in ipsilateral infraclavicular (level III axillary) lymph node(s) with or without level I, II axillary lymph node involvement; or in clinically detected* ipsilateral internal mammary lymph node(s) with clinically evident level I, II axillary lymph node metastases; or metastases in ipsilateral supraclavicular lymph node(s) with or without axillary or internal mammary lymph node involvement
N3a	Metastases in ipsilateral infraclavicular lymph node(s)
N3b	Metastases in ipsilateral internal mammary lymph node(s) and axillary lymph node(s)
N3c	Metastases in ipsilateral supraclavicular lymph node(s)

**Note: Clinically detected* is defined as detected by imaging studies (excluding lymphoscintigraphy) or by clinical examination and having characteristics highly suspicious for malignancy or a presumed pathologic macrometastasis based on fine needle aspiration biopsy with cytologic examination. Confirmation of clinically detected metastatic disease by fine needle aspiration without excision biopsy is designated with an (f) suffix, for example, cN3a(f). Excisional biopsy of a lymph node or biopsy of a sentinel node, in the absence of assignment of a pT, is classified as a clinical N, for example, cN1. Information regarding the confirmation of the nodal status will be designated in site-specific factors as clinical, fine needle aspiration, core biopsy, or sentinel lymph node biopsy. Pathologic classification (pN) is used for excision or sentinel lymph node biopsy only in conjunction with a pathologic T assignment.

Table 9.3 The American Joint Committee on Cancer Staging System: Metastases

Distant Metastases (M)	
M0	No clinical or radiographic evidence of distant metastases
cM0(i+)	No clinical or radiographic evidence of distant metastases, but deposits of molecularly or microscopically detected tumor cells in circulating blood, bone marrow, or other nonregional nodal tissue that are no larger than 0.2 mm in a patient without symptoms or signs of metastases
M1	Distant detectable metastases as determined by classic clinical and radiographic means and/or histologically proven larger than 0.2 mm

Used with permission of the American Joint Committee on Cancer (AJCC), Chicago, Illinois. The original source for this material is the *AJCC Cancer Staging Manual*, Seventh Edition (2010) published by Springer Science and Business Medial LLC, www.springer.com.

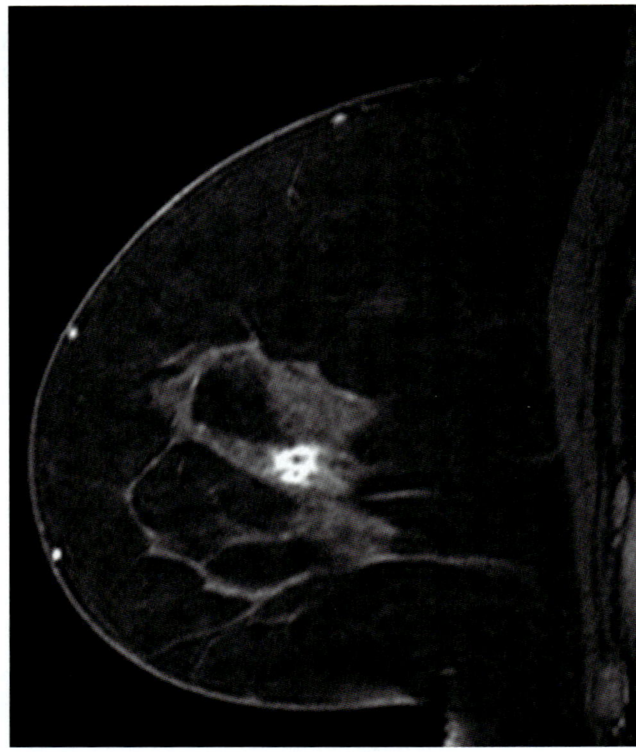

FIGURE 9.1 Fat-suppressed, postcontrast, sagittal image demonstrates a unifocal invasive ductal carcinoma (IDC) with heterogenous rim enhancement.

Table 9.4

Anatomic Stage/Prognostic Groups			
Stage 0	Tis	N0	M0
Stage IA	T1*	N0	M0
Stage IB	T0	N1mi	M0
	T1*	N1mi	M0
Stage IIA	T0	N1**	M0
	T1*	N1**	M0
	T2	N0	M0
Stage IIB	T2	N1	M0
	T3	N0	M0
Stage IIIA	T0	N2	M0
	T1*	N2	M0
	T2	N2	M0
	T3	N1	M0
	T3	N2	M0
Stage IIIB	T4	N0	M0
	T4	N1	M0
	T4	N2	M0
Stage IIIC	Any T	N3	M0
Stage IV	Any T	Any N	M1

Notes:
*T1 includes T1mi
**T0 and T1 tumors with nodal micrometastases only are excluded from Stage IIA and are classified Stage IB.
M0 includes M0(i+).
The designation of pM0 is not valid; any M0 should be clinical.
If a patient presents with M1 prior to neoadjuvant systemic therapy, the stage is considered stage IV and remains stage IV regardless of response to neoadjuvant therapy.
Stage designation may be changed if postsurgical imaging studies reveal the presence of distant metastases, provided that the studies are carried out within 4 months of diagnosis in the absence of disease progression and provided that the patient has not received neoadjuvant therapy.
Postneoadjuvant therapy is designated with "yc" or "yp" prefix. Of note, no stage group is assigned if there is a complete pathologic response (CR) to neoadjuvant therapy, for example, ypT0ypN0cM0.
Used with permission of the American Joint Committee on Cancer (AJCC), Chicago, Illinois. The original source for this material is the *AJCC Cancer Staging Manual*, Seventh Edition (2010) published by Springer Science and Business Medial LLC, www.springer.com.

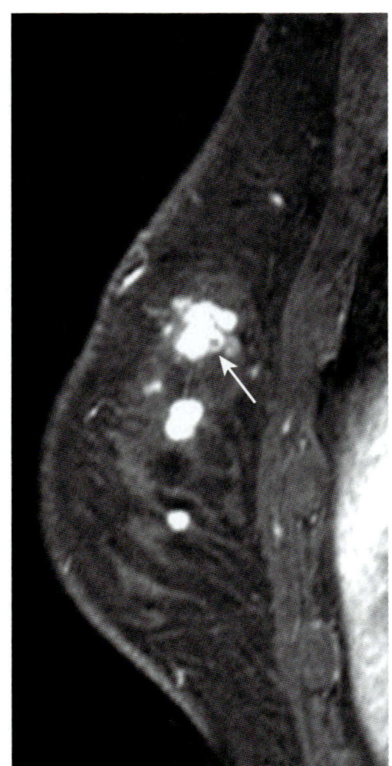

FIGURE 9.2 Fat-suppressed, postcontrast, sagittal image demonstrates a known index malignancy in the superior breast (*arrow*). Two additional, otherwise occult masses are present, one in the same quadrant (multifocal) and another in the inferior breast (multicentric).

and underestimation of disease may occur more often with low-grade invasive tumors and low-grade DCIS.[3,9] Also, there is a greater tendency for tumor size overestimation for tumors larger than 2 cm in size than for tumors smaller than 2 cm.[10]

Multifocal and Multicentric Disease

Multifocal and/or multicentric malignancy may be present at the time of diagnosis but undetected by conventional mammographic and sonographic imaging. This may consist of one or more discrete enhancing masses separate from the known index tumor and/or nonmasslike enhancement, typical for DCIS (Figures 9.3 and 9.4). The preoperative identification of additional sites of malignancy in the breast provides information for surgical planning. It has been consistently shown that breast MRI detects additional unsuspected malignancy within the ipsilateral breast.[2,11-14] A recent meta-analysis of 50 studies found that MRI identified occult multicentric or multifocal malignancy in 20% of preoperative MRIs with a positive predictive value (PPV) of 75% and accuracy of 93% when using at least 1.5 Tesla (T) MRI.[15] The same meta-analysis examined 26 studies (n = 4839) that gave information about surgical impact. They found an appropriate change in surgical management occurred in 12.8% of patients with confirmed additional malignancy, 8.3% of whom were converted to receive mastectomy and 4.5% of whom were converted to receive a wider local excision. On the other hand, overestimation of disease (false positives) resulted in inappropriate alteration in surgical management in 6.3% of patients, 4.6% of whom had a wider local excision and 1.7% of whom had mastectomies.[15] The importance of not subjecting patients to unnecessary extensive surgery, combined with the known risk of overestimation of disease with MRI, emphasizes the need to obtain histologic confirmation of suspicious MRI findings before changing surgical treatment. This was not done in all of the studies included in the meta-analysis. Given a PPV of 75%, one in four patients with suspicious findings will, in fact, have benign disease. Additionally, given the imperfect specificity of MRI and limited data regarding the appropriate use of the American College of Radiology Breast Imaging Reporting and Data System (BI-RADS) category 3 in MRI, it is generally not acceptable to recommend short-term follow-up MRI imaging for suspicious lesions in the ipsilateral breast that may alter surgical treatment. Proceeding with an image-guided biopsy is often prudent in these cases.

Several studies have shown that diffusion-weighted imaging (DWI) and spectroscopy have shown promise in increasing the PPV of MRI.[16-20] Further studies on these techniques are warranted.

False negatives, in which additional tumor is present but not detected, are also known to occur with MRI. Background diffuse parenchymal enhancement of normal tissue

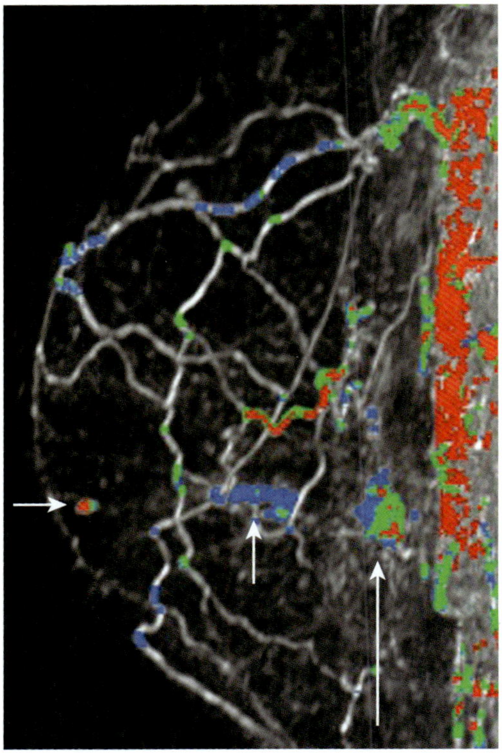

FIGURE 9.3 Sagittal maximum-intensity projection (MIP) with computer-aided detection (CAD) color overlay demonstrates an irregular mass with heterogeneous enhancement corresponding to a known index IDC in the posterior breast (*long vertical arrow*). Occult DCIS is seen as a separate area of linear nonmasslike enhancement (*short vertical arrow*). A second, small 5-mm mass with wash-out kinetics farther anteriorly (>4 cm away) was confirmed as IDC by MRI-guided biopsy (*short horizontal arrow*).

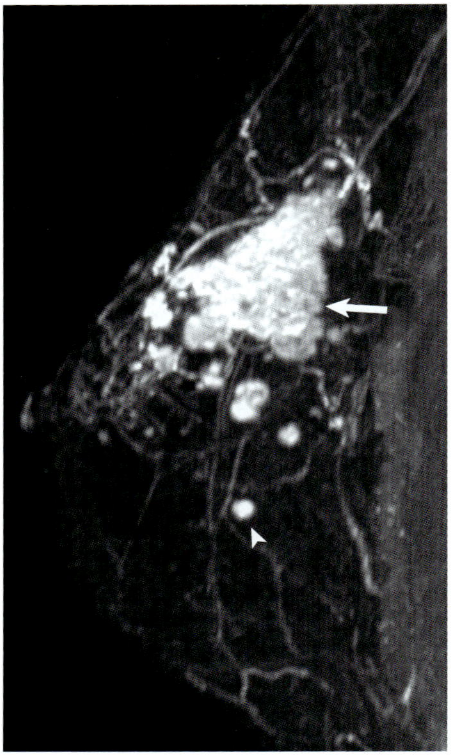

FIGURE 9.4 Sagittal MIP image demonstrates a large enhancing mass corresponding to an index ICD in a young patient with dense breast tissue (*long arrow*). MRI demonstrates multiple additional small masses. Biopsy of the mass in lower breast confirmed multicentric malignancy (*arrowhead*).

obscuring lesion enhancement is a common reason for false-negative imaging.[2,21,22] Moderate and marked background enhancement can reduce the sensitivity for multifocal and multicentric lesions that are small and lack distinguishing morphologic features.[23,24] Even extensive nonmasslike enhancement, which occurs with DCIS, is difficult to detect in the presence of moderate/marked background enhancement. Background parenchymal enhancement is hormonally mediated and does not correlate with mammographic density. Scheduling the patient's MRI study during the first half of her menstrual cycle and discontinuing exogenous hormone therapy for several months before the study decrease the risk of excessive background enhancement. However, this is often not possible in patients with newly diagnosed malignancy, who need to avoid treatment delays.

Pectoral Muscle and Chest Wall Involvement

Tumors located posteriorly in the breast may invade the pectoral muscles and/or chest wall. Chest wall invasion by breast cancer is defined as tumor infiltrating the ribs, intercostal muscles, and/or serratus anterior muscle (Figure 9.5). Tumors with chest wall invasion are classified as T4a, regardless of size (see Table 9.1).[1] This results in a minimum TNM classification of at least stage IIIb disease (see Table 9.4), which correlates with a worse prognosis compared with the prognosis for patients who have tumors of comparable size without chest wall invasion. Preoperative treatment with chemotherapy and/or chest wall radiation, followed by more extensive surgery, including chest wall resection, is typically performed.[25] Alternatively, a tumor that invades only the pectoralis muscle does not change the disease stage; however, it alters the surgical treatment. When a tumor superficially invades the pectoralis muscle, a portion of the muscle may be resected, or when deep muscle invasion is present, a radical mastectomy with removal of the entire muscle may be required[25] (Figures 9.6 and 9.7).

Mammography and ultrasound are typically limited in making the diagnosis of muscle or chest wall invasion.[26,27] Posterior tumors are often difficult to include in the

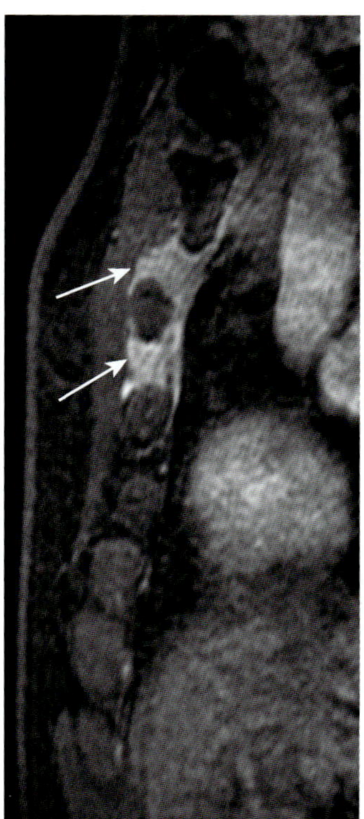

FIGURE 9.5 Sagittal, postcontrast, fat-suppressed, T1 image at the parasternal level in a patient being evaluted for breast cancer recurrance. An enhancing mass infiltrating the intercostal muscles and surrounding the first rib (*arrows*) was found to represent a chest wall metastasis.

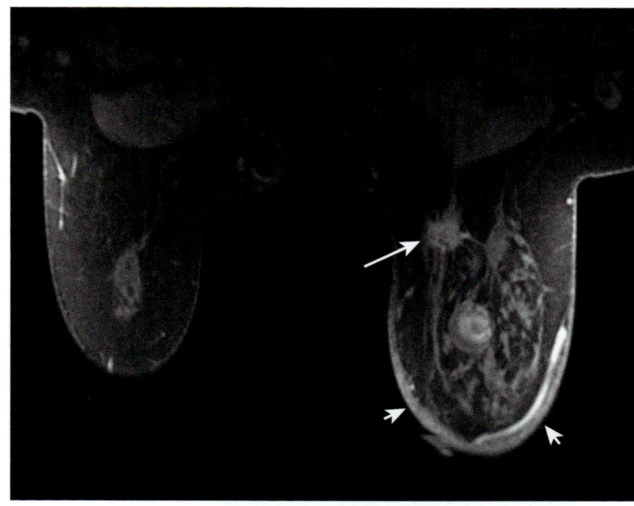

FIGURE 9.6 Axial, fat-suppressed, T1 image demonstrates a known IDC (*arrow*) with associated desmoplastic tenting of the pectoral muscle. No muscle enhancement is present at this level to indicate muscle invasion. Hematoma from a recent biopsy is seen as a heterogeneous mass more anteriorly. Diffuse skin thickening and enhancement raise suspicion for inflammatory carcinoma (*arrowheads*).

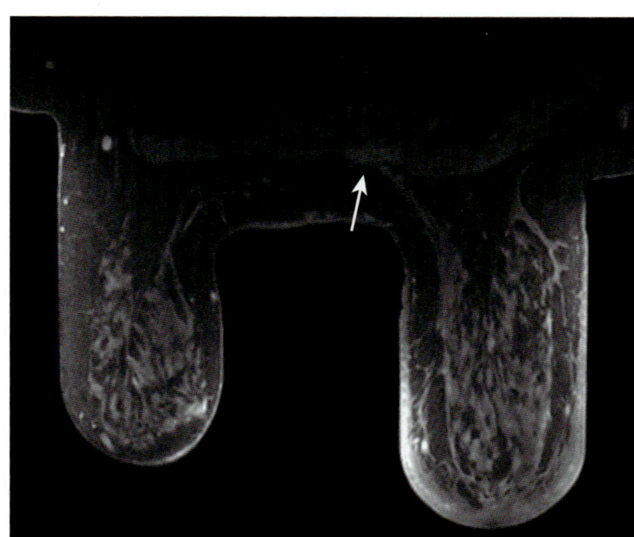

FIGURE 9.7 Axial, fat-supressed T1 image in the same patient as in Figure 9.1 at more superior level demonstrates ill-defined enhancement through the entire thickness of the medial aspect of the pectoral muscle abutting the sternum.

mammographic image, particularly when they are affixed to the muscle. Acoustic shadowing caused by many tumors interferes with the sonographic visualization of the posterior border of the mass and underlying muscle. Even when tumors are palpable and clinically suspected to invade the underlying muscle, the ability to preoperatively determine the extent of invasion is limited.[28] Breast MRI is superior in making this diagnosis.[28] The pectoral muscle and chest wall are well visualized on breast MRI. It has been shown that contrast enhancement of the pectoral muscles or chest wall muscles is the only reliable finding to predict invasion.[28,29] The enhancement may appear infiltrative with preservation of the muscular architecture or it may be masslike.[28] It should be noted that muscle enhancement related to a recent biopsy can result in a false-positive MRI appearance.[29] Loss of fat planes or close proximity of the tumor mass to the muscle are not reliable indicators of invasion.[28,29] Also, vessels feeding the tumor, which course through the muscle, are commonly visualized and do not indicate invasion.

Skin Involvement

Breast cancers invading the skin are classified as T4b (see Table 9.1), also resulting in at least stage IIIb disease (see Table 9.4). Skin invasion is defined as skin ulceration or tumor nodules within the skin. Involvement of the dermis alone does not meet the criteria for skin invasion to increase the tumor stage.[1] Inflammatory breast carcinoma is a separate entity in which peau d'orange changes involve greater than one third of the breast, resulting from tumor micrometastases within the dermal lymphatics (to be discussed later). However, peau d'orange changes that do not involve more than one third of the breast—which would meet the criteria for inflammatory breast carcinoma—are also classified as T4b.[1] Locally advanced breast cancer is at times associated with direct skin invasion, which is typically contiguous with the underlying mass and localized to the skin overlying the mass (Figure 9.8). Skin enhancement demonstrated on MRI with this pattern suggests skin involvement.[30,31] Skin edema and skin thickening (>3mm) may also occur as the result of lymphatic obstruction with or without malignant involvement.

Nipple Involvement

Malignant involvement of the nipple related to an underlying malignancy is an important factor for treatment planning because resection of the nipple areola complex (NAC) is required, usually with a mastectomy. The identification of NAC involvement by MRI can be difficult because of the normal physiologic enhancement of the nipple. Both a lack of nipple enhancement and bilaterally symmetric nipple enhancement are normal, while unilateral nipple enhancement raises suspicion for nipple involvement[32] (Figure 9.9). Findings most suggestive of malignant nipple involvement include unilateral nipple enhancement, which is contiguous with the underlying index tumor[32] (Figures 9.10 and 9.11). Other patterns of unilateral nipple enhancement that may suggest malignant involvement include adjacent skin enhancement and diffuse nipple enhancement. Rim enhancement or linear/periductal enhancement within the nipple may be seen with DCIS[32] (Figures 9.12 and 9.13). Although the sensitivity of MRI to detect nipple involvement is imperfect, it is important to report both the size of the tumor and its distance from the nipple. Tumor size greater than 2 cm and tumor-to-nipple distance of less than 2 cm may be significant factors in predicting nipple involvement.[33]

Skin and nipple retraction are often obvious on clinical exam. However, subtle changes may not be appreciated. Retraction occurs as the result of tumor desmoplasia, which is identified on MRI as fine linear bands extending from the tumor to the skin or nipple, resulting in retraction. This finding may be best appreciated on the non–fat-suppressed T1 sequence. Although this should be reported, without corresponding abnormal enhancement of the skin, nipple, or muscle, it neither implies invasion nor alters the clinical stage.

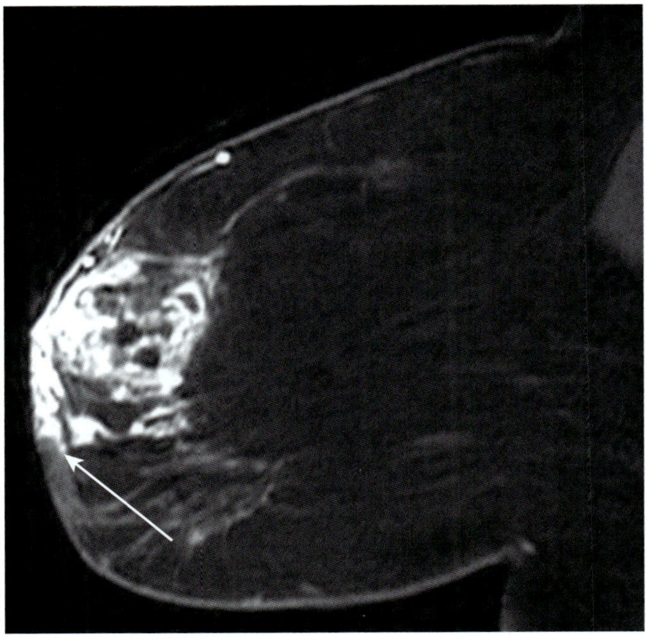

FIGURE 9.8 Fat-suppressed, postcontrast T1 sagittal image in a patient with known IDC demonstrates localized skin thickening and enhancement (*arrow*) overlying the tumor consistent with skin invasion.

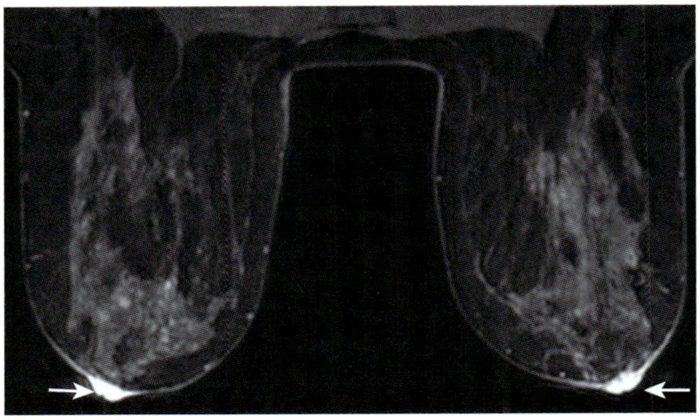

FIGURE 9.9 Axial, fat-suppressed, postcontrast image demonstrates normal, bilaterally symmetric nipple enhancement (*arrows*).

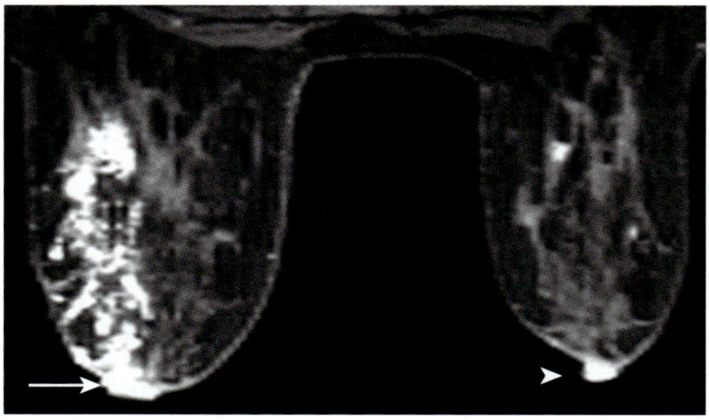

FIGURE 9.10 Reconstructed, axial, fat-suppressed, postcontrast image demonstrates segmental, clumped, nonmasslike enhancement of DCIS. The extent of disease is greater than expected mammographically. Abnormal, asymmetric nipple enhancement contiguous with the underlying DCIS is suspicious for malignant nipple involvement (*arrow*). Note the normal physiologic enhancement of the contralateral nipple (*arrowhead*).

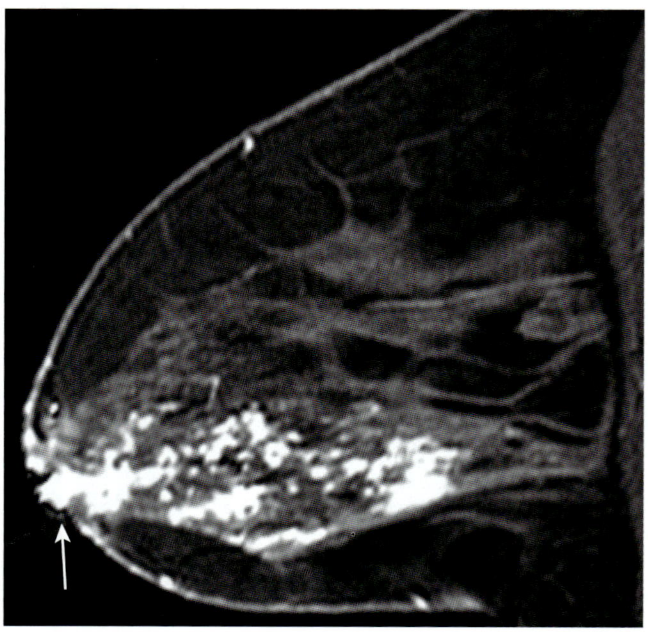

FIGURE 9.11 Sagittal, fat-suppressed, postcontrast image demonstrates segmental, clumped, nonmasslike enhancement of DCIS (*arrow*) in the left breast extending into the nipple in the same patient as in Figure 9.10.

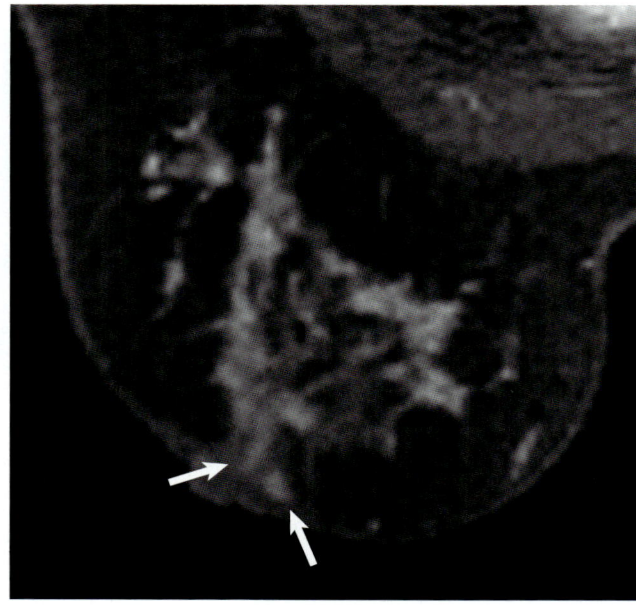

FIGURE 9.12 Axial, postcontrast, T1 image in a patient with newly diagnosed IDC demonstrates nipple retraction with linear and nodular areas of enhancement involving the nipple (*arrow*).

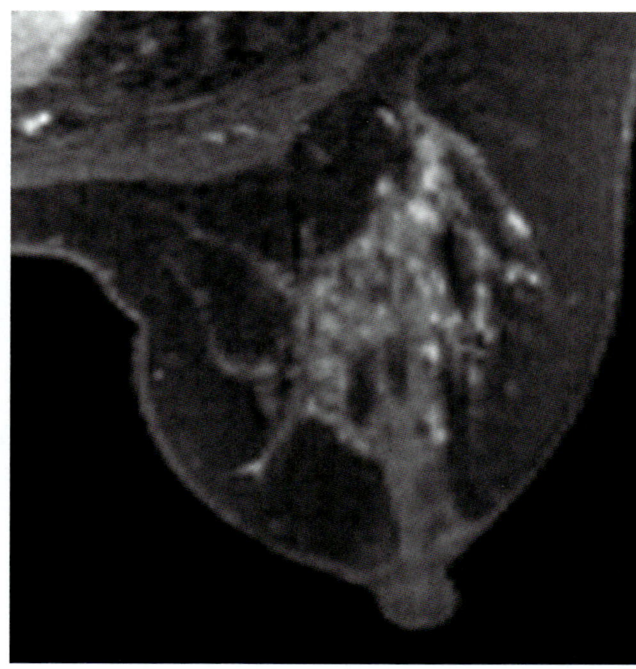

FIGURE 9.13 The normal nipple on the contralateral breast in the same patient as in Figure 9.12 demonstrates no enhancement.

Patient Selection for MRI Evaluation of the Ipsilateral Breast

Determining which patients are most likely to benefit from preoperative breast MRI has been the focus of a number of studies. Several studies have suggested that breast MRI may be most useful in women with mammographically dense breasts (>50% density).[34-36] This is intuitive, given the known decrease in mammographic sensitivity related to breast density suggesting a higher likelihood of occult disease in these patients (Figures 9.14 and 9.15). However, there may still be benefit for MRI in patients with nondense breasts (<50% density) because additional studies have found an equal number of occult malignancies in patients with newly diagnosed breast cancer with nondense breasts.[14,37,38] Therefore preoperative MRI should not be reserved only for those patients with high mammographic density.

MRI has high sensitivity in detecting and evaluating invasive breast cancer. Evidence suggests that preoperative breast MRI is particularly useful in patients with a new diagnosis of invasive lobular carcinoma. Although invasive lobular

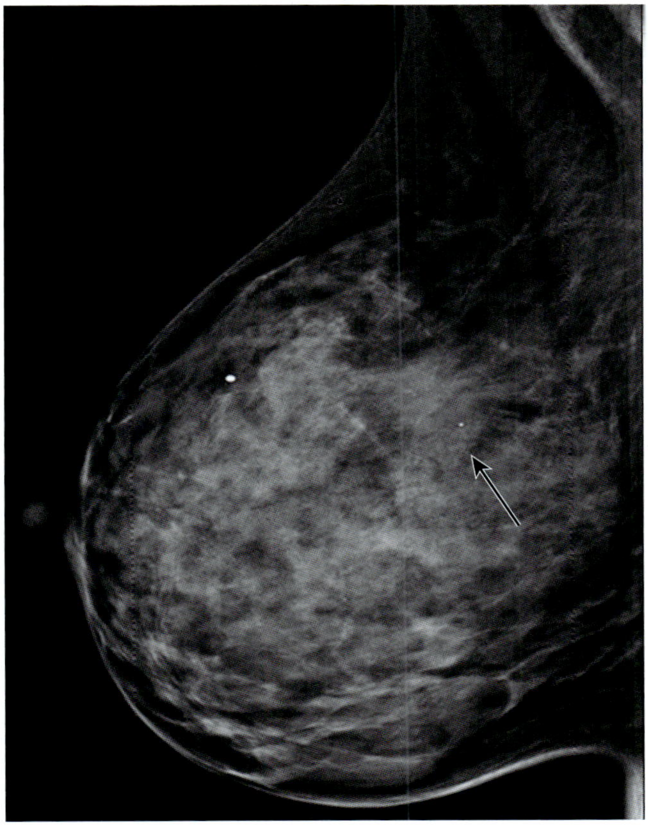

FIGURE 9.14 Mediolateral oblique-view mammogram shows only a subtle index tumor (*black arrow*). Multicentric malignancy identified by MRI is not visible in this patient with heterogeneously dense breasts.

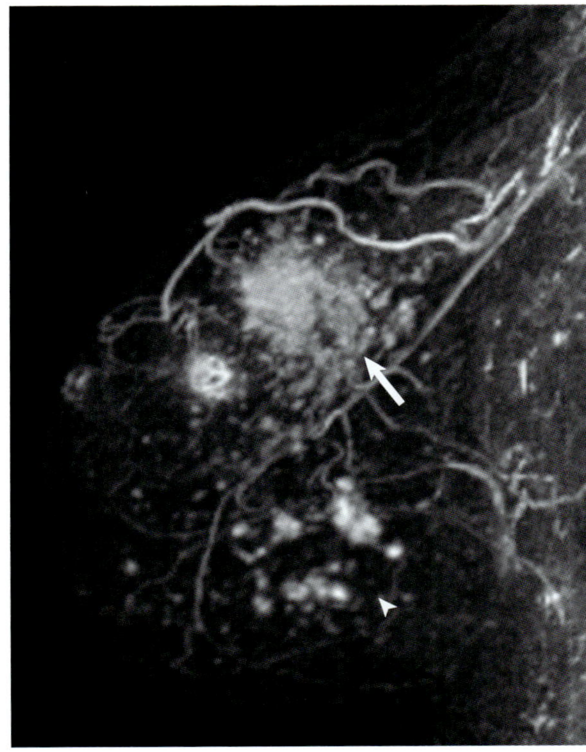

FIGURE 9.15 Sagittal MIP image demonstrates a large irregular enhancing mass in the posterior, superior breast corresponding to an index invasive lobular carcinoma that was detected by mammography (*white arrow*) in the same patient as in Figure 9.14. The mass is much larger than expected, and multiple additional mammographically occult, enhancing masses are also present both near the mass and in the inferior breast (*arrowhead*). Ultrasound-guided biopsy of an inferior mass confirmed multicentric malignancy.

carcinomas can be elusive on mammography because of their tendency for an infiltrative growth pattern, they most commonly appear on MRI as an enhancing mass. Reported mammographic sensitivities for invasive lobular carcinoma range from 34% to 81%, with MRI sensitivity range of 93% to 96%.[2,39,40] MRI has also been shown to assess tumor size with higher accuracy than mammography.[39,41] Lower reexcision rates for positive margins have been demonstrated when MRI is used preoperatively in patients with invasive lobular carcinoma.[41-44] This is attributed to both the improved sensitivity of MRI over mammography in detecting invasive cancers and the known decreased sensitivity of mammography in detecting invasive lobular carcinoma (Figure 9.16).

Although early reports asserted that DCIS was not well detected on MRI, more recent studies have shown that MRI is, in fact, superior to mammography in detecting DCIS.[9] DCIS most commonly presents on MRI as clumped nonmasslike enhancement in a segmental, linear, or regional distribution. DCIS lesions produce a variety of kinetic curve shapes, including plateau and persistent curves. Thus the diagnosis should be suspected based on morphology rather than enhancement kinetics. Kuhl and colleagues found that MRI allows prospective diagnosis of DCIS even when the disease is undetected by mammography.[9] In their study, MRI detected more cases of DCIS, including low, intermediate, and high grade, than did mammography. Of note, the sensitivity of MRI was higher with higher nuclear-grade DCIS, whereas mammographic sensitivity decreased with higher-grade DCIS. MRI sensitivity for high-grade DCIS was 98% compared with mammography sensitivity at 52%. Overall, the sensitivity for diagnosing all types of DCIS on MRI was 92% compared with 56% for mammography. This suggests that preoperative MRI should be useful to evaluate the extent of disease in patients with newly diagnosed DCIS, particularly with high-grade disease, as well as for invasive cancers with an extensive intraductal component (Figures 9.17 and 9.18).

As less-invasive treatments such as partial breast radiation and nipple-sparing mastectomies are being used in the treatment of breast cancers, breast MRI may add substantial value. Although limited data are available, preoperative MRI is beneficial for patients intending to undergo partial breast radiation. This treatment is being used with increased frequency to treat early-stage breast cancers. Eligibility criteria are based on clinical exam and conventional imaging with mammography and ultrasound.[45] However, several single-site studies (n range 79-260) have shown benefit with preoperative breast MRI for appropriate patient selection.[46-50] Studies using breast MRI in patients with presumed limited disease who are considered candidates for partial breast irradiation (PBI) have demonstrated additional sites of ipsilateral breast malignancy with a range of 4.2% to 38%, thereby excluding these patients for PBI.[46-50] Among these patients, it seems that the incidence of occult disease is higher when

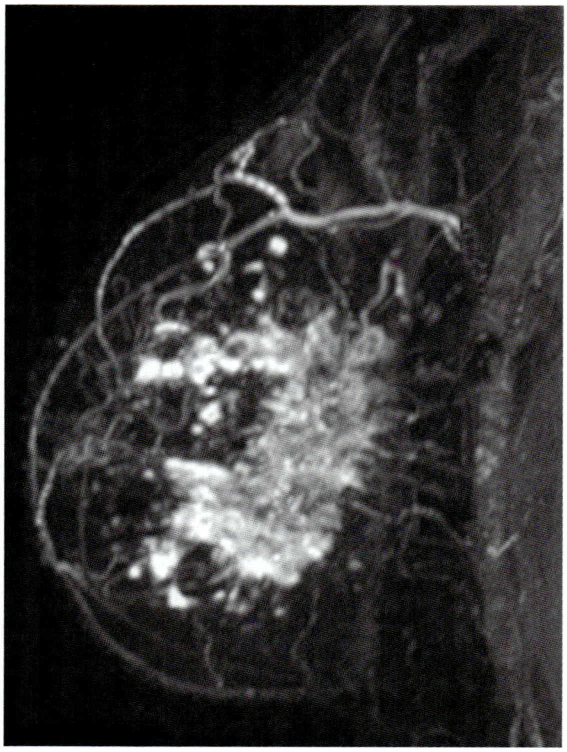

FIGURE 9.16 Subtraction, postcontrast, sagittal MIP image demonstrates a large enhancing mass with spiculated margins and multiple surrounding satellite masses that corresponds to an invasive lobular carcinoma that is much larger than had been suspected based on earlier mammographic results.

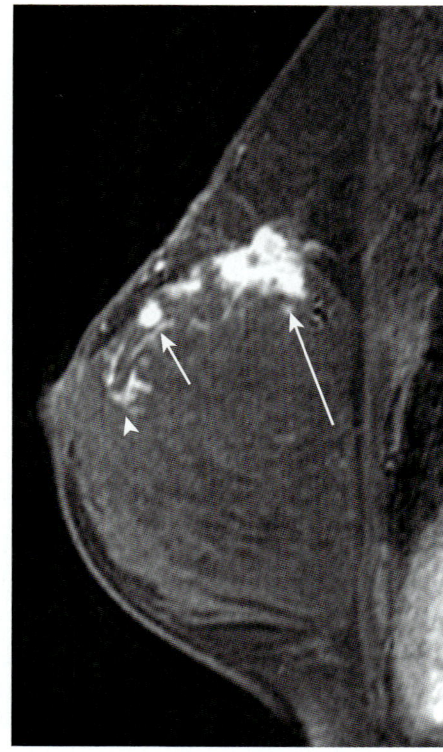

FIGURE 9.17 Fat-suppressed, postcontrast, sagittal image demonstrates an irregular enhancing mass corresponding to a known index IDC in the posterior, superior breast (*long arrow*). Occult DCIS (extensive intraductal component) is seen as linear nonmasslike enhancement extending to near the nipple in a segmental distribution (*arrowhead*). A second (multifocal) invasive mass is also identified (*short arrow*).

the primary malignancy consists of DCIS (20%) or invasive lobular carcinoma (18%).[47,48]

Nipple-sparing mastectomy (NSM) is essentially a skin-sparing mastectomy with preservation of the nipple-areolar complex. This procedure is now used to treat select breast cancer patients because it offers good cosmetic outcome without the need for multiple reconstructive surgical procedures.[51] However, given concerns for increased cancer recurrence risk, caution must be taken when selecting patients for an NSM. Factors that have been shown to increase the risk of occult nipple involvement include a distance of less than 2 cm between the nipple and tumor, large tumor size (>2-3 cm), lymph node metastasis, lymphovascular invasion, and multicentricity or multifocality.[52-61] MRI adds additional information that may aid in patient selection for NSM. Tumor size greater than 2 cm and tumor-to-nipple distance of less than 2 cm on MRI have been shown to be significantly related to histopathologically proven nipple involvement.[33] A low rate of nipple involvement (2.2%, 2 out of 89 patients) has been reported in high-risk patients undergoing NSM, with a negative preoperative breast MRI assessment.[62]

Evaluation of Regional Lymph Nodes

The presence of regional lymph node metastases is an important component of breast cancer staging and the most significant prognostic factor.[63] Regional lymph nodes are composed of ipsilateral axillary, ipsilateral internal mammary, ipsilateral intramammary, and ipsilateral supraclavicular nodes. Ipsilateral axillary lymph nodes are divided into three levels (Figure 9.19):

- Level I is composed of low axillary lymph nodes, lateral to the lateral border of the pectoralis minor muscle. For staging and N classification purposes, intramammary lymph nodes are grouped with level I axillary nodes.
- Level II is composed of mid-axillary lymph nodes between the medial and lateral borders of the pectoralis minor muscle as well as interpectoral lymph nodes (located between the pectoralis major and minor muscles).
- Level III is composed of apical axillary lymph nodes, medial to the medial margin of the pectoralis minor muscle and inferior to the clavicle (infraclavicular).

Ipsilateral internal mammary lymph nodes (parasternal) are located along the margin of the sternum in the intercostal spaces. All three axillary levels and the internal mammary region are typically included in the field of view on breast MRI. Abnormal lymph nodes identified by MRI should be described by location and axillary level. Metastases in ipsilateral internal mammary or level III lymph nodes result in clinical stage III disease (see Tables 9-2 and 9.4).

Ipsilateral supraclavicular lymph nodes are located in the supraclavicular fossa. Lymph nodes that lie outside the supraclavicular fossa but adjacent to this region are considered lower cervical nodes. These regions are usually not within the field

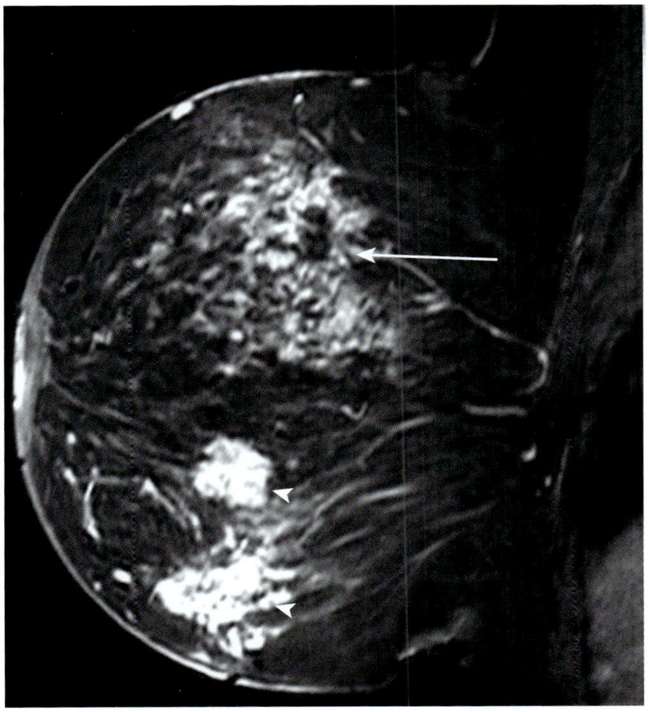

FIGURE 9.18 Fat-suppressed, postcontrast, sagittal image demonstrates two irregular enhancing masses corresponding to known index IDC (*arrowheads*). Clumped, nonmasslike enhancement with a segmental distribution in the superior breast was found to represent occult DCIS (*long arrow*).

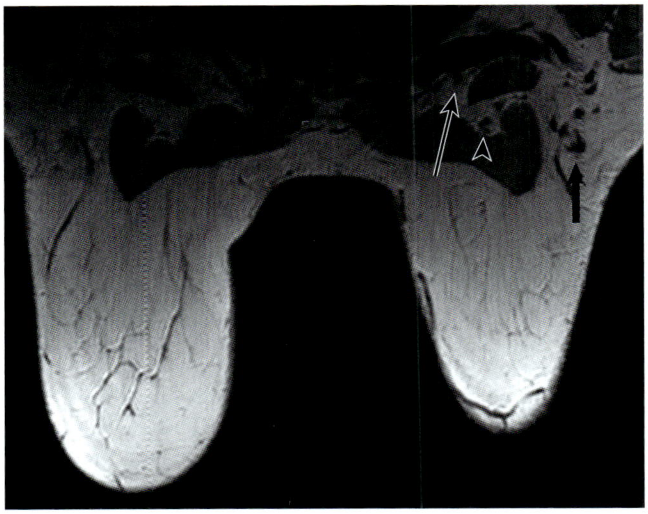

FIGURE 9.19 Normal axillary lymph nodes: level 1 (*black arrow*), level 2 (*arrowhead*), level 3 (*long arrow*).

of view using current breast MRI coils. Metastases to cervical, contralateral internal mammary, and contralateral axillary lymph nodes are considered distant metastases (see Table 9.2).

The ability of MRI to predict metastatic lymph node involvement is limited, with sensitivities reported to range from 36% to 88%, and specificities ranging from 73% to 100%.[64-68] Morphologic features are used for predicting lymph node positivity. Findings that suggest the possibility of metastatic involvement include the following: loss

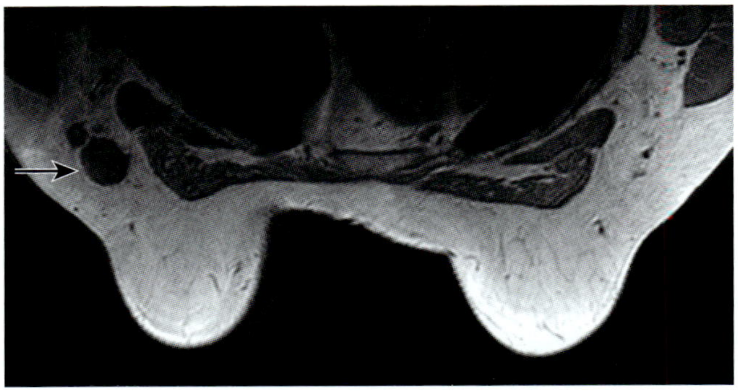

FIGURE 9.20 Non–fat-suppressed, precontrast, axial, T1 image of a patient with breast cancer demonstrates an abnormal axillary lymph node with loss of hilar fat and cortical thickening.

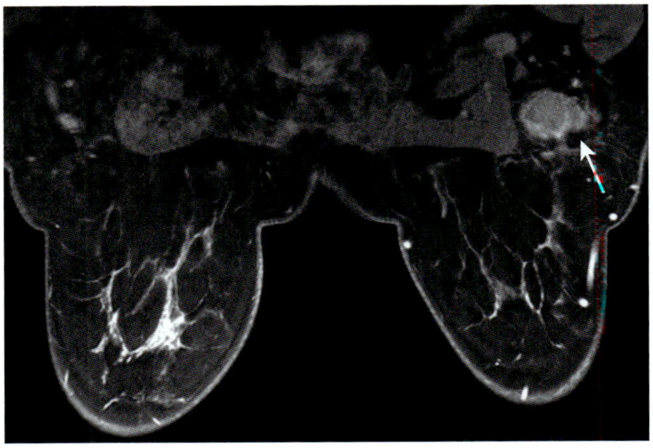

FIGURE 9.21 Fat-suppressed, postcontrast, axial, T1 image of a patient with breast cancer demonstrates an abnormal axillary lymph node (*arrow*) with loss of hilar fat, heterogenous internal enhancement, and surrounding edema.

of a fatty hilum, increased cortical thickness (>3 mm), eccentric or focal cortical thickening, irregular margins, edema surrounding the lymph node, and asymmetry of these characteristics when the node is compared with the contralateral axialla.[63,65,69,70] The visualization of a fatty hilum and cortical thickening are best appreciated on a high resolution noncontrast, non–fat-suppressed imaging sequence.[63] Enhancement kinetics are not useful because normal lymph nodes are highly vascular and demonstrate intense, rapid enhancement, often with wash-out kinetics. Both normal and abnormal lymph nodes may be high in T2 signal (Figures 9.20 and 9.21).

Normal internal mammary lymph nodes are typically not visible on MRI. Thus, when visualized, they should be reported and viewed with suspicion. Internal mammary lymph nodes have been shown to be more likely to contain metastases when 5 mm or larger in size[71] (Figure 9.22). However, it is notable that additional adenopathy typically accompanies internal mammary metastases. Isolated internal mammary metastases are very rare, found in only 1% of sentinel lymph node biopsies.[72-77]

Small recent studies have suggested that DWI may be helpful in diagnosing metastatic lymph nodes, with modest sensitivity and specificity.[78,79] Also, imaging with ultrasmall super-paramagnetic iron oxide–enhanced MRI has shown

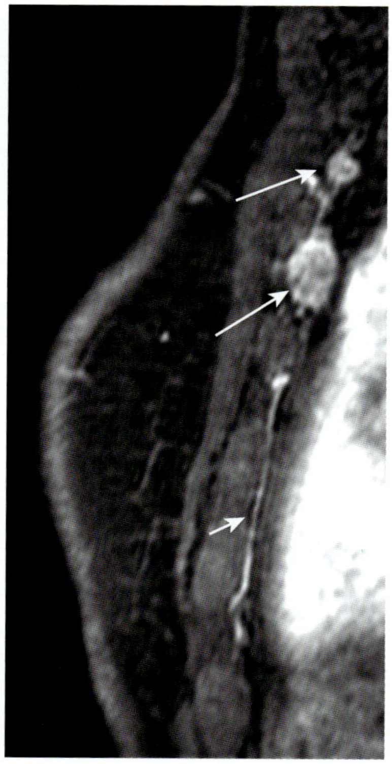

FIGURE 9.22 Sagittal, postcontrast, fat-suppressed image in a patient with breast cancer at the level of the internal mammary vessels (*short arrow*). Two enlarged internal mammary lymph nodes (*long arrows*) raise suspicion for metastatic involvement.

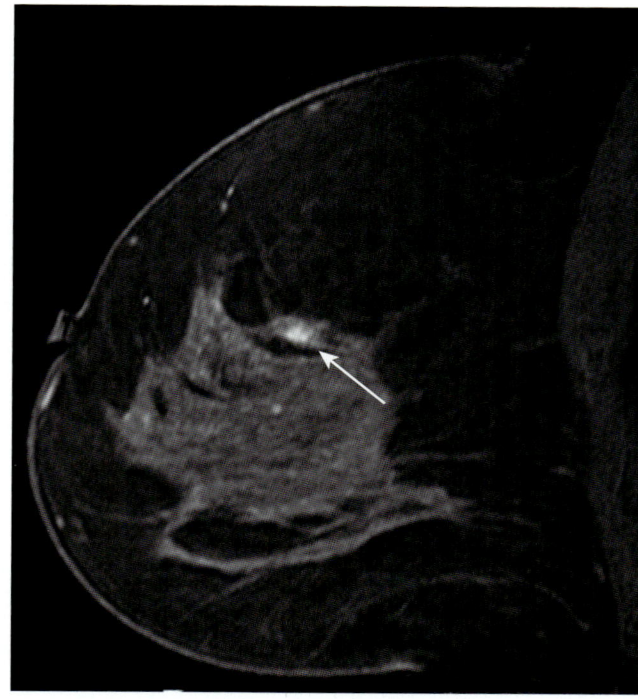

FIGURE 9.23 Fat-suppressed, postcontrast, sagittal image demonstrates a small, irregular, enhancing mass (*arrow*). This was found to represent an occult synchronous IDC in the contralateral breast of a young patient with known breast cancer.

high sensitivity (98%) and specificity (96%) for detecting lymph node metastases.[68]

Adding ultrasound-guided lymph node sampling increases the specificity of MRI in predicting metastatic involvement.[66,80] Thus, when abnormal lymph nodes are suspected on MRI, these may be further imaged and sampled using ultrasound techniques. However, it should be noted that although the specificity of a positive lymph node fine-needle aspiration or core biopsy is very high (100%), the negative predictive value is relatively low (70%).[81,82]

Traditionally, efforts were made to identify axillary metastases preoperatively in order to spare patients an unnecessary sentinel lymph node biopsy, allowing them to proceed directly to lymph node dissection. However, this approach has come into question after an American College of Surgery, Obstetrics, and Gynecology (ACOSOG) Z 0011 trial. This trial suggested that patients with T1 and T2 tumors who are clinically node negative and have only one or two positive sentinel lymph nodes may not benefit from axillary lymph node dissection.[83] However, there are several issues with the design of the study that are beyond the scope of this chapter, and practice patterns may vary among institutions.[84-86] Thus close collaboration with the surgeons in each institution is recommended.

Screening the Contralateral Breast

Current dedicated breast MRI coils allow rapid three-dimensional volume acquisition images of both breasts to be obtained, and the majority of MRI exams include both breasts. This provides useful information for interpreting the images regarding bilateral breast symmetry. It also provides a screening tool for the contralateral breast in patients with newly diagnosed breast cancer, useful because they are known to be at increased risk. Contralateral breast cancer is diagnosed in up to 10% of women, despite negative initial mammographic and clinical evaluations.[87-90] MRI has been shown to identify otherwise occult synchronous contralateral breast cancer in 3.0% to 5.5% of these patients (3% in a study of 969 women by Lehman and 5.5% based on a meta-analysis by Plana, including 30 studies [n = 703]).[15,91] However, the PPV of MRI for contralateral findings was found to be lower than for findings in the ipsilateral breast (21% by Lehman and 40% by Plana using 1.5 T).[15,91] Thus histologic confirmation is imperative before altering surgical treatment. Lehman also identified a negative predictive value of 99%, showing that negative MRI findings indicate with high accuracy that there is no malignancy present in the contralateral breast. When those studies are considered in the meta-analysis, an appropriate change to bilateral surgery was performed in 2.6% of patients and inappropriate bilateral surgery was performed in 0.4% of patients. When contralateral malignancy is found by MRI, it is most often early-stage disease, either DCIS or T1 tumors with negative lymph node status.[91,92] This raises the question of overdetection, and the effect of contralateral tumor detection on overall survival is unclear. However, it does allow appropriate and timely treatment of the malignancy in the contralateral breast, such that a second round of surgery and chemotherapy may be avoided. The knowledge of bilateral malignancy may also prove useful in stratifying patients for genetic testing (Figure 9.23).

Special Cases

Inflammatory Breast Carcinoma

Inflammatory breast carcinoma is a rare aggressive variant of breast cancer that carries a poor prognosis. It accounts for approximately 2% of breast cancer cases.[93] The classic clinical presentation includes rapidly progressive unilateral breast erythema, edema, and warmth. Rapid enlargement of the breast is often seen, at times doubling or tripling in size over several weeks. The skin edema is associated with exaggerated hair follicles resulting in the characteristic peau d'orange appearance. A palpable underlying breast mass may or may not be evident. Although this is often a clinically apparent abnormality, the diagnosis can be difficult to distinguish from neglected locally advanced breast carcinoma or acute mastitis. The rapid onset and progression often differentiates inflammatory cancer from noninflammatory breast carcinoma. Infectious symptoms and severe pain may signify acute mastitis. However, differentiating the two at the initial patient presentation can be challenging. Patients are often treated empirically with antibiotics, in which case clinical improvement within 48 hours is expected. Given the aggressive nature of inflammatory breast carcinoma, the diagnosis should not be delayed. Any patient with presumed mastitis whose symptoms do not resolve within 2 weeks should be suspected to have malignancy, and the situation warrants further evaluation.

The diagnostic criteria for inflammatory breast carcinoma, as defined by the American Joint Committee on Cancer, are both clinical and pathologic, including rapid onset of breast edema; edema and/or peau d'orange changes of the skin and/or warmth of the breast, with or without an underlying palpable mass; duration of the symptoms of no more than 6 months; skin edema occupying at least one third of the breast; and pathologic confirmation of invasive carcinoma.[94] Although the pathologic hallmark of the disease is that of tumor emboli occluding the dermal lymphatics of the breast, this is not a requisite for diagnosis because of the recognition of sampling errors with skin biopsy. Along with the clinical findings, a diagnosis of malignancy is required that may arise from tumor within the skin or from within the breast.

The diagnosis of inflammatory breast carcinoma results in a minimum classification as stage IIIB (T4 tumor). Recognized as a unique entity, this is assigned a separate T stage of T4d regardless of the primary tumor size (see Tables 9-1 and 9-4). In contrast, breast cancer is considered locally advanced when the largest tumor size is greater than 5 cm (T3) or in cases in which there is tumor invasion of the chest wall and/or skin (T4a-c) or extensive lymph node involvement (N2 or N3). This also results in a diagnosis of stage IIIB or IIIC.[1]

Mammography and ultrasound are recommended for the initial work-up in patients with suspected inflammatory breast carcinoma. Characteristic mammographic findings relate to breast edema including diffuse skin thickening, trabecular thickening, and diffuse increased density. The mammographic evaluation is often limited by the increased breast density and the patient's inability to tolerate optimal compression of the symptomatic breast, interfering with identification of the primary malignancy. The sensitivity of mammography to identify an underlying primary breast carcinoma has been reported to range from 43% to 68%.[95,96] Breast ultrasound shows improved sensitivity in identifying the primary malignancy, in the range of 94% to 95%.[95,96] Thus ultrasound is the first-line examination along with mammography. Ultrasound should be performed for patients who cannot tolerate mammography. Not uncommonly, however, diffuse tissue edema may obscure the identification of a primary breast malignancy with ultrasound. MRI has shown superior sensitivity for identifying the underlying malignancy (98% to 100%), as well as superior accuracy, often demonstrating an increased number of tumors compared with number of tumors found on ultrasound.[95,96]

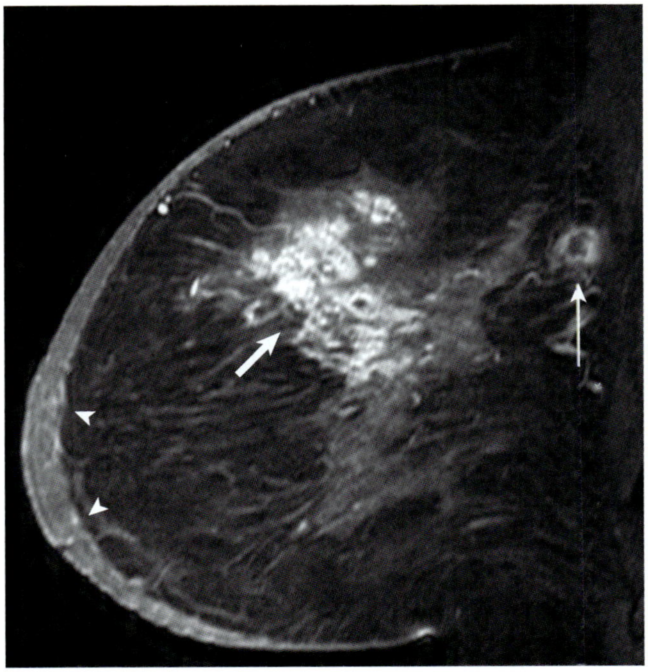

FIGURE 9.24 Fat-suppressed, sagittal, postcontrast, T1 image of a patient with clinically suspected inflammatory breast carcinoma. Primary IDC is identified as multiple, small, confluent, enhancing masses and nonmasslike enhancement in the superior breast (*large arrow*). Diffuse skin thickening and heterogenous skin enhancement are also present (*arrowheads*). A necrotic lymph node is also noted (*thin arrow*).

The primary malignancy involved with inflammatory carcinoma is most often invasive ductal carcinoma (84%) with poorly differentiated carcinoma (6%) and invasive lobular carcinoma (5%) found less often.[96] Multicentric or multifocal disease is more common than a unifocal mass. MRI findings typically consist of multiple masses or nonmasslike enhancement. Most commonly, MRI demonstrates multiple, small, irregularly shaped, heterogeneously enhancing masses, which are often confluent or interconnected by nonmasslike enhancement.[96] Nonmasslike enhancement is often diffuse, with heterogeneous or reticular dendritic enhancement, with a median size of 8 cm reported[30,31,96] (Figure 9.24). Rapid uptake and wash-out delayed kinetics are most often seen with both masses and nonmasslike enhancement.[96] Diffuse unilateral breast enlargement is more often described (68%) than diffuse breast retraction (14%).[96] Ipsilateral axillary lymphadenopathy is observed by MRI in more than 80% of cases.[95,97-99]

Additional MRI findings include those related to malignant involvement of the skin and breast edema. Breast edema is identified as high signal on fat-suppressed T2-weighted images. This can be subtyped into focal or peritumoral, cutaneous/subcutaneous, prepectoral, or intramuscular edema. Peritumoral edema occurring adjacent to the primary tumor is variably present in both inflammatory and noninflammatory breast carcinoma, while the other patterns of edema are more often seen with inflammatory carcinoma than with noninflammatory cancers. Diffuse edema appears as high T2 signal thickened strands throughout the breast parenchyma.[96] Prepectoral edema results from lymphatic obstruction of the retromammary lymphatic system, which runs along the prepectoral fascia, following penetrating vessels through the pectoral and intercostal muscles.[100] Diffuse, intramuscular, high T2 signal indicating chest wall edema may also be seen. Skin and subcutaneous edema results in skin thickening and high T2 signal in the subcutaneous fat (Figure 9.25). Skin thickening is defined as greater than 3 mm, which is best measured on non-fat-suppressed images (Figure 9.26). This is often diffuse and greatest in the periareolar region. Skin thickening is identified in 90% to 100% of cases of inflammatory breast cancer.[95-99,101] Skin enhancement is also often present, reported in 84% to 100% of cases. The enhancement is usually heterogenous and may consist of small (1-6 mm) enhancing nodular or irregular foci[96] (Figure 9.27; see Figure 9.24). It should be noted that varying edema patterns may also be present in acute mastitis, which may not be distinguishable from inflammatory carcinoma by imaging in the absence of an identifiable malignant tumor mass.

Paget Disease of the Breast

Paget disease in an uncommon form of breast cancer accounting for 1% to 3% of breast cancer cases.[102,103] It is characterized by infiltration of the nipple epidermis by large malignant adenocarcinoma cells, termed Paget cells, which contain abundant cytoplasm with enlarged pleomorphic and hyperchromatic nuclei. The disease typically arises with symptoms related to the nipple, such as itching, erythema, eczema, scaling, erosion, ulceration, nipple retraction, bloody nipple discharge, or any combination.[102] Underlying DCIS or invasive malignancy in the breast is reported in more than 90% of cases.[102,104,105] Three classifications for Paget disease have been described, including no underlying DCIS, associated with DCIS in the lactiferous ducts underlying the nipple-areolar complex, and associated with DCIS or invasive carcinoma located elsewhere in the breast, at least 2 cm from the nipple areolar complex.[106] The diagnosis is usually suspected on the basis of clinical findings, with the diagnostic gold standard being a full thickness surgical biopsy of the nipple and areola. Imaging is required to identify and characterize the extent of disease of an underlying malignancy. Mammography and ultrasound should be performed initially. However, imaging is normal in 22% to 50% of cases with mammography alone, and in 13% of cases in which both mammography and ultrasound are performed.[107-110]

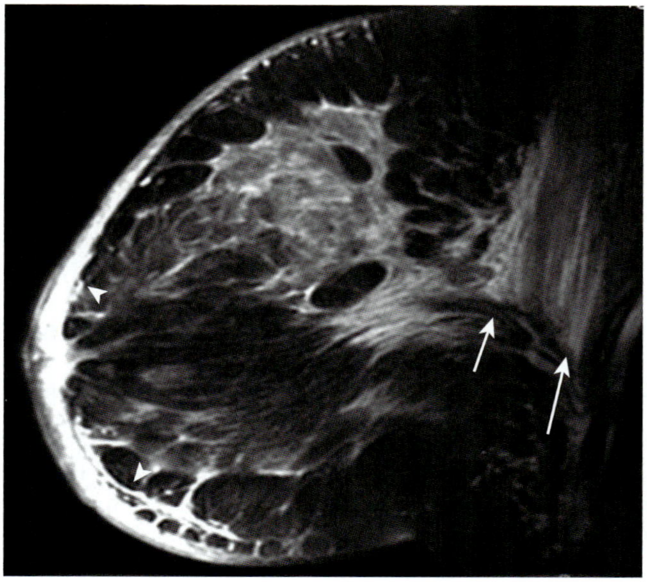

FIGURE 9.25 Sagittal, T2 image of a patient with inflammatory breast carcinoma demonstrates edema: cutaneous/subcutaneous (*arrowheads*), diffuse, prepectoral (*medium arrow*) and intramuscular (*long thin arrow*).

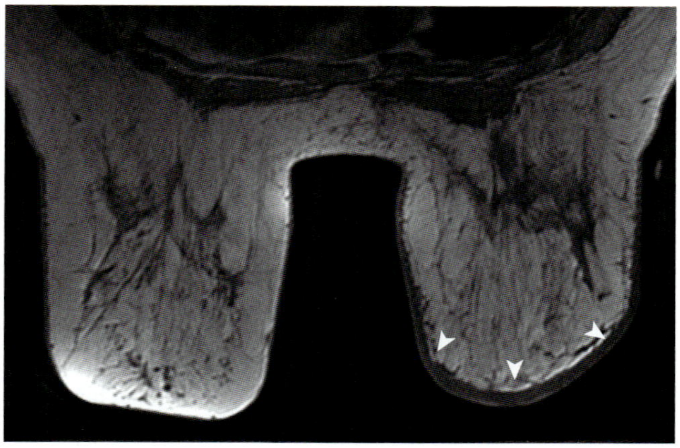

FIGURE 9.26 Axial, noncontrast, non-fat-suppressed, T1 image of the same patient as in Figure 9.25 with inflammatory breast carcinoma demonstrates diffuse skin thickening (*arrowheads*).

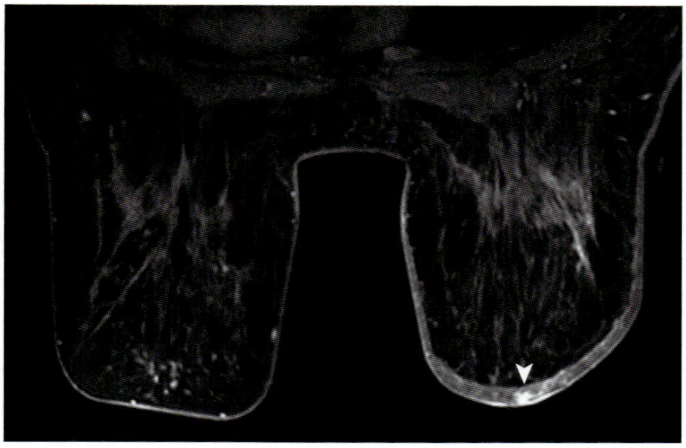

FIGURE 9.27 Axial, contrast-enhanced, fat-suppressed, T1 image of the same patient as in Figures 9.25 and 9-26 with inflammatory breast carcinoma demonstrates diffuse skin thickening and heterogeneous enhancement including small, focal, enhancing nodules (*arrowhead*).

Mammography also tends to underestimate the extent of disease in up to 43% of cases.[107,111] The addition of breast MRI in the preoperative evaluation of patients with Paget disease is useful for identifying and depicting the extent of disease of an underlying malignancy, especially when mammography and ultrasound are normal.[105]

Nipple enhancement, with or without thickening of the nipple-areolar complex, may be seen by MRI in Paget disease. Abnormal nipple enhancement is recognized by asymmetry. Normal enhancement of the nipples, although variable, should be bilaterally symmetric.[112,113]

MRI findings of an underlying malignancy include nonmasslike enhancement, typical of DCIS or an enhancing mass caused by invasive carcinoma. Defining the location and extent of disease is important, particularly for patients planning conservative therapy. Classically, mastectomy has been the standard treatment for Paget disease. However, because approximately two thirds of patients have tumor confined to the central breast, central lumpectomy involving complete resection of the nipple areolar complex followed by radiation therapy has been adopted more recently, with similar survival rates.[106,111,114-116] MRI helps determine the appropriate surgical approach by more accurately identifying when malignancy is present more than 2 cm from the nipple. It also identifies the presence of multifocal and multicentric malignancy, which has been reported in 41% and 43% of cases, respectively.[111] However, negative MRI scans do not reliably exclude the presence of underlying malignancy.[105]

Metastatic Breast Cancer with an Unknown Primary Malignancy

Breast cancer rarely presents as isolated metastatic axillary lymphadenopathy without a known primary tumor. When unilateral lymphadenopathy is identified, lymph node sampling with ultrasound guidance is indicated. When a malignant diagnosis suggestive of a breast primary is made with no identifiable tumor in the breast on clinical exam, mammography, or ultrasound, breast MRI should be the next step. In the case of negative lymph node sampling with no inflammatory explanation, surgical lymph node biopsy should be considered. Because of the rarity of this entity, only a few studies have reported the ability of MRI to identify the occult breast malignancy; it ranges from 62% to 86% of cases.[117,118] Often the primary tumors are found to be of less than 2 cm in size.[117] Identifying the primary tumor allows the patient the benefit of a histologic diagnosis to provide targeted chemotherapeutic and hormonal treatments, as well as breast conservation surgery. In cases in which no primary tumor is identified in the breast or elsewhere in the body, patients have traditionally been treated with mastectomy and axillary lymph node dissection. No primary tumor is still identified in the mastectomy specimen in one third of the cases after pathologic evaluation. However, a high percentage of patients were found to develop ipsilateral breast cancer when treated with axillary dissection alone.[119-121] More recently, some patients are being treated with axillary lymph node dissection and whole breast radiation rather than mastectomy. There are limited data regarding the efficacy of this treatment. However, many of these patients did not undergo breast MRI, and further study of the long-term outcomes of this treatment option with the addition of breast MRI is indicated.[119,122]

Evaluation of the Breast Cancer Patient with Positive Surgical Margins

When breast conservation surgery is performed for breast cancer and malignancy is found extending to the margins of the lumpectomy tissue specimen, tumors are considered to have positive surgical margins. This indicates that there may be residual malignancy remaining within the breast. These patients are typically treated with a repeat excision of the involved margins. Ultimately, if negative pathologic margins cannot be obtained, a mastectomy may be required. Positive surgical margins are reported to occur in 19% to 50% of patients.[123-125] Breast MRI is useful in these patients to guide the repeat surgical excision, as well as to prospectively identify patients with extensive residual disease who would ultimately require mastectomy. This is typically most useful in those patients who did not have a preoperative MRI. Granulation tissue at the lumpectomy bed often demonstrates enhancement. Thus MRI is not sensitive to detect minimal or microscopic disease at the surgical margin. In general, a relatively uniform and thin rim of enhancement surrounding a postoperative seroma is expected. The goal of MRI is to identify bulky residual malignancy at the lumpectomy site, as well as multifocal or multicentric disease elsewhere in the breast. Enhancing masses or linear areas of clumped nonmasslike enhancement radiating from the surgical bed may suggest residual invasive malignancy or DCIS (Figure 9.28). Sensitivities have been reported ranging from 61% to 86% for MRI in detecting residual malignancy.[126-128]

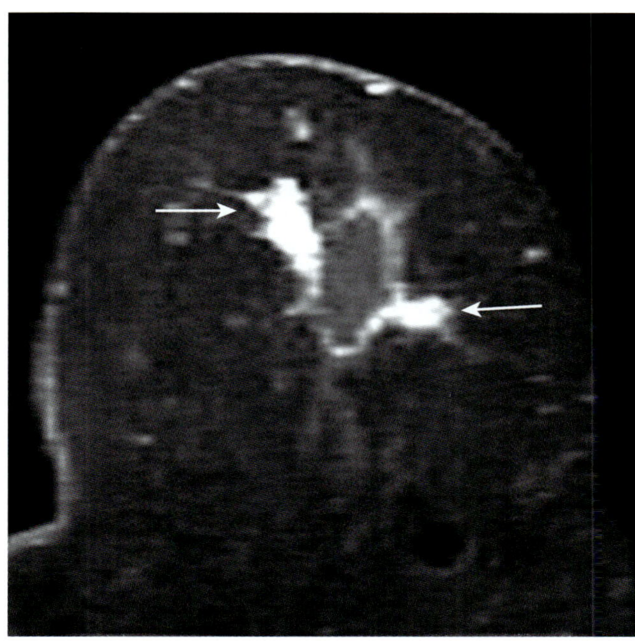

FIGURE 9.28 Reconstructed, axial, fat-suppressed, postcontrast, T1 image of a patient found to have positive surgical margins after lumpectomy for IDC. Two areas of bulky masslike enhancement present adjacent to the seroma cavity represent residual malignancy (*arrows*). Note the expected thin rim of enhancement surrounding the remainder of the fluid collection.

Evaluation of the Breast Cancer Patient Treated with Neoadjuvant Chemotherapy

Adjuvant systemic chemotherapy is used to decrease the risk of recurrence and improve survival from invasive breast carcinoma. The use of neoadjuvant chemotherapy (NACT) (chemotherapy prior to surgery for local regional control) has become more widely adopted. Although NACT is the current standard recommended treatment for locally advanced breast carcinoma (stage III B and C), it is also an option for operable stage II and III A disease.[129] Two large clinical trials with reported 16-year follow-up (NSABP 18 and 27) showed no statistically significant difference in relapse-free and overall survival between adjuvant and neoadjuvant treatment groups, although there was a trend in favor of the NACT group in women younger than 50 years of age. Change in the primary tumor size during NACT was positively associated with improved survival. Additionally, more women in the NACT group were able to achieve breast conservation.[130] Achieving negative axillary nodes after treatment and pathologic complete response (pCR; measured as no invasive tumor remaining in the breast at the time of surgery) clearly predicted favorable long-term outcomes. Using change in tumor size as a measure of tumor response is predictive of patient survival and clinically useful. This benefit, along with increased likelihood of successful breast conservation, has resulted in more widespread use of NACT in stage II and III A disease.

Breast MRI has been shown to better correlate with pathologic response after the completion of NACT versus conventional methods, with a wide range of reported accuracies: for clinical exam, 19% to 60%; for ultrasound, 35% to 75%; for mammography, 26% to 70%; and for MRI, 71% to 90%.[131-137] however, limitations of MRI are recognized. A recent meta-analysis, including 30 studies evaluating the accuracy of MRI to predict pathologic response, showed an overall combined sensitivity of 68% (57% to 77%) with a specificity of 91% (87% to 94%).[138] The limited sensitivity of MRI is due to underestimation of disease—that is, underestimation of residual tumor size or no tumor visible on MRI when residual disease is subsequently proved by pathology (Figures 9.29 and 9.30). Multiple studies have shown that the variable diagnostic accuracy of MRI is affected by both tumor biology and the chemotoxic effects on vascularity. Underestimation of residual disease has been particularly reported with invasive lobular carcinomas and DCIS.[133,135,139,141] This may be because of the low degree of angiogenesis often seen with these tumors, as well as the hard-to-detect infiltrative nature of lobular carcinomas.[133,141] Several studies have shown MRI to have better diagnostic accuracy for residual disease when assessing tumors with more aggressive biologies. These include tumors with high proliferation indices (Ki67 >40%); tumors expressing *HER2*/neu receptors (Her2+); and those expressing no estrogen, progesterone, or *HER2*/neu receptors (triple-negative or basal subtypes). These subtypes are more accurately evaluated with MRI for residual disease following NACT compared with MRI evaluation of luminal subtypes (*HER2*-negative/ER-positive).[142-147]

It has also been shown that the manner in which invasive tumors regress in response to NACT is variable. Some tumors exhibit a concentric decrease in size that results in

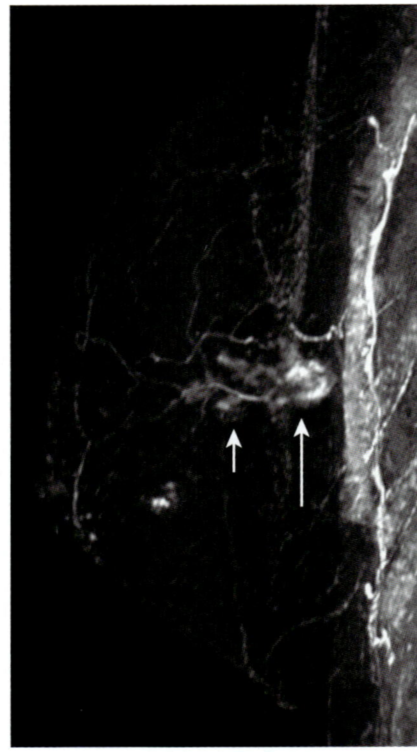

FIGURE 9.29 Sagittal MIP image of a patient with newly diagnosed IDC (*long arrow*). Occult DCIS was also identified by MRI (*short arrow*).

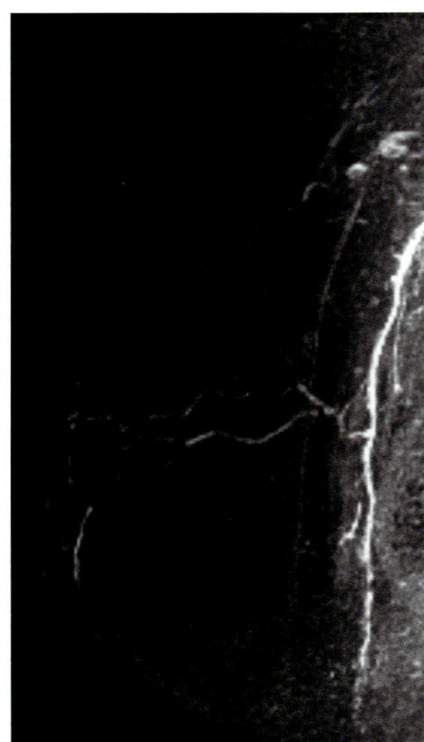

FIGURE 9.30 Same patient as in Figure 9.29 after completing NACT. No residual disease is visible on MRI. However, residual DCIS was present in the pathologic specimen.

better pathologic and MRI concordance. However, others demonstrate heterogeneous tumor regression, with residual tumor micronodules scattered in the tumor bed. This is not well demonstrated on MRI and may explain some of the false-negative MRI cases.[133,137,141,148] Additionally, medication effects may play a role in limiting the visualization of tumor vascularity, seen as enhancement on MRI. The antiangiogenic effect of tamoxifen has been implicated and high false-negative rates have also been seen in patients treated with the antiangiogenic medication bevacizumab (Avastin).[137,149]

Overestimation of disease by MRI, including overestimation of residual tumor size and the appearance of residual tumor on MRI but not identified in the pathologic specimen, occurs in approximately 5% of cases, much less frequently than underestimation.[133,141] Although the exact cause is not known, granulation tissue in the tumor bed has been implicated.[141] DWI has shown high sensitivity in the neoadjuvant setting. A meta-analysis of six studies showed an overall 93% (82% to 97%) sensitivity and 82% (70% to 90%) specificity for predicting the pathologic response after NACT using DWI alone.[138] Thus adding DWI to the current dynamic contrast-enhanced MRI techniques may improve diagnostic accuracy in the neoadjuvant setting.

Besides identifying residual disease following treatment, identifying which patients will respond to NACT early in their treatment course is also valuable. The use of MRI for this purpose is promising. Recently published results from the American College of Radiology Imaging Network's (ACRIN) multicenter trial (6657), titled the Investigation of Serial Studies to Predict Your Therapeutic Response with Imaging And moLecular Analysis (I-SPY TRIAL) showed the MRI measurements of tumor volume and longest tumor diameter to be superior to clinical exam for predicting pCR and in-breast residual cancer burden (pathologic index including tumor size and cancer cell density).[150] In these patients undergoing anthracycline-based NACT, changes in tumor volume showed the greatest predictive value for response after the first cycle of NACT. Scans performed following the first cycle of NACT carry the greatest opportunity for clinical impact. Early recognition of patients not responding to the NACT regimen allows treatment alterations to be made in a timely manner, sparing the patient exposure to ineffective and toxic therapy. The study found the highest predictive value for pCR after the completion of NACT to be obtained using a combination of clinical and MRI measurements. The study indicates that serial MRI exams combined with clinical exam offers high accuracy for monitoring treatment response (Figures 9.31 through 9.34). Additionally, an ongoing part of this trial is investigating single-voxel MR spectroscopy measurement of choline and tumor volume measurements as predictors of early treatment response.

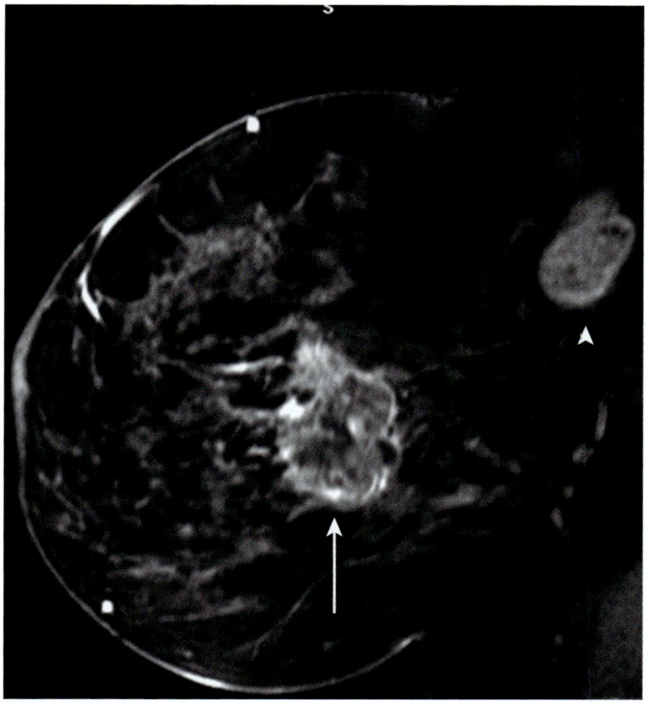

FIGURE 9.31 Sagittal, postcontrast, T1 image of a patient with newly diagnosed, high-grade IDC (*long arrow*) and axillary lymph node metastasis (*arrowhead*).

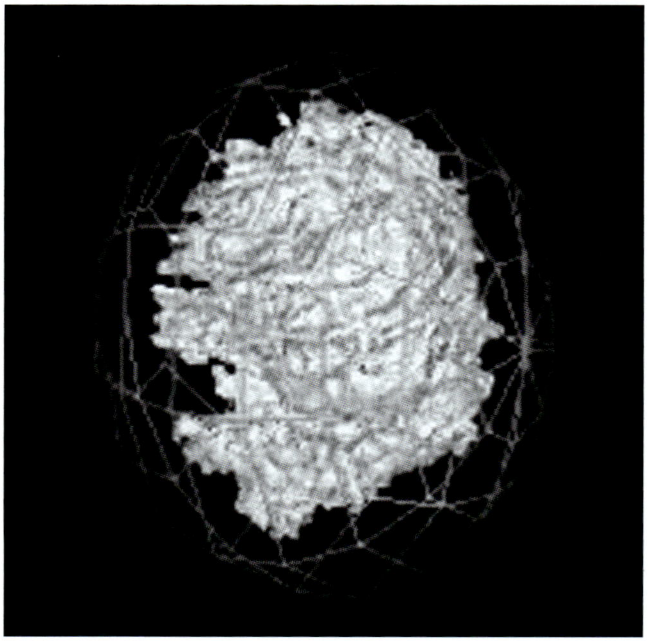

FIGURE 9.32 Volumetric measurement of the tumor mass (Figure 9.31) produced by the CAD system. Tumor volume is 64.6 cc.

Extramammary Findings on Breast MRI in the Patient with Breast Cancer

Although breast MRI is performed with a small field of view focusing on the breast and axilla, other structures, including portions of the lungs, mediastinum, chest wall, spine, and upper abdomen are also visible. The skeleton, lung, and liver are common sites for breast cancer metastases. Thus both incidental benign and metastatic lesions may be demonstrated. Extramammary lesions are best seen on axial postcontrast images. Vertebral fractures and lesions may also be evident on the sagittal localizing sequence; these are commonly overlooked.[151] Bone metastases appear low in signal on T1-weighted sequences and high in signal on T2-weighted sequences, and enhancement may be visualized. A recent retrospective review of 1535 breast MRI

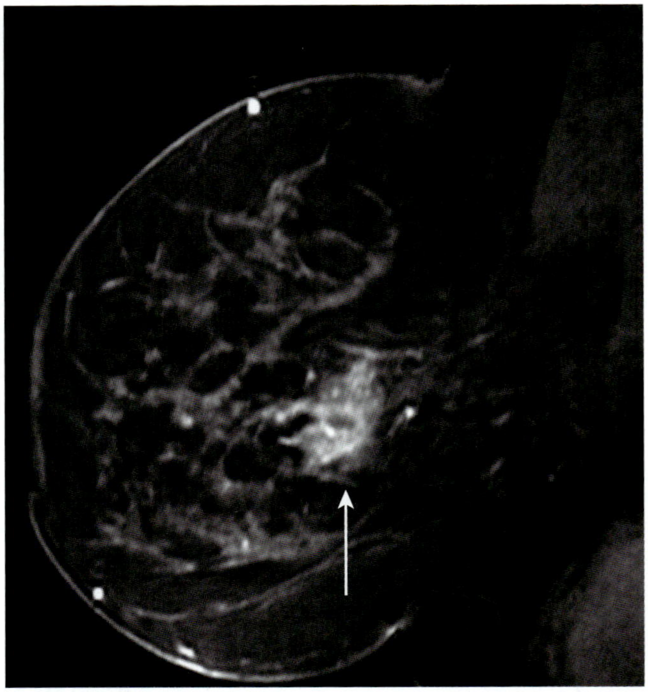

FIGURE 9.33 MRI scan from the same patient as in Figure 9.31 after completing NACT, showing that the tumor size has decreased.

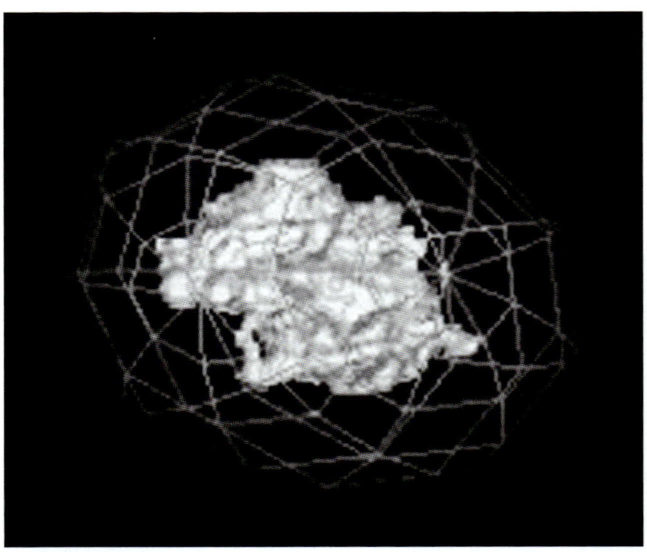

FIGURE 9.34 Volumetric measurement of the tumor mass (Figure 9.31) has decreased from 64.6 to 7.02 cc, indicating response to NACT.

studies identified incidental extramammary findings in 228 breast cancer patients. Most of these were located in the liver, followed by the lungs, bone, mediastinal lymph nodes, pleura, and pericardium.[152] In this study, PPVs for the MRI-detected lesions to represent metastases were as follows: for osseous lesions, 89%; for mediastinal lymph nodes of more than 1 cm in the short axis, 83%; for lung nodules, 59%. On the other hand, the PPV for metastases was low if the lesions were located in the liver (9%) or consisted of pleural or pericardial effusions (6%)[152] (Figures 9.35 through 9.38).

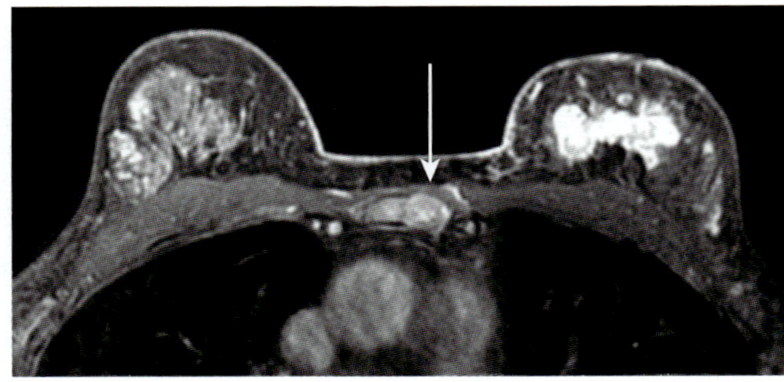

FIGURE 9.35 Delayed, postcontrast, fat-suppressed, axial image demonstrates an enhancing sternal mass (*arrow*) that was found to represent metastatic disease. This was first identified on a staging MRI in a patient with newly diagnosed breast cancer.

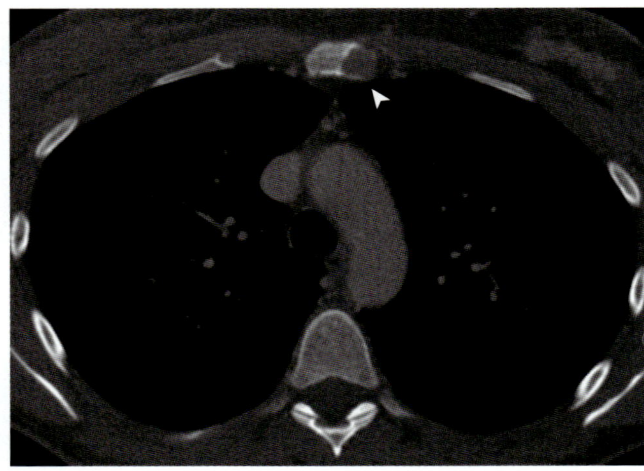

FIGURE 9.36 Bone algorithm chest computed tomography (CT) image in the same patient as in Figure 9.35 subsequently demonstrated the corresponding lytic osseous metastatic lesion.

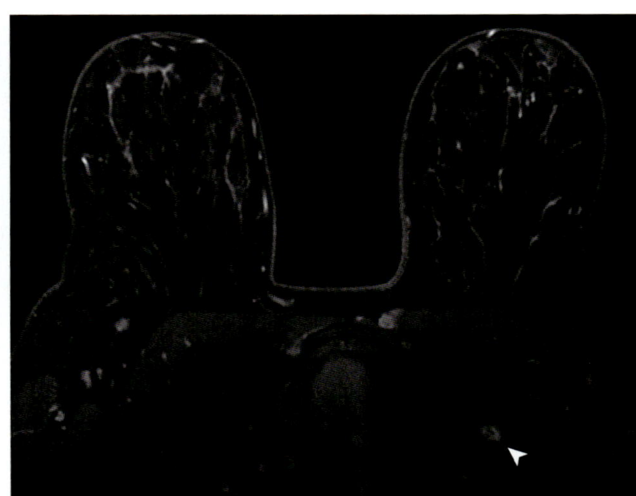

FIGURE 9.37 Enhancing lung nodule identified on a delayed axial postcontrast image (*arrowhead*).

Benign incidental pleural effusions are commonly identified on breast MRI. Benign pleural effusions were identified in 87% of 200 patients without breast cancer undergoing screening MRI. Both bilateral and unilateral effusions, with a normal reference range of up to 7 mm on the right and

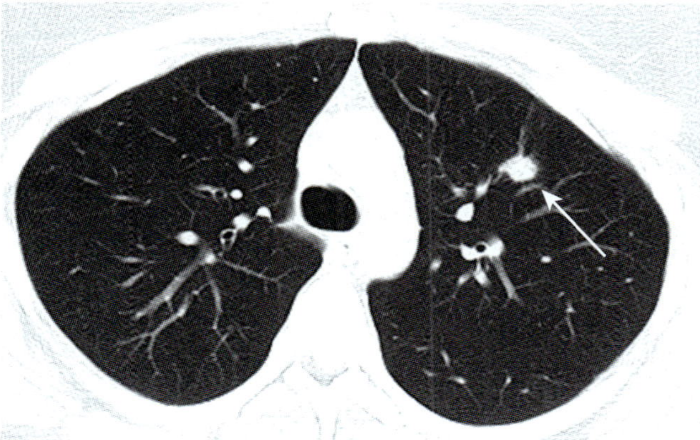

FIGURE 9.38 Subsequent axial CT in the same patient as in Figure 9.37 confirms a noncalcified lung nodule (*arrow*).

5 mm on the left, were identified.[153] Although specific studies have not been performed in patients with known breast cancer, Rinaldi and colleagues found 2 of 32 pleural/pericardial effusions among breast cancer patients to be malignant.[152] Findings that may increase suspicion for a malignant pleural effusion include the size of the effusion, circumferential or mediastinal pleural involvement, pleural nodularity, and pleural enhancement. It should be noted that pericardial or pleural fluid will layer anteriorly on breast MRI images because the patient is in the prone position.

When incidental extramammary lesions are identified on breast MRI in patients with breast cancer, further specific imaging studies are often required. Correlation with earlier images should always be performed to evaluate the stability of these findings before suggesting further imaging.

Benefits of Using Breast MRI in Patients with Breast Cancer

This chapter has reviewed MRI evaluation of the extent of disease in patients with newly diagnosed breast cancer. Breast MRI clearly provides benefit in some patients with breast cancer, particularly those whose primary breast tumor is unidentified. This includes patients with metastatic axillary lymphadenopathy, Paget disease of the nipple, and inflammatory breast carcinoma. Breast MRI is also useful for evaluating the extent of residual disease after NACT, and shows promise in predicting response to NACT early in the treatment cycle. It may also be useful for patients without a preoperative MRI found to have positive surgical margins after breast conservation surgery. The most common indication is evaluation of the extent of disease in patients with newly diagnosed breast cancer.

Breast MRI provides superior sensitivity and accuracy in evaluating the tumor burden in patients with newly diagnosed breast cancer. A large meta-analysis showed MRI to depict additional sites of occult malignancy in the ipsilateral breast in 20% of newly diagnosed patients and superior accuracy in depicting primary tumor size.[6,7,15] Thus preoperative MRI can be beneficial in planning surgical treatment for breast cancer with the following objectives: decreasing surgical reexcisions for positive margins, decreasing breast cancer recurrences, and prospectively identifying which patients should be treated with a mastectomy. The data to prove that MRI can meet these objectives are conflicting. Also, no survival benefit from preoperative MRI has been demonstrated.

The ability of MRI to decrease the occurrence of positive surgical margins and thus decrease reoperation rates was evaluated in one randomized controlled trial. The Comparative Effectiveness of MRI in Breast Cancer (COMICE) trial (n = 1623), reported in 2010, found no difference in reoperation rates with the addition of MRI in patients planning to undergo wide excision.[123] Re-excision rates were 19% for both the MRI and non-MRI groups. A criticism of this trial is that MRI-guided biopsy techniques were not widely available, so many women underwent mastectomy without pathologic verification of malignancy (28% of mastectomies in the MRI group). MRI-guided biopsy techniques were not widely available at the time of this trial, as is also true for earlier metaanalyses.[123,154] It is not known whether MRI would have performed better if the extent of disease was confirmed using currently available biopsy techniques. A smaller, more recent, study in which biopsies were performed to confirm malignant disease found a significant improvement in reoperation rates using preoperative breast MRI. In this retrospective study by Grady and colleagues (n = 184), patients in the MRI group had a lower reoperation rate of 11% versus 25% of those in the non-MRI group. Also, mastectomy rates among the MRI group were not increased.[125] Numerous studies have found significantly lower reoperation rates when using breast MRI in the preoperative evaluation of invasive lobular carcinomas.[41-44]

Given the improved sensitivity of breast MRI to detect occult sites of malignancy over mammography, an intended benefit is to prospectively select patients with multicentric malignancy for mastectomy. There has also been concern that the use of preoperative breast MRI would lead to an increase in mastectomy rates, which has not occurred.[155-157] It has not been shown that preoperative MRI results in unnecessary mastectomies. As discussed earlier, a large meta-analysis identified an appropriate change to mastectomy in 8.3% of patients, with an inappropriate change to mastectomy in only 1.7% of patients.[15] The rate of inappropriate mastectomies should decrease by obtaining biopsy confirmation of malignancy before changing treatment, which was not done in all of these studies. It has also been shown that patients are electing to undergo mastectomies independent of breast MRI. A retrospective study of 310 patients found that 44% of women younger than 50 years of age and 41% of those 50 years or older chose mastectomy, although they were given the option of breast conservation.[158] There is no clear explanation for this trend, although it may be related to patient anxiety.

Presumably, recognition of occult sites of malignancy in the breast by preoperative MRI would improve local control (decreasing breast cancer recurrences). However, retrospective studies evaluating local control rates by Solin and colleagues[159] (n = 756, 8-year follow-up) and Hwang[160] (n = 472, 4.5-year median follow-up) found no significant difference in 8-year local failure rates with or without MRI (Solin, 3% with MRI vs. 4% without; Hwang 2% with MRI vs. 3% without).[159,160] Alternatively, Fischer and colleagues[161] found a significant decrease in local recurrences using MRI (1%, n = 121) compared with local recurrences in patients without MRI (7%, n = 225; $P < .001$). However, this study is limited by a short median follow-up of only 3.4 years. The potential benefit for MRI to improve local control is expected to be low, given the already low recurrence rates of 5% to 10% at 10 years, using the standard treatment of whole breast radiation therapy following lumpectomy.[162,163] To show improvement in these already excellent results would require very long-term follow-up, which has not yet been evaluated. It is known that residual disease is often present in the breast, found in 20% to 63% of mastectomy specimens.[164-168] This residual disease is usually effectively treated by radiation therapy, given the current low recurrence rates. However, this may not be the case for patients who undergo partial breast irradiation, in which no more than one quadrant of the breast is treated. Additional sites of occult malignancy take on greater significance in these patients because radiation therapy cannot be relied upon as adjunctive treatment.[46-50]

References

1. Edge S, Byrd D, Compton, Fritz A, Greene F, Trotti A: *American Joint Committee on Cancer Staging manual*, ed 7, 2010, pp 347–376.
2. Berg WA, Gutierrez L, Nes Aiver MS, et al: Diagnostic accuracy of mammography, clinical examination, US, and MR imaging in preoperative assessment of breast cancer, *Radiology* 233:830–849, 2004.
3. Bassett LW, Dhaliwal SG, Eradat J, et al: National trends and practices in breast MRI, *AJR Am J Roentgenol* 191:332–339, 2008.
4. Fisher ER, Sass R, Fisher B: Pathologic findings from the National Surgical Adjuvant Project for Breast Cancers (protocol no. 4). X. Discriminants for tenth year treatment failure, *Cancer* 53 (suppl 3) 712–723, 1984.
5. Morrow M, Strom E, Bassett LW, et al: Standard for breast conservation therapy in the management of invasive breast carcinoma, *CA Cancer J Clin* 52:277–300, 2002.
6. VanGoethem M, Schelfout K, Kersschot E, et al: Enhancing area surrounding breast carcinoma on MR mammography: comparison with pathological examination, *Eur Radiol* 14:1363–1370, 2004.
7. Boetes C, Mus RD, Holland R, et al: Breast tumors: comparative accuracy of MR imaging relative to mammography and US for demonstrating extent, *Radiology* 197:743, 1995.
8. Blair S, Mcelroy M, Middleton M, et al: The efficacy of breast MRI in predicting breast conservation therapy, *J Surg Oncol* 94:220–225, 2006.
9. Kuhl CK, Schrading S, Bieling HB, et al: MRI for diagnosis of pure ductal carcinoma in situ: a prospective observational study, *Lancet* 370:435–492, 2007.
10. Onest JK, Mangus BE, Helmer SD, et al: Breast cancer tumor size: Correlation between magnetic resonance imaging and pathology measurements, *Am J Surg* 196:844–848, 2008 (discussion 849-850).
11. Bedrosian I, Mick R, Orel SG, et al: Changes in the surgical management of patients with breast carcinoma based on preoperative magnetic resonance imaging, *Cancer* 98:468–473, 2003.
12. Liberman L, Morris EA, Dershaw DD, et al: MR imaging of the ipsilateral breast in women with percutaneously proven breast cancer, *AJR Am J Roentgenol* 180:901–910, 2003.
13. Schelfout K, Van Goethem M, Kersschot E, et al: Contrast-enhanced MRI imaging of breast lesions and effect on treatment, *Eur J Surg Oncol* 30:501–507, 2004.
14. Schnall MD, Blume J, Bluemke DA, et al: MRI detection of distinct incidental cancer in women with primary breast cancer studied in IBMC 6883, *J Surg Oncol* 92:32–38, 2005.
15. Plana MN, Carreira C, Muriel A, et al: Magnetic resonance imaging in the preoperative assessment of patients with primary breast cancer: systematic review of diagnostic accuracy and meta-analysis, *Eur Rad* 22(1):26–38, 2012.
16. Bogner W, Gruber S, Pinker K, Grabner G, Stadlbauer A, Weber M, Moser E, Helbich TH, Trattnig S: Diffusion-weighted MR for differentiation of breast lesions at 3.0 T: how does selection of diffusion protocols affect diagnosis? *Radiology* 253:341–351, 2009.
17. Partridge SC, Mullins CD, Kurland BF, Allain MD, DeMartini WB, Eby PR, Lehman CD: Apparent diffusion coefficient values for discriminating benign and malignant breast MRI lesions: effects of lesion type and size, *AJR Am J Roentgenol* 194:1664–1673, 2010.
18. Ei Khouli RH, Jacobs MA, Mezban SD, Huang P, Kamel IR, Macura KJ, Bluemke DA: Diffusion-weighted imaging improves the diagnostic accuracy of conventional 3.0-T breast MR imaging, *Radiology* 256: 64–73, 2010.
19. Bartella L, Thakur SB, Morris EA, et al: Enhancing nonmass lesions in the breast: evaluation with proton (1H) MR spectroscopy, *Radiology* 245:80–87, 2007.
20. Bartella L, Morris EA, Dershaw DD, et al: Proton MR spectroscopy with choline peak as malignancy marker improves positive predictive value for breast cancer diagnosis: preliminary study, *Radiology* 239:686–692, 2006.
21. Rosen EL, Smith-Foley SA, DeMartini WB, et al: BI-RADS MRI enhancement characteristics of ductal carcinoma in situ, *Breast J* 13:545–550, 2007.
22. Obdeijin IM, Loo CE, Rijnsburger AJ, et al: Assessment of false-negative cases of breast MR imaging in women with familial or genetic predisposition, *Breast Cancer Res Treat* 119:399–407, 2010.
23. Morris EA: Diagnosis breast MR imaging: current status and future directions, *Radiol Clin North Am* 45:863–880, 2007.
24. Kuhl CK: The current status of breast MR imaging. Part 1. Choice of technique, image interpretation, diagnostic accuracy, and transfer to clinical practice, *Radiology* 244:356–378, 2007.
25. Harris JR, Lippman ME, Veronesi U, et al: Breast cancer, *N Engl J Med* 327:390–398, 1992.
26. Wolfe JN: Analysis of 462 breast carcinomas, *AJR Am J Roentgenol* 121:846–853, 1974.
27. Bassett LW, Pagani JJ, Gold RH: Pitfalls in mammography, *Radiology* 136:641–645, 1980.
28. Morris EA, Schwartz LH, Drotman MB, et al: Evaluation of pectoralis major muscle in patients with posterior breast tumors on breast MR images: Early experience, *Radiology* 214:67–72, 2000.
29. Kazama T, Nakamura S, Doi O, et al: Prospective evaluation of pectoralis muscle invasion of breast cancer by MR imaging, *Breast Cancer* 12:312–316, 2005.
30. Renz DM, Baltzer PA, Bottcher J, Thaher F, Gajda M, Camara O, et al: Inflammatory breast carcinoma in magnetic resonance imaging: a comparison with locally advanced breast cancer, *Acad Radiol* 15:209–221, 2008.
31. Girardi V, Carbognin G, Camera L, Bonetti F, Manfrin E, Pollini G, et al: Inflammatory breast carcinoma and locally advanced breast carcinoma: characterisation with MR imaging, *Radiol Med* 116:71–83, 2011.
32. Sakamoto N, Toazki M, Hoshi K, Fukuma E. Is MRI useful for the prediction of nipple involvement? *Breast Cancer*, published online February 7, 2012. Available at DOI 10.1007/s12282-012-0338-1. Accessed May 31, 2013.
33. Steen S, Chung A, Han S, et al: Predicting nipple-areolar involvement using preoperative breast MRI and primary tumor characteristics, *Ann Surg Oncol* 20:633–639, 2013.
34. Liberman L, Morris EA, Dershaw DD, Abramson AF, Tan LK: MR imaging of the ipsilateral breast in women with percutaneously proven breast cancer, *AJR Am J Roentgenol* 180:901–910, 2003.
35. Hlawatsch A, Teifke A, Schmidt M, Thelen M: Preoperative assessment of breast cancer: sonography versus MR imaging, *AJR Am J Roentgenol* 179:1493–1501, 2002.
36. Sardanelli F, Giuseppetti GM, Panizza P, et al: Sensitivity of MRI versus mammography for detecting foci of multifocal, multicentric breast cancer in fatty and dense breasts using the whole breast pathologic examination as a gold standard, *AJR Am J Roentgenol* 183:1149–1157, 2004.
37. Gutierrez R, DeMartini W, Silbergeld J, et al: High cancer yield and positive predictive value: outcomes at a center routinely using preoperative breast MRI for staging, *AJR Am J Roentgenol* 196:W93–W99, 2011.
38. Forrest W: *ARRS: Breast density may not influence need for preop MRI; Aunt Minnie Web site*. Available at www.auntminnie.com/index.aspx?sec=supsub=mri&pag=dis&ItemID=99244. May 4, 2012. Accessed November 5, 2012.
39. Krecke KN, Gisvold JJ: Invasive lobular carcinoma of the breast: mammographic findings and extent of disease at diagnosis in 184 patients, *AJR Am J Roentgenol* 161:957–960, 1993.
40. Mann RM, Hoogeveeri YL, Blickman JG, Boetes C: MRI compared to conventional diagnostic work-up in the detection and evaluation of invasive lobular carcinoma of the breast: a review of existing literature, *Breast Cancer Res Treat.* 107:1–14, 2008.
41. Rodenko GN, Harris SE, Prurieda JM, et al: MR imaging in the management before surgery of lobular carcinoma of the breast: correlation with pathology, *AJR Am J Roentgenol* 167:1415–1419, 1996.

42. Mann RM, Loo CE, Wobbes T, et al: The impact of preoperative breast MRI on the re-excision rate in invasive lobular carcinoma of the breast, *Breast Cancer Res Treat* 119:415–422, 2010.
43. McGhan LJ, Wasif N, Gray RJ, et al: Use of preoperative magnetic resonance imaging for invasive lobular cancer: good, better, but maybe not the best? *Ann Surg Oncol* 17:S255–S262, 2010.
44 Dillon MF, Hill AD, Fleming FJ, et al: Identifying patients at risk of compromised margins following breast conservation for lobular carcinoma, *Am Surg* 191:201–205, 2006. 17.
45. Smith BD, Arthur DW, Buchholz TA, et al: Accelerated partial breast irradiation consensus statement from the American Society for Radiation Oncology (ASTRO), *J Am Coll Surg* 209:269–277, 2009.
46. Al-Hallaq HA, Mell LK, Bradley JA, et al: Magnetic resonance imaging identifies multifocal and multicentric disease in breast cancer patients who are eligible for partial breast irradiation, *Cancer* 113:2408–2414, 2008.
47. Kowalchik K, Vallow L, McDonough M, et al: The role of preoperative bilateral breast magnetic resonance imaging in patient selection for partial breast irradiation in ductal carcinoma in situ, *Int J Surg Oncol* 1–6, 2012.
48. Tendulkar RD, Chellman-Jeffers M, Rybicki LA, et al: Preoperative breast magnetic resonance imaging in early breast cancer: implications for partial breast irradiation, *Cancer* 115:1621–1630, 2009.
49. Kühr M, Wolfgarten M, Stölzle M, et al: Potential impact of preoperative magnetic resonance imaging of the breast on patient selection for accelerated partial breast irradiation, *Int J Radiat Oncol Biol Phys* 81:e541–e546, 2011.
50. Godinez J, Gombos EC, Chikarmane SA, Griffin GK, Birdwell R: Breast MRI in the evaluation of eligibility for accelerated partial breast irradiation, *AJR Am J Roentgenol* 191:272–277, 2008.
51. Spear S, Hannan C, Willey S, Cocilovo C: *Nipple-sparing mastectomy. plastic & reconstructive surgery* 123(6):1665–1673, June 2009.
52. Smith J, Payne WS, Carney JA: Involvement of the nipple and areola in carcinoma of the breast, *Surg Gynecol Obstet* 143:546–548, 1976.
53. Lagios MD, Gates EA, Westdahl PR, Richards V, Alpert BS: A guide to the frequency of nipple involvement in breast cancer. A study of 149 consecutive mastectomies using a serial subgross and correlated radiographic technique, *Am J Surg* 138:135–142, 1979.
54. Vlajcic Z, Zic R, Stanec S, Lambasa S, Petrovecki M, Stanec Z: Nipple-areola complex preservation: predictive factors of neoplastic nipple-areola complex invasion, *Ann Plast Surg* 55:240–244, 2005.
55. Wertheim U, Ozzello L: Neoplastic involvement of nipple and skin flap in carcinoma of the breast, *Am J Surg Pathol* 4:543–549, 1980.
56. Morimoto T, Komaki K, Inui K, Umemoto A, Yamamoto H, Harada K, et al: Involvement of nipple and areola in early breast cancer, *Cancer* 15:2459–2463, 1985.
57. Luttges J, Kalbfleisch H, Prinz P: Nipple involvement and multicentricity in breast cancer. A study on whole organ sections, *J Cancer Res Clin Oncol* 113:481–487, 1987.
58. Santini D, Taffurelli M, Gelli MC, Grassigli A, Giosa F, Marrano D, et al: Neoplastic involvement of nipple-areolar complex in invasive breast cancer, *Am J Surg* 158:399–403, 1989.
59. Vyas JJ, Chinoy RF, Vaidya JS: Prediction of nipple and areola involvement in breast cancer, *Eur J Surg Oncol* 24:15–16, 1998.
60. Laronga C, Kemp B, Johnston D, Robb GL, Singletary SE: The incidence of occult nipple-areola complex involvement in breast cancer patients receiving a skin-sparing mastectomy, *Ann Surg Oncol* 6:609–613, 1999.
61. Maxwell G, Storm-Dickerson T, Whitworth P, Rubano C, Gariel A: Advances in nipple-sparing mastectomy: oncological safety and incision selection, *Aesthet Surg J* 31:310–319, 2011.
62. Sakamoto N, Fukuma E, Higa K, Ozaki S, Sakamoto M, Abe S, et al: Early results of an endoscopic nipple-sparing mastectomy for breast cancer, *Ann Surg Oncol* 16:3406–3413, 2009.
62a. D'Alonzo M, Martinchich L, Biglia N, et al. Clinical and radiological predictors of nipple-areola complex involvement in breast cancer patients, *Eur J Cancer* 2012;48:2311-2318.
63. Scaranelo AM, Eiada R, Jacks L, Kulkarni S, Crysta P: Accuracy of unenhanced MRI imaging in the detection of axillary lymph node metastasis: study of reproducibility and reliability, *Radiology* 262:425–434, 2011.
64. Mumataz H, Hall-Craggs MA, Davidson T, et al: Staging of symptomatic primary breast cancer with MRI imaging, *AJR Am J Roentgenol* 169:417–419, 1997.
65. Valente SA, Levine GM, Silver MJ, et al: Accuracy of predicting axillary lymph node positivity by physical examination, mammography, ultrasongraphy and magnetic resonance imaging, *Ann Surg Oncol* 19:1825–1830, 2012.
66. Fernandez AG, Fraile M, Gimenez N, et al: Use of axillary ultrasound, ultrasound-fine needle aspiration biopsy and magnetic resonance imaging in the preoperative triage of breast cancer patients considered for sentinel node biopsy, *Ultrasound Med. Biol.* 37:16–22, 2011.
67. Yoshimura G, Sakurai T, Oura S, et al: Evaluation of axillary lymph node status in breast cancer with MRI, *Breast Cancer* 6:249–258, 1999.
68. Harnan SE, Cooper KI, Meng Y, et al: Magnetic resonance for assessment of axillary lymph node status in early breast cancer: a systematic review and meta-analysis, *Eur J Surg Oncol* 37:928–939, 2011.
69. Mortellaro VE, Marshall J, Singer L, et al: Magnetic resonance imaging for axillary staging in patients with breast cancer, *J Magn Reson Imaging* 30:309–312, 2009.
70. Balzer PA, Dietzel M, Burmeister HP, et al: Application of MR mammography beyond local staging: is there a potential to accurately assess axillary lymph nodes? Evaluation of an extended protocol in an initial prospective study, *AJR Am J Roentgenol* 196:W641–W647, 2011.
71. Kinoshita T, Odagiri K, Andoh K, et al: Evaluation of small internal mammary lymph node metastases in breast cancer by MRI, *Radiat Med* 17:189–193, 1999.
72. Van der Ent FW, Kengen RA, van der Pol HA, Povel JA, Stroeken HJ, Hoofwijk AG: Halsted revisited: internal mammary sentinel lymph node biopsy in breast cancer, *Ann Surg* 234:79–84, 2001.
73. Estourgie SH, Tanis PJ, Nieweg OE, Valdes Olmos RA, Rutgers EJ, Kroon BB: Should the hunt for internal mammary chain sentinel nodes begin? An evaluation of 150 breast cancer patients, *Ann Surg Oncol* 10:935–941, 2003.
74. Farrus B, Vidal-Sicart S, Velasco M, Zanon G, Fernandez PL, Munoz M, et al: Incidence of internal mammary node metastases after a sentinel lymph node technique in breast cancer and its implication in the radiotherapy plan, *Int J Radiat Oncol Biol Phys* 60:715–721, 2004.
75. Leidenius MH, Krogerus LA, Toivonen TS, Leppanen EA, von Smitten KA: The clinical value of parasternal sentinel node biopsy in breast cancer, *Ann Surg Oncol* 13:321–326, 2006.
76. Madsen E, Gobardhan P, Bongers V, Albregts M, Burgmans J, De HP, et al: The impact on post-surgical treatment of sentinel lymph node biopsy of internal mammary lymph nodes in patients with breast cancer, *Ann Surg Oncol* 14:1486–1492, 2007.
77. Heuts EM, Van der Ent FWC, von Meyenfeldt MF, Voogd AC: Internal mammary lymph drainage and sentinel node biopsy in breast cancer e a study on 1008 patients, *Eur J Surg Oncol (EJSO)* 35(3):252–257, 2009.
78. Fornasa F, Nesoti MV, Bovo C, Bonavina MG: Diffusion-weighted magnetic resonance imaging in the characterization of axillary lymph nodes in patients with breast cancer, *J Magn Reson Imaging* 36:858–864, 2012.
79. Junping W, Tongguo S, Yunting Z, Chunshui Y, Renju B: Discrimination of axillary metastatic from nonmetastatic lymph nodes with PROPELLER diffusion-weighted MR imaging in a metastatic breast cancer model and its correlation with cellularity, *J Magn Reson Imaging* 36:624–631, 2012.
80. Park SH, Kim MJ, Park BW, Moon HJ, Kwak JY, Kim EK: Impact of preoperative ultrasonography and fine-needle aspiration of axillary lymph nodes on surgical management of primary breast cancer, *Ann Surg Oncol* 18:738–744, 2011.
81. Leenders MW, Broeders M, Croese C, et al: Ultrasound and fine needle aspiration cytology of axillary lymph nodes in breast cancer. To do or not to do? *Breast* 21:578–583, 2012.
82. Solon JG, Power C, Al-Azawi D, Duke D, Hill AD: Ultrasound-guided core biopsy: an effective method of detecting axillary nodal metastases, *J Am Coll Surg* 214:12–17, 2012.
83. Yi M, Giordano SH, Meric-Bernstam F, Mittendorf EA, Kuerer HM, Hwang RF, Bedrosian I, Rourke L, Hunt KK: Trends in and outcomes from sentinel lymph node biopsy (SLNB) alone vs. SLNB with axillary lymph node dissection for node-positive breast cancer patients: experience from the SEER database, *Ann Surg Oncol* Suppl 3(3):343–351, 2010.
84. Cody H, Houssami N: Axillary management in breast cancer: what's new for 2012? *The Breast* 21:411–415, 2012.
85. Nathanson DS: Ultrasound-Guided Core Needle biopsy of axillary lymph nodes in breast cancer, *J Am Coll Surg* 214:871–872, 2012.
86. Caudle AS, Hunt KK, Kuerer HM, Meric-Bernstam F, Lucci A, Bedrosian I, et al: Multidisciplinary considerations in the implementation of the findings from the American College of Surgeons Oncology Group (ACOSOG) Z0011 study: a practice-changing trial, *Ann Surg Oncol* 18:2407–2412, 2011.
87. Schwartz GF, Mansfield CM: Bilateral breast carcinoma: risk factors and outcomes for patients with synchronous and metachronous disease, *Cancer* 88:2739–2750, 2000.

88. Poggi MM, Danforth DN, Sciuto LC, et al: Eighteen-year results in the treatment of early breast carcinoma with mastectomy versus breast conservation therapy: the National Cancer Institute randomized trial, *Cancer* 98:697–702, 2003.
89. Samant RS, Olivotto IA, Jackson JS, Mates D: Diagnosis of metachronous contralateral breast cancer, *Breast J* 7:405–410, 2001.
90. Veronesi U, Cascinelli N, Mariani L, et al: Twenty-year follow-up of a randomized study comparing breast-conserving surgery with radical mastectomy for early breast cancer, *N Engl J Med* 347, 2002.
91. Lehman CD, Gatsonis C, Kuhl CK, et al: MRI evaluation of the contralateral breast in women with recently diagnosed breast cancer, *N Engl J Med* 356:1295–1303, 2007.
92. Brennan ME, Houssami N, Lord S, et al: Magnetic resonance imaging screening of the contralateral breast in women with newly diagnosed breast cancer: systematic review and meta-analysis of incremental cancer detection and impact on surgical management, *J Clin Oncol* 27:5640–5649, 2009.
93. Hance KW, Anderson WF, Devesa SS, Young HA, Levine PH: Trends in inflammatory breast carcinoma Incidence and survival: the surveillance, epidemiology, and end results program at the National Cancer Institute, *J Natl Cancer Inst* 97:966–975, 2005.
94. Dawood S, Merajver SD, Viens P, Vermeulen PB, Swain SM, Buchholz TA, et al: International expert panel on inflammatory breast cancer: consensus statement for standardized diagnosis and treatment, *Ann Oncol* 22:515–523, 2011.
95. Yang WT, Le-Petross HT, Macapinlac H, et al: Inflammatory breast cancer: PET/CT, MRI, mammography, and sonography findings, *Breast Cancer Res Treat* 109:417–426, 2008.
96. Le-Petross HT, Cristofanilli M, Carkaci S, et al: MRI features of inflammatory breast cancer, *AJR Am J Roentgenol* 197:W769–W776, 2011.
97. Chow CK: Imaging in inflammatory breast carcinoma, *Breast Dis* 22:45–54, 2005.
98. Belli P, Costantini M, Romani M, et al: Role of magnetic resonance imaging in inflammatory carcinoma of the breast, *Rays* 27:299–305, 2002.
99. Le-Petross HT, Charnsangavej C, Cristofanilli C, et al: *Inflammatory breast cancer (IBC): magnetic resonance imaging (MRI) characteristics at 1.5 and 3.0T*. Presented at the Annual Meeting of the Radiological Society of North America, 2007, November 26-30, Chicago, IL.
100. Takayoshi Uematsu: MRI findings of inflammatory breast cancer, locally advanced breast cancer, and acute mastitis: T2 weighted images can increase the specificity of inflammatory breast cancer, *Breast Cancer* 19:289–294, 2012.
101. Lee KW, Chung SY, Yang I, et al: Inflammatory breast cancer: imaging findings, *Clin Imaging* 29:22–25, 2005.
102. Ashikari R, Park K, Huvos AG, Urban JA: Paget's disease of the breast, *Cancer* 26:680–685, 1970.
103. Kollmorgen DR, Varanasi JS, Edge SB, Carson WE 3rd: Paget's disease of the breast: a 33-year experience, *J Am Coll Surg* 187:171–177, 1998.
104. Paone JF, Baker RR: Pathogenesis and treatment of Paget's disease of the breast, *Cancer* 48:825–829, 1981.
105. Morrogh M, Morris EA, Liberman L, Van Zee K, Cody HS 3rd, King TA: MRI identifies otherwise occult disease in select patients with Paget disease of the nipple, *J Am Coll Surg* 206:316–321, 2008.
106. Chen CY, Sun LM, Anderson BO: Paget disease of the breast: changing patterns of incidence, clinical presentation, and treatment in the U.S, *Cancer* 107:1448–1458, 2006.
107. Ikeda DM, Helvie MA, Frank TS, Chapel KL, Andersson IT: Paget disease of the nipple: radiologic-pathologic correlation, *Radiology* 189:89–94, 1993.
108. Sawyer RH, Asbury DL: Mammographic appearances in Paget's disease of the breast, *Clin Radiol* 49:185–188, 1994.
109. Ceccherini AF, Evans AJ, Pinder SE, Wilson AR, Ellis IO, Yeoman LJ: Is ipsilateral mammography worthwhile in Paget's disease of the breast? *Clin Radiol* 51:35–38, 1996.
110. Günhan-Bilgen I, Oktay A: Paget's disease of the breast: clinical, mammographic, sonographic and pathologic findings in 52 cases, *Eur J Radiol* 60:256–263, 2006.
111. Kothari AS, Beechey-Newman N, Hamed H, et al: Paget disease of the nipple: a multifocal manifestation of higher-risk disease, *Cancer* 95:1–7, 2002.
112. Friedman EP, Hall-Craggs MA, Mumtaz H, Schneidau A: Breast MR and the appearance of the normal and abnormal nipple, *Clin Radiol* 52:854–861, 1997.
113. Da Costa D, Taddese A, Cure ML, Gerson D, Poppiti R Jr, Esserman LE: Common and unusual diseases of the nipple-areolar complex, *RadioGraphics* 27(spec no):S65–S77, 2007.
114. Pierce LJ, Haffty BG, Solin LJ, et al: The conservative management of Paget's disease of the breast with radiotherapy, *Cancer* 80:1065–1072, 1997.
115. Bijker N, Rutgers EJ, Duchateau L, Peterse JL, Julien JP, Cataliotti L: Breast-conserving therapy for Paget disease of the nipple: a prospective European Organization for Research and Treatment of Cancer study of 61 patients, *Cancer* 91:472–477, 2001.
116. Dalberg K, Hellborg H, Wärnberg F: Paget's disease of the nipple in a population based cohort, *Breast Cancer Res Treat* 111:313–319, 2008.
117. Orel SG, Weinstein SP, Schnall MD, et al: Breast MR imaging in patients with axillary node metastases and unknown primary malignancy, *Radiology* 212:543–549, 1999.
118. Buchanan CL, Morris EA, Doru PL, et al: Utility of breast magnetic resonance imaging in patients with occult primary breast cancer, *Am Surg Oncol* 12:1045–1053, 2005.
119. Vlastos G, Mrina JE, Attiqa N, et al: Feasibility of breast preservation in the treatment of occult primary carcinoma presenting with axillary metastases, *Ann Surg Oncol* 8:425–431, 2001.
120. Abbruzzese JL, Abbruzzese MC, Hess KR, et al: Unknown primary carcinoma: natural history and prognostic factors in 657 consecutive patients, *J Clin Oncol* 12:1272–1280, 1994.
121. Hainsworth JD, Greco AF: Treatment of patients with cancer of an unknown primary site, *N Engl J Med* 329:257–263, 1993.
122. Masinghe SP, Faluyi OO, Kerr GR, Kunkler IH: Breast radiotherapy for occult breast cancer with axillary nodal metastases-does it reduce the local recurrence rate and increase overall survival? *Clin Oncol (R Coll Radiol)* 23:95–100, 2011.
123. Turnbull L, Brown S, Harvey L, et al: Comparative effectiveness of MRI in breast cancer (COMICE) trial: a randomized controlled trial, *Lancet* 375:563–571, 2010.
124. Dillon MF, Hill AD, Fleming FJ, et al: Identifying patients at risk of compromised margins following breast conservation for lobular carcinoma, *Am J Surg* 191:201–205, 2006.
125. Grady I, Gorsuch-Rafferty H, Hadley P: Preoperative staging with magnetic resonance imaging, with confirmatory biopsy, improves surgical outcomes in women with breast cancer without increasing rates of mastectomy, *Breast J* 18:214–218, 2012.
126. Frei KA, Kinkel K, Bonel HM, et al: MR imaging of the breast in patients with positive margins after lumpectomy: Influence of the time interval between lumpectomy and MR imaging, *AJR Am J Roentgenol* 175:1577–1584, 2000.
127. Orel SG, Reynolds C, Schnall MD, et al: Breast carcinoma MR imaging before re-excisional biopsy, *Radiology* 205:429–439, 1997.
128. Lee JM, Orel SG, Czerniecki BJ, et al: MRI before re-excision surgery in patients with breast cancer, *AJR Am J Roentgenol* 182:473–480, 2004.
129. Kaufmann M, von Minckwitz G, Bear HD, et al: Recommendations from an international expert panel on the use of neoadjuvant (primary) systemic treatment of operable breast cancer: new perspectives 2006, *Ann Oncol* 18:1927–1934, 2007.
130. Rastogi P, Anderson SJ, Bear HD, et al: Preoperative chemotherapy: updates of National Surgical Adjuvant Breast and Bowel Project Protocols B-18 and B-27, *J Clin Oncol* 26:778–785, 2008.
131. Akazawa K, Tamaki Y, Taguchi T, et al: Preoperative evaluation of residual tumor extent by three-dimensional magnetic resonance imaging in breast cancer patients treated with neoadjuvant chemotherapy, *Breast J* 12:130–137, 2006.
132. Segara D, Krop IE, Garber JE, et al: Does MRI predict pathologic tumor response in women with breast cancer undergoing preoperative chemotherapy? *J Surg Oncol* 96:474–480, 2007.
133. Yeh E, Slanetz P, Kopans D, et al: Prospective comparison of mammography, sonography and MRI in patients undergoing neoadjuvant chemotherapy for palpable breast cancer, *AJR Am J Roentgenol* 184:868–877, 2005.
134. Partridge S, Gibbs J, Yin L, et al: Accuracy of MR imaging for revealing residual breast cancer in patients who have undergone neoadjuvant chemotherapy, *AJR Am J Roentgenol* 179:1193–1199, 2002.
135. Belli P, Consantini M, Malaspina C, et al: MRI accuracy in residual disease evaluation in breast cancer patients treated with neoadjuvant chemotherapy, *Clin Rad* 61:946–953, 2006.

136. Chagpar AB, Middleton LP, Sahin AA, et al: Accuracy of physical examination, ultrasonography, and mammography in predicting residual pathologic tumor size in patients treated with neoadjuvant chemotherapy, *Ann Surg* 243:257–264, 2006.
137. Chen JH, Feig B, Agrawal G, et al: MRI evaluation of pathologically complete response and residual tumors in breast cancer after neoadjuvant chemotherapy, *Cancer* 112:17–26, 2008.
138. Wu L, Hu J, Gu H, et al: Can diffusion-weighted MR imaging and contrast-enhanced MRI imaging precisely evaluate and predict pathological response to neoadjuvant chemotherapy in patients with breast cancer? *Breast Cancer Res Treat* 135:17–28, 2012.
139. Londero V, Bazzocchi M, Del Frate C, et al: Locally advanced breast cancer: comparison of mammography, sonography and MR imaging in evaluation of residual disease in women receiving neoadjuvant chemotherapy, *Eur Radiol* 14:1371–1379, 2004.
140. Rieber A, Brambs HJ, Gabelmann A, Heilmann V, Kreienberg R, Kuhn T: Breast MRI for monitoring response of primary breast cancer to neo-adjuvant chemotherapy, *Eur Radiol* 12:1711–1719, 2002.
141. Woodhams R, Kakita S, Hata H, et al: Identification of residual breast carcinoma following neoadjuvant chemotherapy: diffusion-weighted imaging—comparison with contrast-enhanced MR imaging and pathologic findings, *Radiology* 254:357–366, 2010.
142. Chen JH, Bahri S, Mehta RS, et al: Breast cancer: evaluation of response to neoadjuvant chemotherapy with 3.0-T MR imaging, *Radiology* 261:735–743, 2011.
143. Gomez-Raposo C, Andreu M, Suarez-Garcia I, et al: Relevance of breast cancer subtypes for magnetic resonance imaging response monitoring during neoadjuvant chemotherapy, *Clin Transl Oncol* 14: 486–488, 2012.
144. Kuzucan A, Chen JH, Bahri S, et al: Diagnostic performance of magnetic resonance imaging for assessing tumor response in patients with HER2-negative breast cancer receiving neoadjuvant chemotherapy is associated with molecular biomarker profile, *Clin Breast Cancer* 12:110–118, 2012.
145. McGuire KP, Toro-Burguete J, Dang H, et al: MRI staging after neoadjuvant chemotherapy for breast cancer: does tumor biology affect accuracy? *Ann Surg Oncol* 18:3149–3154, 2011.
146. Nakahara H, Yasuda Y, Machida Y, et al: MR and US for breast cancer patients who underwent conservation surgery after neoadjuvant chemotherapy: comparison of triple negative breast cancer and other intrinsic subtypes, *Breast Cancer* 18:152–160, 2011.
147. Loo CE, Straver ME, Rodenhuis S, et al: Magnetic resonance imaging response monitoring of breast cancer during neoadjuvant chemotherapy: relevance of breast cancer subtype, *J Clin Oncol* 29:660–666, 2011.
148. Kim TH, Kang DK, Yim H, et al: Magnetic resonance imaging patterns of tumor regression after neoadjuvant chemotherapy in breast cancer patients: correlation with pathological response grading system based on tumor cellularity, *J Comput Assist Tomogr* 36:200–206, 2010.
149. Marson LP, Kurian KM, Miller WR, Dixon JM: The effect of tamoxifen on breast tumor vascularity, *Breast Cancer Res Treat* 66:9–15, 2001.
150. Hylton N Blume J, Bernreuter W, et al: Locally advanced breast cancer: MR imaging for prediction of response to neoadjuvant chemotherapy—results from ACRIN 6657/I-SPY Trial, *Radiology* 263:-663–672, 2010.
151. Bazzocchi A, Spinnato P, Garzillo G, et al: Detection of incidental vertebral fractures in breast imaging: the potential role of MR localisers, *Eur Radiol* 22:2617–2623, 2012.
152. Rinaldi P, Costantini M, Belli P, et al: Extra-mammary findings in breast MRI, *Eur Radiol* 21:2268–2276, 2011.
153. Nguyen J, Nicholson BT, Patrie JT, Harvey JA: Incidental pleural effusions detected on screening breast MRI, *AJR Am J Roentgenol* 199:W142–W145, 2012.
154. Morris EA: Should we dispense with preoperative breast MRI? *Lancet* 375:528–530, 2010.
155. Angarita FA, Acuna SA, Fonseca A, et al: Impact of preoperative breast MRIs on timing of surgery and type of intervention in newly diagnosed breast cancer patients, *Ann Surg Oncol* 17:S273–S279, 2010.
156. Lim HI, Choi JH, Yang JH, et al: Does pre-operative breast magnetic resonance imaging in addition to mammography and breast ultrasonography change the operative management of breast carcinoma? *Breast Cancer Res Treat* 119:163–167, 2010.
157. Carpenter SG, Stucky CC, Dueck AC, et al: Scientific Presentation Award: The impact of magnetic resonance imaging on surgical treatment of invasive breast cancer, *Am J Surg* 198:475–481, 2009.
158. Fisher CS, et al: Fear of recurrence and perceived survival benefit are primary motivators for choosing mastectomy over breast-conservation therapy regardless of age, *Ann Surg Oncol* 19:3246–3250, 2012.
159. Solin LJ, Orel SG, Hwang WT, et al: Relationship of breast magnetic resonance imaging to outcome after breast-conservation treatment with radiation for women with early-stage invasive breast carcinoma or ductal carcinoma in situ, *J Clin Oncol* 26:386–391, 2008.
160. Hwang N, Schiller DE, Crystal P, et al: Magnetic resonance imaging in the planning of initial lumpectomy for invasive breast carcinoma: its effect on ipsilateral breast tumor recurrence after breast-conservation therapy, *Ann Surg Oncol* 16:3000–3009, 2009.
161. Fischer U, Zachariae O, Baum F, et al: The influence of preoperative MRI of the breasts on recurrence rate in patients with breast cancer, *Eur Radiol* 14:1725–1731, 2004.
162. Recht A, Solin LJ: Breast-conserving surgery and radiotherapy in early stage breast cancer: the importance of local control, *Semin Radiat Oncol* 21:3–9, 2011.
163. Clarke M, Collins R, Darby S, et al: Effects of radiotherapy and of differences in the extent of surgery for early breast cancer on local recurrence and 15-year survival: an overview of the randomized trials, *Lancet* 366:2087–2106, 2005.
164. Rosen PP, Fracchia AA, Urban JA, et al: "Residual" mammary carcinoma following simulated partial mastectomy, *Cancer* 35:739–747, 1975.
165. Lagios MD: Multicentricity of breast carcinoma demonstrated by routine correlated serial subgross and radiographic examination, *Cancer* 40:1726–1734, 1977.
166. Holland R, Veling SH, Mravunac M, et al: Histologic multifocality of Tis, T1-2 breast carcinomas: implications for clinical trials of breast conserving surgery, *Cancer* 56:979–990, 1985.
167. Anastassiades O, Iakovou E, Stavridou N, et al: Multicentricity in breast cancer. A study of 366 cases, *Am J Clin Pathol* 99:238–243, 1993.
168. Vaidya J, Vyas J, Chinoy R, et al: Multicentricity of breast cancer: Whole-organ analysis and clinical implications, *Br J Cancer* 74:820–824, 1996.

CHAPTER 10

MRI of the Postoperative Breast

Patricia Poole
Haydee Ojeda-Fournier

The breast undergoes significant anatomic and histologic changes after intervention. Posttreatment imaging findings have been thoroughly described for mammography and breast ultrasound,[1-6] but only isolated descriptions of postsurgical breast changes seen on dynamic contrast enhanced (DCE) breast magnetic resonance imaging (MRI) are found in the literature.[7-9] New or recurrent cancer can be difficult to detect in the postsurgical breast by physical examination, breast ultrasound, and mammography. DCE breast MRI has emerged as an important adjunct study in the evaluation of the breast in postsurgical patients. Therefore it is critical for radiologists to understand the common surgical procedures performed on the breast and to be able to recognize their expected appearance on DCE breast MRI.

Understanding which findings are usual in the postsurgical and postradiation setting is of utmost importance in distinguishing between suspicious findings and expected changes after intervention. In addition to high risk screening and evaluation of extent of disease, the American College of Radiology practice guidelines included additional evaluation of clinical or imaging findings.[10] Many of the patients referred to DCE breast MRI have had previous breast interventions. Although DCE breast MRI postsurgical findings can have similar morphologic appearance to those seen with mammography and ultrasound, there are also postprocedural changes specific to breast MRI.

Drawing on our experience as well as a thorough literature review, we wrote this chapter to catalog the most common changes attributable to prior breast surgical intervention, including image-guided biopsy, lumpectomy, radiation, mastectomy, and reconstructive and cosmetic surgery as well as other regional surgical changes.

Our Experience

After obtaining Institutional Review Board approval, we reviewed 719 breast MRIs performed between July 1, 2008, and June 30, 2009. The cohort of patient underwent breast MRI at the University of California San Diego department of radiology, an academic center with a breast MRI volume of more than 700 patients annually. Of the 719 patients imaged, 881 breasts on 590 patients (82%) had undergone earlier surgical or image-guided procedures. We identified patients who had undergone prior core biopsy, excisional biopsy, lumpectomy, mastectomy, breast reconstruction, breast reduction, breast implants, and nodal dissection. Using these data, we identified the most common postoperative changes seen on DCE breast MRI. Breast MRI changes observed included susceptibility artifacts, skin thickening, architectural distortion, implant-related changes, postoperative fluid collection, skin enhancement, skin retraction, scar progression, edema, fat necrosis, nipple retraction, hematoma, hemosiderin deposition, and chest wall changes (Table 10.1).

Image-Guided Interventions

The paradigm of breast cancer diagnosis has changed from radical surgeries to minimally invasive procedures. In the United States, about 1.6 million biopsies of breast tissue are performed every year; of these 75% will be benign.[11,12] Minimally invasive procedures for tissue diagnosis are performed using devices including spring-loaded and vacuum-assisted devices of varying gauges. Stereotactic, ultrasound, and MRI-guided large-core (>14-gauge) biopsies have reduced the number of surgical biopsies and are indicated for histologic tissue diagnosis of palpable findings and/or imaging abnormalities.[12] Most image-guided core biopsies are performed parallel to the chest wall, to prevent intrathoracic injury. A tissue marker should be left in place to document the location of the procedure.

Although minimally invasive, these procedures disrupt the breast tissue, resulting in imaging findings easily identified on breast MRI. Depending on how recently the procedure was performed, the biopsy tract may be visualized by MRI. Figure 10.1 demonstrates a biopsy tract adjacent to an area of nonmasslike enhancement, diagnosed as invasive ductal carcinoma.

Tissue Markers

As mentioned, a tissue marker is routinely placed after core biopsy. Susceptibility artifacts of varying degrees may be noted and are typically more pronounced at higher field strengths (3 Tesla [T] vs. 1.5 T) and on T1-weighted sequences. Depending on the marker composition, identifying the marker may be challenging. Tissue markers are

Table 10.1 Percentage of Postoperative Changes Identified on Review of 881 Breasts on 590 Patients Who Underwent Breast MRI

Finding	Total	Percent
Susceptibility artifact	321	36.44%
Skin thickening	70	7.95%
Architectural distortion	61	6.92%
Seroma	61	6.92%
Implants	39	4.43%
Edema	13	1.48%
Chest wall changes	12	1.36%
Fat necrosis	12	1.36%
Hematoma	11	1.25%
Skin retraction	9	1.02%
Nipple retraction	8	0.91%
Hemosiderin	4	0.45%
Skin enhancement	3	0.34%
Scar progression	2	0.23%
"Benign postprocedural"	405	45.97%

Note. This study was done in an academic facility with interpreter variability in reporting of visualized findings. This is reflected in the large number of patients (45.7%) with reported "benign postoperative changes" with no further specific description. In cases in which "benign postoperative changes" were reported, the phrase was noted to be directly dependent on a single interpreting radiologist. Therefore despite this large percentage, our experience accurately catalogs the most common changes attributable to prior breast surgical intervention.

often best identified on the non–fat-saturated T1-weighted sequence, as seen in Figure 10.2. Magnetic susceptibility is discussed further under the postsurgical findings of hemosiderin and metal.

Seroma/Hematoma

Seromas or hematomas are less common and usually less prominent by minimally invasive image-guided intervention than by surgical intervention. However, even large hematomas can be caused by image-guided interventions, as seen in Figure 10.3. In this case, a delayed hematoma developed after stereotactic biopsy in a patient who was feeling well enough to exercise after the biopsy procedure. The stereotactic biopsy was positive for minimal ductal carcinoma in situ (DCIS). The hematoma, which had not been present immediately after stereotactic biopsy, was identified at the time of preoperative MRI to assess the extent of disease. Because seroma/hematoma findings are identical in both image-guided and surgical procedures, they are discussed further in the postlumpectomy findings in the next section.

Surgical Interventions

Lumpectomy

Lumpectomy is the most common form of breast cancer surgery and consists of removal of the tumor and immediate surrounding tissue. Randomized clinical trials have shown that breast conservation surgery with lumpectomy plus radiation therapy will yield the same disease-free and overall survival rates as mastectomy.[13] However, after lumpectomy only, positive margins are present in the breast in 32% to 63% of patients[14] and MRI is the primary imaging modality to evaluate for residual or recurrent tumor in the postoperative breast.

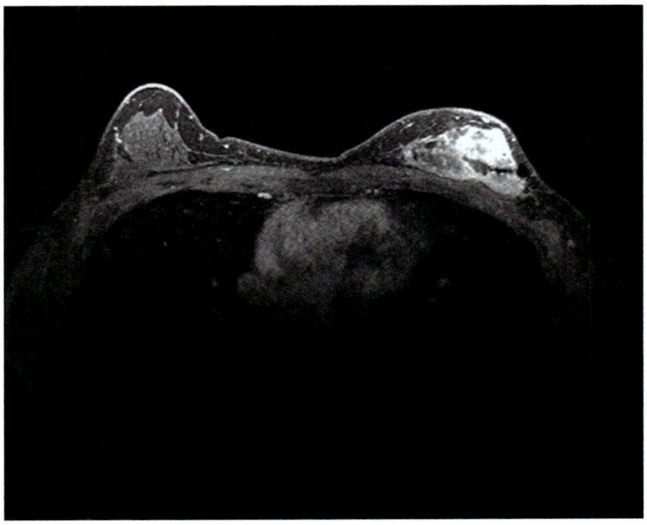

FIGURE 10.1 A tract from a minimally invasive image-guided core biopsy is shown in a T1-weighted fat-saturated postcontrast image demonstrates extensive nonmasslike enhancement resulting from invasive ductal carcinoma. A hemosiderin tract is seen laterally in the posterior third of the left breast at the site of biopsy.

Although it is not always possible to differentiate postsurgical changes from recurrent or residual tumor on MRI, it is crucial for the interpreting physician to be familiar with the imaging findings related to surgery, to distinguish them from tumor, and refrain from unnecessary intervention.

As with mammography, postsurgical changes identified at MRI are expected. These include enhancement of the postoperative seroma rim, architectural distortion, skin thickening, and retraction. Most of these changes diminish over time. In the case of positive surgical margins following breast conserving surgery, MRI can be beneficial in identifying clumped or masslike enhancement. This information can aid the surgeon in directing the region of reexcision.

Fat Necrosis

Fat necrosis results from a vascular injury to fat cells within the breast and can be seen with any trauma to the breast, including invasive procedures such as needle or surgical biopsy, lumpectomy, mastectomy, reconstructive surgery, and radiation therapy to the breast.[15] The imaging findings of fat necrosis have been well described in multiple modalities.[16-18] Similar to other imaging modalities, the appearance on MRI can be variable, including oil cysts, architectural distortion, or a spiculated mass. Figure 10.4 demonstrates the classic appearance of fat necrosis by mammography and by DCE breast MRI. The most common MRI appearance is a round or oval mass with hyperintense T1-weighted signal that saturates on fat-saturated images and is compatible with a lipid cyst.[15] Oil cysts may contain internal fat-fluid levels. Identifying central T1 hyperintensity on non–fat-saturated images helps confirm the diagnosis of fat necrosis. Fat necrosis will calcify over time, and therefore comparison with mammograms is often helpful in evaluating suspected fat necrosis and required for accurate interpretation of breast MRI. Overall, the MRI signal characteristics of fat necrosis typically follow that of fat elsewhere in the breast.

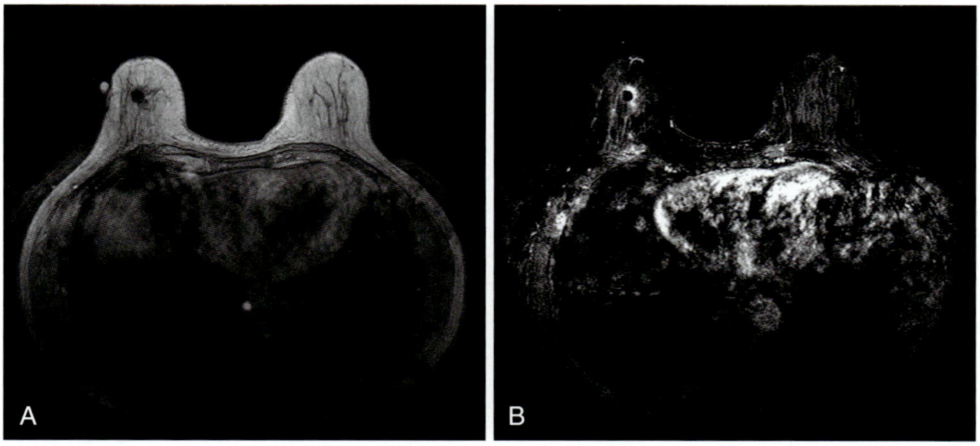

FIGURE 10.2 Susceptibility artifact caused by a tissue marker placed at the time of biopsy is shown. **A,** A T1-weighted image demonstrating magnetic susceptibility at the site of the tissue marker. **B,** A subtraction image showing a "blooming" artifact around the tissue marker. The artifact almost entirely obscures the known invasive ductal carcinoma.

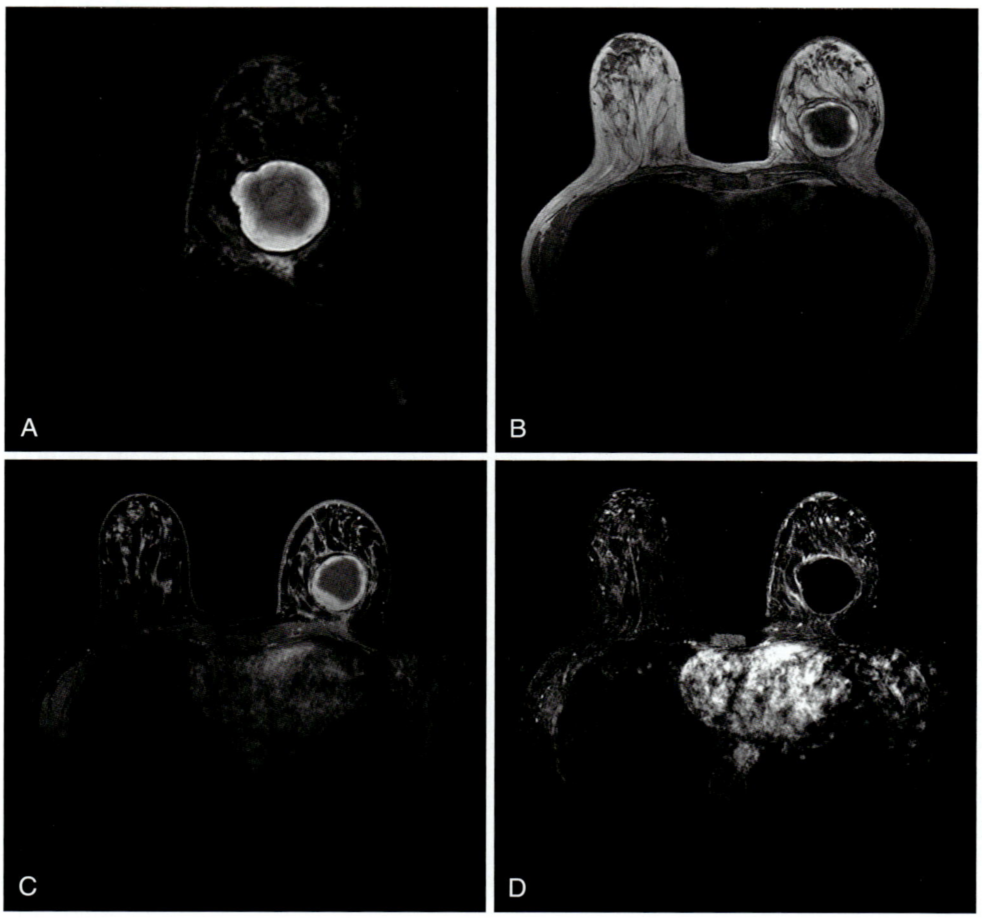

FIGURE 10.3 Post stereotactic-guided biopsy with delayed hematoma identified at preoperative DCE breast MRI. A subacute hematoma imaged with DCE breast MRI scans is seen in a T2-weighted fat saturated image (**A**), a T1-weighted non–fat-saturated image (**B**), a precontrast image (**C**), and a postconstrast image (**D**).

The enhancement pattern of fat necrosis is also widely variable. Kinetic assessment may demonstrate either benign or malignant type curves. The pattern of enhancement often correlates with the stage of fat necrosis evolution. The most malignant appearing enhancement occurs early after the inciting event and is secondary to acute inflammatory changes. As the inflammatory changes become chronic, granulation tissue develops, and the pattern of enhancement can change to reflect this evolution, with persistent or plateau delayed kinetics.[15] However, fat necrosis is a great mimic of cancer, not only on MRI but also on all other imaging modalities. Therefore, if the lesion in question has suspicious morphologic or kinetic features, biopsy will be indicated. Two additional examples of fat necrosis are illustrated in the *Reconstructive and Cosmetic Surgery* section later.

Seroma/Hematoma

A hematoma is characterized by heterogeneous signal intensity and lack of contrast enhancement. However, hematomas can have rim enhancement secondary to

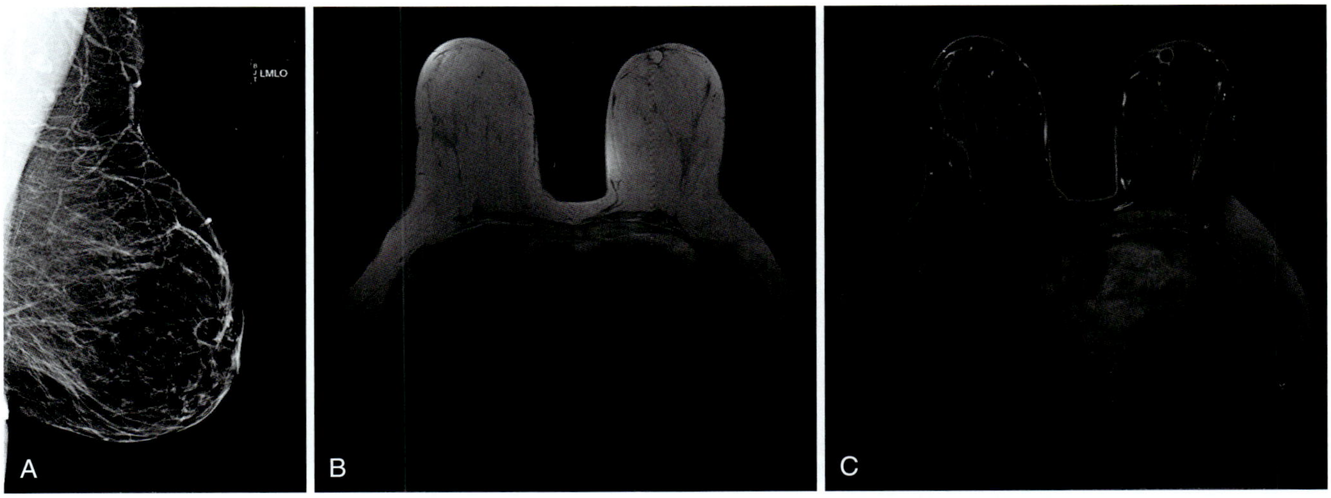

FIGURE 10.4 Classic imaging appearance of fat necrosis by mammogram (**A**) and DCE breast MRI (**B** and **C**) in a patient after lumpectomy for breast cancer. The mammogram demonstrates a lucent fat-containing oval mass with circumscribed margins. The non–fat-saturated T1 sequence (**B**) demonstrates a fat-containing oval mass that correlates with the mammographic finding. On the DCE breast MRI scan with fat saturation (**C**), the signal intensity of the lesion follows fat signal.

Table 10.2 Blood Signal on MRI Varies with its Age and the Pulse Sequence

Stage	T1 Enhancement	T2 Enhancement
Hyperacute	Intermediate	Bright
Acute	Intermediate	Dark
Subacute:		
Early	Bright	Dark
Late	Bright	Bright
Chronic	Dark	Dark

surrounding inflammatory changes. The signal of blood varies depending on its age and the pulse sequence used for imaging (Table 10.2). Chronic hematomas can demonstrate a low-signal intensity rim of hemosiderin on T1-weighted images.

Seromas typically appear as fluid collections, with high signal intensity on T2-weighted sequences and low signal intensity on T1-weighted sequences and no internal enhancement (Figure 10.5). Rarely, seromas can have rim enhancement, which is related to postprocedural inflammation, or focal or nodular enhancement that may represent residual disease, as is demonstrated in Figure 10.6. Seromas usually resorb over time. However, the findings may also persist for months or even years. One study showed that 3.7% of women had a seroma persisting at 6 years or more after surgery.[19] In the rare case in which DCE breast MRI is obtained in the immediate postsurgical period, air and fluid levels may be present in the dependent portions of the lumpectomy cavity. This is demonstrated in Figure 10.7 in a patient 2 days after surgery.

Hemosiderin and Metal

Postsurgical changes often include hemosiderin deposition from old blood products and iatrogenic metal such as surgical clips or tissue markers. Both hemosiderin and metal cause magnetic susceptibility artifacts. An example of magnetic susceptibility artifact is presented in Figure 10.2. Hemosiderin deposition tends to have less prominent magnetic susceptibility artifact than iatrogenic metals, seen as 1-to-2 mm areas of signal void as demonstrated in Figure 10.8. In the presence of metal or hemosiderin, the local magnetic field exhibits large changes, causing rapid dephasing of proton spins and resultant signal loss. These foci of magnetic susceptibility can appear as either bright spots or signal dropout, best seen on the T1-weighted non–fat-saturated precontrast images.[9] Additionally, because spatial positioning in an MR image is determined by the magnetic field gradients, the presence of metal or hemosiderin can result in voxel displacement and distortion of the image. These artifacts are most prominent on sequences without a refocusing pulse, such as gradient echo images, but are most commonly identified on T1-weighted images during breast MRI. The image distortion and signal dropout can obscure underlying abnormalities, so close attention to the affected tissue is needed to ensure that a small lesion is not missed.

Focal Skin Thickening and Fibrosis

Focal skin thickening and underlying fibrosis are commonly seen following lumpectomy and surgical biopsy. Compared with patients who have undergone whole breast radiation (discussed later), patients with surgical biopsy and no radiation may demonstrate minimal focal skin thickening. MRI compatible markers placed at the site of previous surgery or palpable abnormality may be helpful in pinpointing skin thickening as being postsurgical, at the site of a scar. The presence of such markers will help correlate the site of clinical interventions with the imaging findings. Figure 10.9 is a typical example of a patient with multiple postsurgical changes, including focal skin thickening.

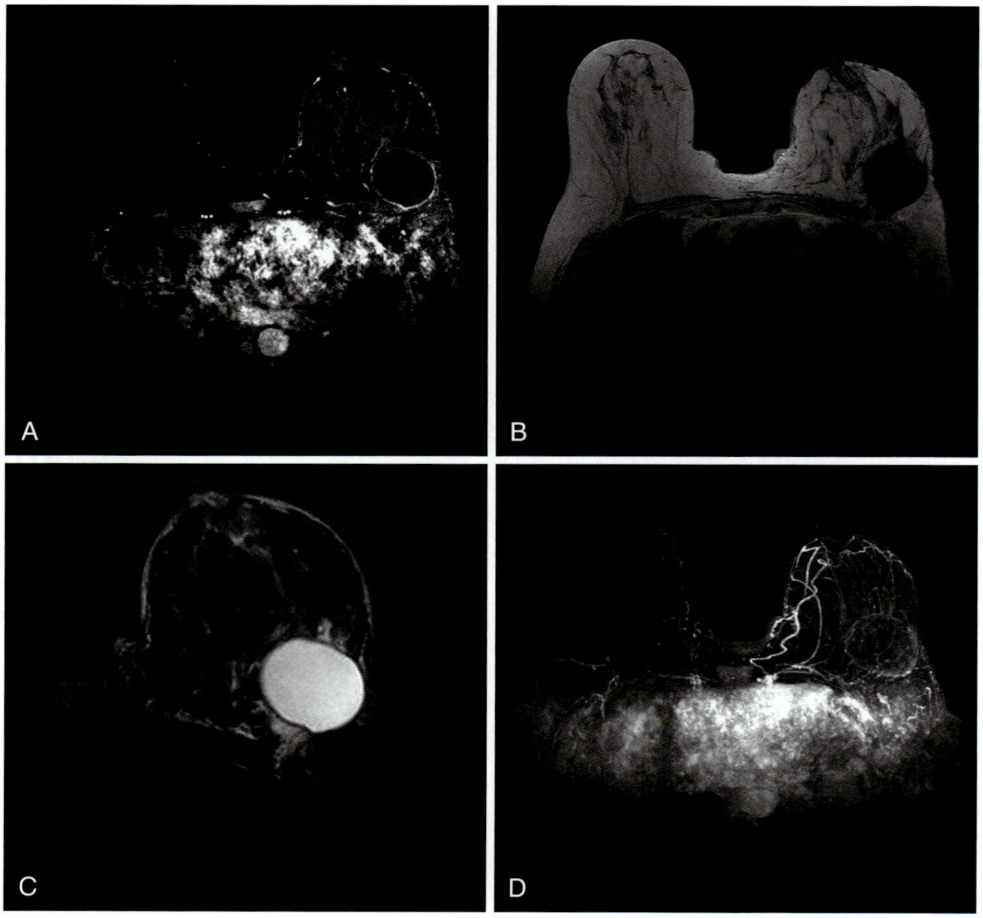

FIGURE 10.5 A postlumpectomy seroma is shown in a patient after lumpectomy for invasive breast cancer. **A,** Subtraction image. **B,** T1-weighted non–fat-saturated image. **C,** T2-weighted image. **D,** DCE breast MRI maximum-intensity projection (MIP) images. Note the homogeneous T2 hyperintensity–T1 hypointensity compatible with a seroma. Note also the minimal peripheral low level enhancement (best seen on the MIP images), most likely related to inflammatory changes.

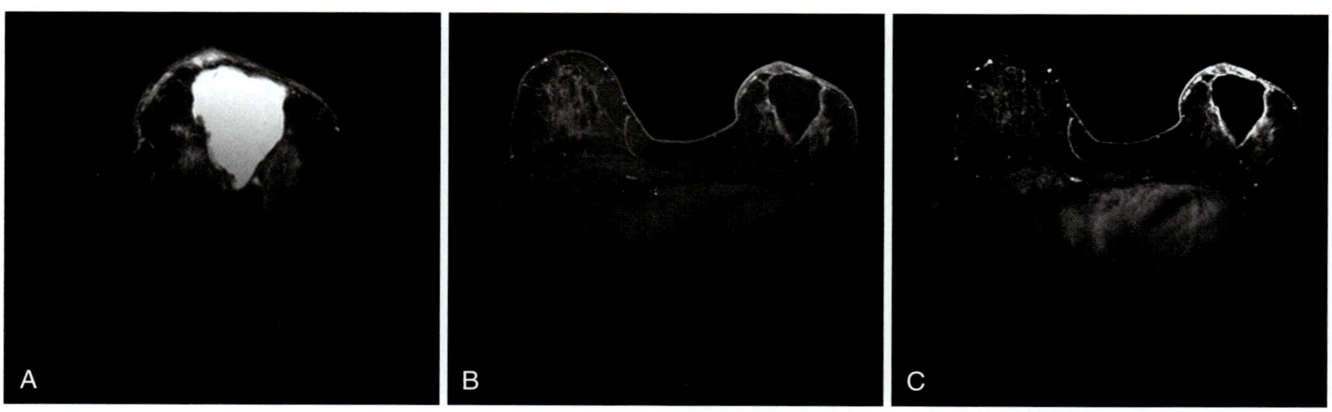

FIGURE 10.6 Postsurgical seroma with associated skin thickening and hemosiderin deposition is shown in a patient after lumpectomy with histologically positive surgical margins. **A,** T2-weighted image. **B,** Precontrast image. **C,** DCE MRI scan. MRI evaluation was requested to assess extent of residual disease. Peripheral nodular enhancement and a large postsurgical seroma are noted. In this case, the reexcised margins revealed no residual disease. Evaluation of positive margins can be difficult because peripheral enhancement can be seen with both inflammatory postsurgical changes and residual neoplastic disease.

Radiation

As discussed, treatment with only lumpectomy results in high recurrence rates, whereas lumpectomy plus radiation therapy will yield the same survival rates as mastectomy. However, adding radiation to surgical changes further complicates evaluation of postprocedural MRI findings. Radiation results in histologic changes to breast tissues that involve the skin, adipose tissue, glandular tissue, vasculature, and supporting ligaments.

Skin Thickening

Normal breast skin thickness is 2 mm or less. Skin thickening is usually apparent and quantification is rarely necessary. This is demonstrated in Figure 10.10, which shows

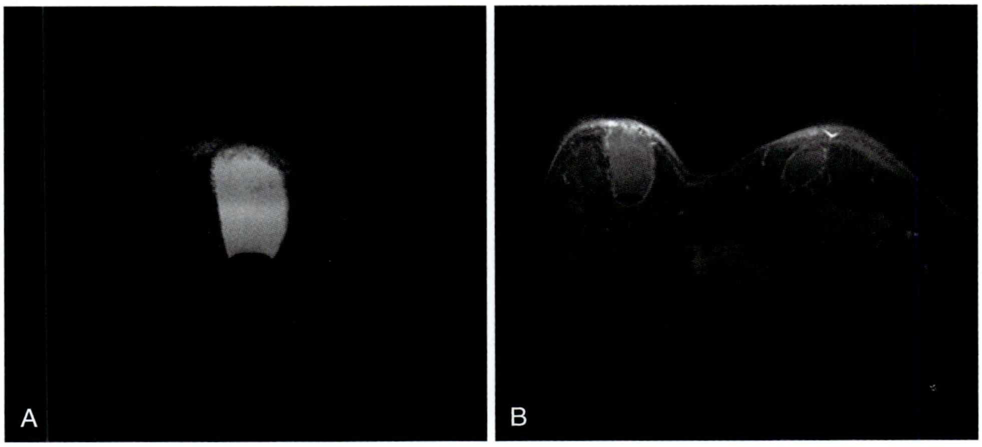

FIGURE 10.7 Postlumpectomy seroma with a fluid-air level is shown. T2-weighted (**A**) and DCE breast MRI (**B**) demonstrate an air-fluid level in a lumpectomy cavity 2 days after surgery. The serous fluid is in the dependent portion of the cavity, and the air bubble rises to the nondependent portion. Note that at our institution, by convention, the breasts are projected as if the women were supine; however, the images are acquired with the patient in a prone position in the breast coil.

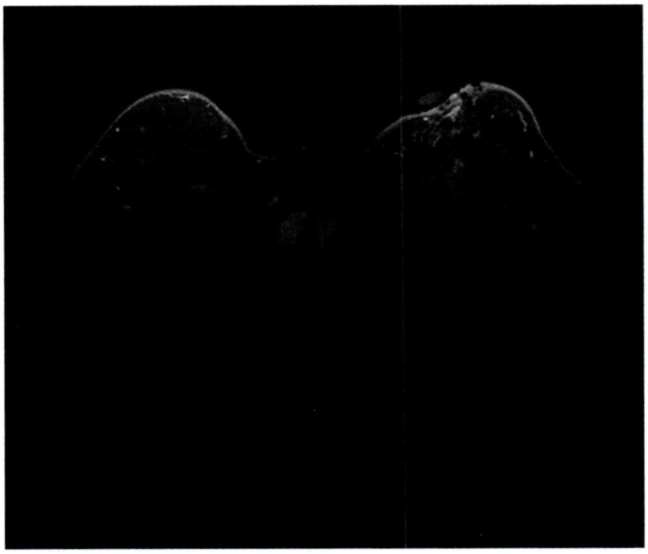

FIGURE 10.8 Hemosiderin deposits are seen in the skin and subcutaneous tissues immediately below the surface skin marker in a patient after lumpectomy for breast cancer in the upper inner left breast.

diffuse, asymmetric, obvious skin thickening of the right breast. Skin thickening may be quantified as outlined in Box 10.1.[20-22] Skin thickening is seen in nearly all postsurgical patients and diminishes over time. Benign skin thickening usually manifests as a diffuse band of T1-dark, T2-bright signal along the surface of the breast.[8] Skin thickening is a nonspecific finding that can be seen with inflammatory breast carcinoma, lymphatic obstruction, infection, radiation changes, and inflammation. The pattern of enhancement can be helpful. With inflammatory cancer, there can be skin enhancement accompanying the skin thickening and underlying trabecular thickening. Radiation therapy may further complicate the appearance of postsurgical skin thickening. After radiation therapy, vasodilatation manifests within the skin and subcutaneous tissues, leading to edema. Additionally, radiation-induced damage to the venous system can result in poor venous outflow and worsening skin and trabecular edema. However, a radiated breast is typically asymmetrically smaller in size, whereas a breast with inflammatory carcinoma is often asymmetrically enlarged, compared with the size of the uninvolved side.

Fibrosis

Fibrosis is a common sequela of radiation therapy, which contributes to the asymmetrically smaller breast size.[8] Fibrotic tissue can complicate postoperative breast MRI interpretation by looking masslike and mimicking a spiculated tumor or by causing nipple retraction (Figure 10.11). However, fibrotic tissue is classically T2-dark, with either no enhancement or low levels of enhancement that persist on the delayed dynamic phase.[8,23,24] During the early postoperative period, new granulation tissue forms, which can be associated with suspicious kinetic enhancement, resulting in false-positive interpretations.[8,23]

Enhancement

Radiation directly affects the enhancement characteristics of the breast parenchyma, resulting in decreased parenchymal enhancement throughout the involved breast, as seen in Figure 10.12. However, in the acute setting, up to 12 months after radiation, there can be increased contrast enhancement throughout the breast secondary to the diffuse edema.[25] Although radiation's effect on contrast enhancement is debated, published literature suggests that the radiation changes do not interfere with the contrast enhancement characteristics of residual or recurrent breast cancers. Therefore using enhancement kinetics along with morphologic features in imaging should not impair diagnostic accuracy in the presence of radiation changes.[26]

AlloDerm

AlloDerm is a human acellular tissue matrix that has been increasingly used in breast reconstruction. It has been used for prosthesis coverage in head and neck reconstructions and in hernia repairs. However, its uses have been expanded to include coverage of breast implants and as a contouring device to fill lumpectomy defects. On MRI, AlloDerm is easily distinguishable from the surrounding tissues. On both non–fat-saturated T1-weighted and T2-weighted sequences, AlloDerm is hypointense to fat, as seen in Figure 10.13. AlloDerm is hypointense to glandular tissue on

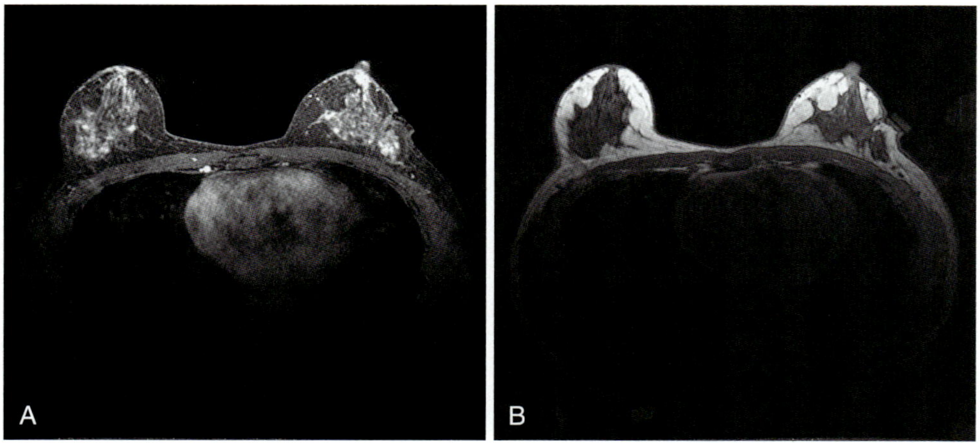

FIGURE 10.9 Focal skin thickening and multiple other associated postsurgical findings are shown. **A,** Note the focal skin thickening and hemosiderin deposition, linear scar, associated architectural distortion, and lack of contrast enhancement at the site of previous lumpectomy. Multiple findings are often seen postsurgically. **B,** A skin marker is usually placed at the surface site of a previous lumpectomy to help correlate the imaging findings with the clinical findings.

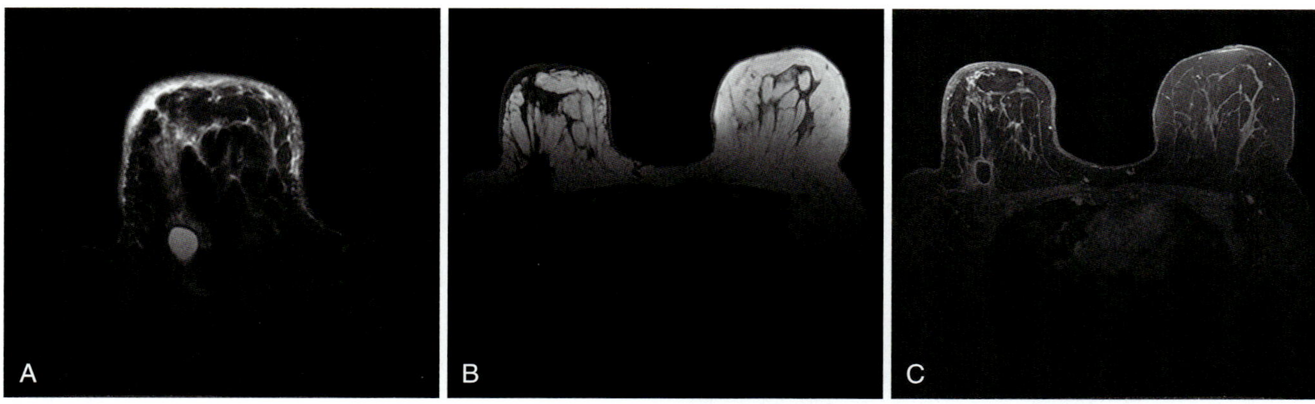

FIGURE 10.10 Postlumpectomy and postradiation changes including diffuse skin thickening are shown. T2-weighted (**A**), T1-weighted non-fat saturated (**B**), and DCE breast scan (**C**) acquired after lumpectomy and radiation therapy for breast cancer. Note the diffuse skin thickening, a sequela of radiation treatment. A more subtle finding is the diffuse trabecular thickening, recognized by the thicker Cooper's ligaments in the right breast as compared with those in the left. A small residual seroma is also seen in the posterior lateral right breast.

Box 10.1 Skin Thickening Grades

Grade	Skin thickening
Mild	Less than 3 mm
Moderate	3-5 mm
Marked	More than 5 mm

T2-weighted sequences and near isointense on non–fat-saturated T1-weighted sequences. Additionally, AlloDerm demonstrates no contrast enhancement, making it easily distinguishable from recurrent or residual tumor.[27]

Mastectomy

Modified radical mastectomy is a surgical procedure that removes the entire breast, including the nipple, for treating breast cancer. Radical mastectomy includes removing the entire breast and nipple, plus removal of both pectoralis muscles. In nipple-sparing mastectomy, the skin and nipple are preserved in the hopes of achieving a more natural-appearing reconstruction. Postsurgical changes seen on MRI following mastectomy are the same as those following lumpectomy, including fibrosis, skin thickening, fat necrosis, hematoma or seroma, or magnetic susceptibility from hemosiderin or metal (Figure 10.14). Although the cancer

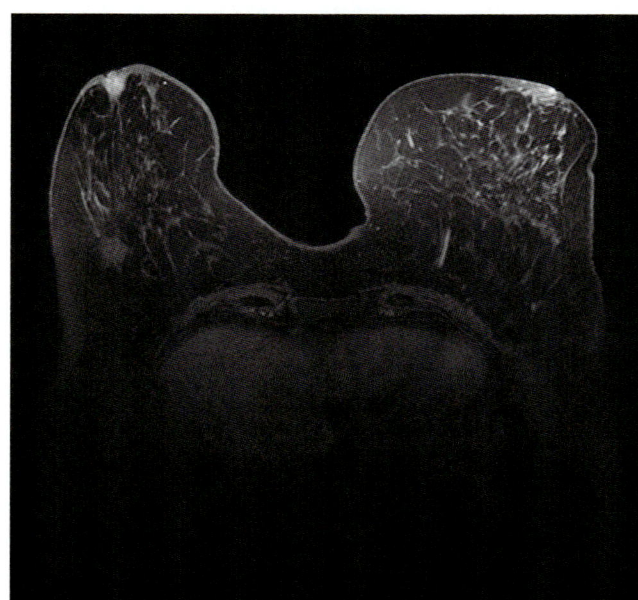

FIGURE 10.11 Associated changes related to surgery and radiation. DCE breast MRI scan demonstrating nipple retraction in a patient after lumpectomy for breast cancer. The lumpectomy site is seen as a nonenhancing mass with associated architectural distortion. Also note the asymmetry in size of the breast and mild skin thickening, due to both radiation and surgical changes.

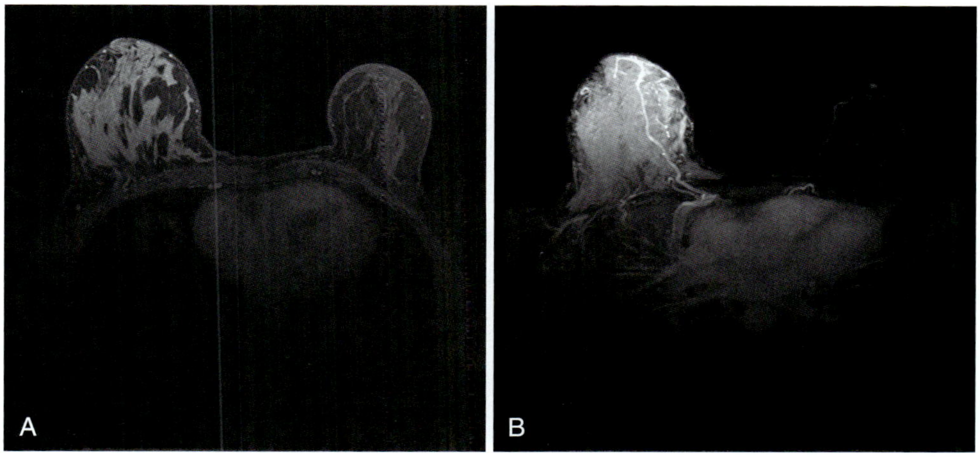

FIGURE 10.12 Postlumpectomy and postradiation changes. **A,** DCE breast MRI scan demonstrates characteristic findings of postradiation changes, including asymmetry in background enhancement, with the radiated breast demonstrating less prominent background enhancement. Diffuse skin and trabecular thickening and smaller size of the radiated breast will also be seen. **B,** MIP of a different patient who is currently lactating and has a history of left breast cancer treated with lumpectomy and radiation therapy. The radiated breast demonstrates no enhancement and is smaller in size than the right breast. The normal breast demonstrates marked diffuse background enhancement attributable to lactational changes.

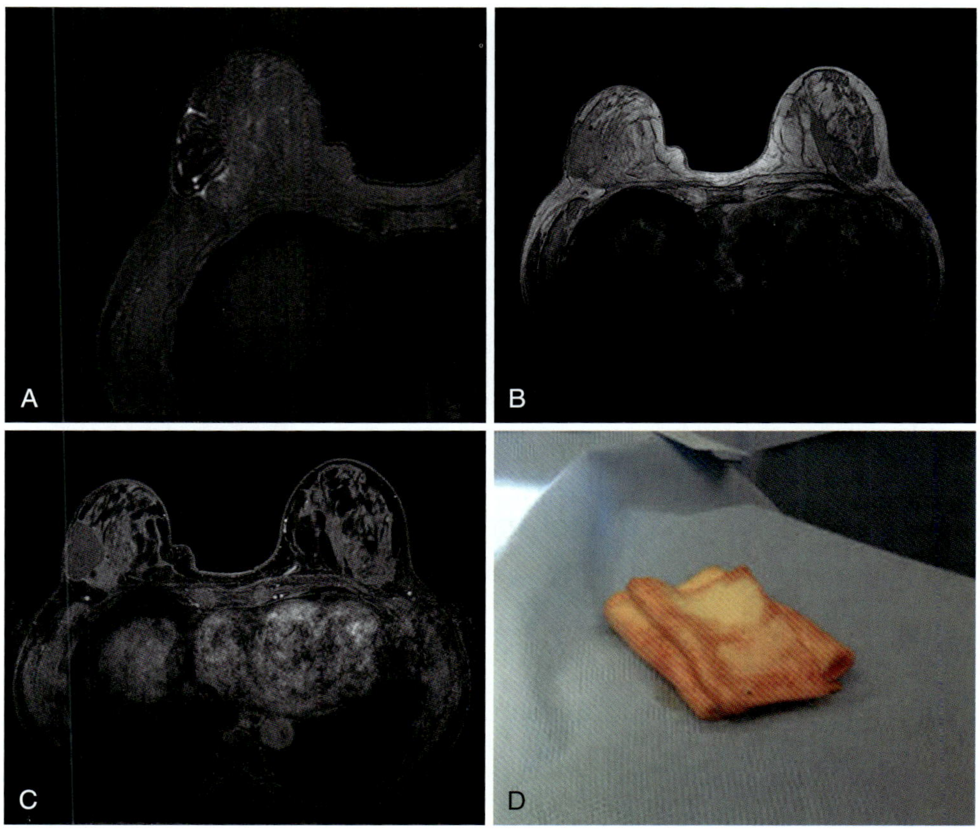

FIGURE 10.13 Human acellular tissue (AlloDerm) can be used for covering implants, defining the inframammary fold, and reconstructing the nipple. It can also be folded or rolled as filler for lumpectomy defects, as is demonstrated in this case. **(A)** T2, **(B)** T1 nonfat-saturated, and **(C)** T1 delayed postcontrast MRI sequences in a patient with AlloDerm rolled to fill a lumpectomy cavity. **D,** A piece of AlloDerm rolled before surgical placement. Note the swirling of the rolled AlloDerm, which was incorrectly identified as a hematoma at the time of initial image interpretation.

recurrence rate in the postmastectomy breast is low because of the theoretical removal of all breast tissue, residual glandular breast tissue can remain after mastectomy with or without breast reconstruction.[28] Recurrence can occur within regional lymph nodes or within the reconstructed breast, with reported rates in the literature of between 5% and 15%.[8] The purpose of MRI in these patients is to evaluate the chest wall in specific cases in which there is concern of chest wall recurrence. Otherwise, the postmastectomy site can be monitored clinically.

Reconstructive and Cosmetic Surgery

After mastectomy or modified radical mastectomy, reconstructive surgery is often performed for cosmetic purposes. Options for reconstruction include autologous tissue

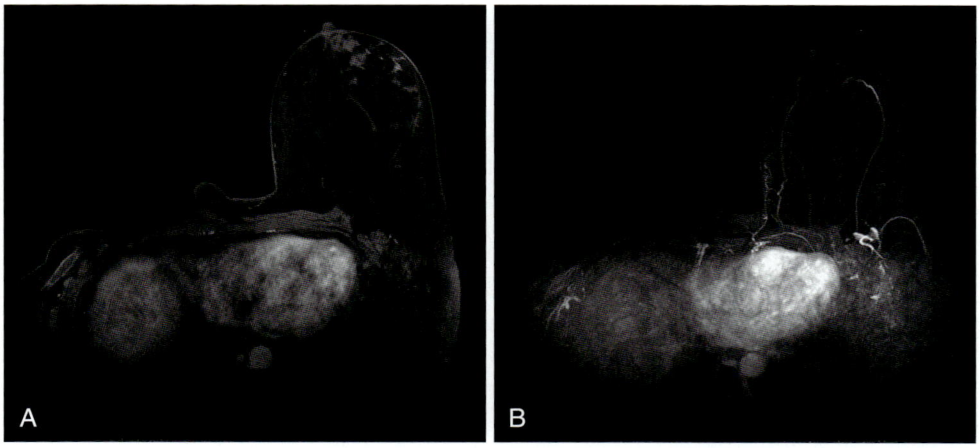

FIGURE 10.14 MRI postmastectomy appearance. Postcontrast (**A**) and MIP DCE breast MRI scan (**B**) in a patient with a right mastectomy for treatment of breast cancer. Deformity of the subcutaneous tissues is noted with no masses or suspicious enhancement of the chest wall.

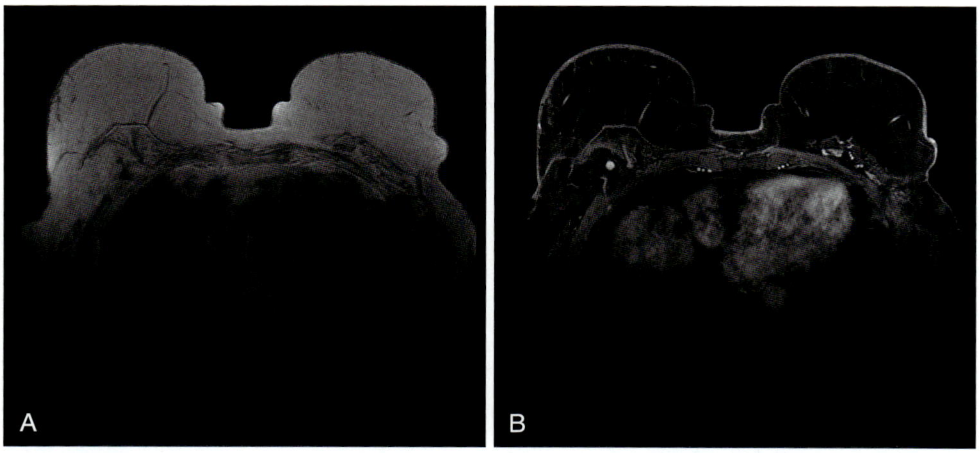

FIGURE 10.15 Autologous tissue breast reconstruction. T1-weighted non–fat-saturated image (**A**) and DCE breast MRI scan (**B**) in a patient with bilateral TRAM flap reconstructions following bilateral mastectomies for breast cancer. Note the muscle/vascular pedicle abutting the chest wall. The reconstructed breast mound is composed entirely of fat.

transfer, tissue expansion/implantation, local tissue rearrangement, or any combination of these. The rectus abdominis, latissimus dorsi, or less frequently gluteus maximus muscles can be used for autologous tissue reconstruction after mastectomy.[29]

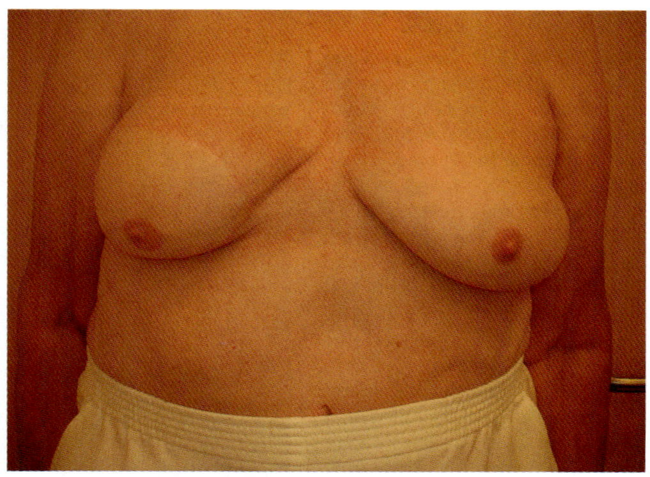

FIGURE 10.16 Photograph of a patient with a history of right mastectomy and TRAM flap reconstruction. The patient has also had a second stage reconstruction of the nipple and tattooing to recreate the areola.

Tissue Expansion and Implantation

The placement of saline or silicone implants has been the standard method of breast augmentation since the 1960s. An older method of augmentation, in which various materials were injected directly into the breast, is still sometimes performed. The most commonly seen materials injected or surgically inserted into the breast are paraffin and direct silicone. Just as it does with mammography, the presence of silicone injections presents a challenge for image interpretation. A complete discussion of implants and injections is included in Chapter 11.

Transverse Rectus Abdominis Myocutaneous Flap

The transverse rectus abdominis myocutaneous (TRAM) flap is one of the most commonly used autologous tissue surgical procedures for breast reconstruction after mastectomy. The rectus abdominis muscle, along with the accompanying subcutaneous tissues and a vascular pedicle, based on either the superior or inferior epigastric vessels, is rotated or transplanted to build a breast mound at the mastectomy defect. This results in lower abdominal fat and an atrophied rectus abdominis muscle visualized within the expected location of normal breast glandular tissue on MRI (Figure 10.15). Further cosmesis can be obtained with rotational flaps and tattooing to reconstruct the nipple and areolar structures, as seen in Figure 10.16.[30]

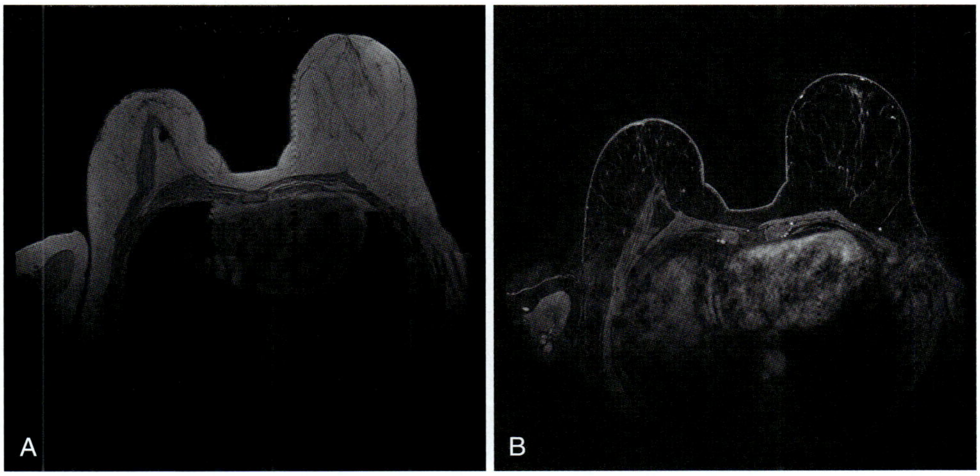

FIGURE 10.17 Autologous tissue reconstruction using a latissimus dorsi flap is illustrated. T1-weighted non–fat-saturated image (**A**) and DCE breast scan (**B**) of a patient with latissimus flap reconstruction following mastectomy for breast cancer. Note the inability of the patient to raise her right arm overhead to perform the study.

Typical postsurgical changes after reconstruction include skin thickening, fat necrosis, seroma/hematoma, magnetic susceptibility, and fibrosis. Fat necrosis is frequently identified and is reported in the literature with rates ranging from 10% to 26%.[8,29,30] The location within the breast can be helpful when diagnosing fat necrosis because it will typically occur at the periphery of the flap, where there is decreased blood supply.[8,15,29] Skin thickening is also commonly seen, secondary to insufficient venous and lymphatic drainage after reconstruction, contributing to fluid accumulation in the skin.

Latissimus Dorsi Flap (Lat Flap)

Another reconstructive strategy is a latissimus dorsi flap, which is often used for smaller reconstructions. This procedure involves bringing the ipsi- or contralateral interpolated myocutaneous latissimus dorsi flap along with the musculovascular pedicle from the thoracodorsal vessels, through a subcutaneous transaxillary tunnel from the back and forming the breast mound at the site of defect.[25] The postsurgical changes are similar to the TRAM flap, including replacement of the breast tissue with adipose tissue and muscle, as seen in Figure 10.17. Often the contact zone between the flap and the native adipose tissue of the breast can be seen as a T1-weighted low signal intensity line. This zone can be especially problematic when evaluating for recurrent tumor because often benign focal contrast enhances along the contact zone,[25] which can be difficult to differentiate from recurrent tumor.

Other Surgical Interventions

Reduction

Reduction mammoplasty can be performed for asymmetry following mastectomy in the contralateral breast, as well as bilaterally for cosmesis of excessive breast tissue. Postreduction scarring usually follows a pattern of circumareolar, horizontal, and sagittal incisions in the inframammary folds, shown in Figure 10.18. Again, typical postsurgical changes include skin thickening, fat necrosis (Figure 10.19), and magnetic susceptibility. Fibrosis and scarring can also be present. Fat necrosis will commonly be seen along the inferior central breast after reduction mammoplasty.[15] Skin thickening can be expected along the scar lines. Involvement of the venous or lymphatic systems is limited in a reduction procedure, making diffuse skin thickening less likely. Occasionally, fat necrosis may be quite exuberant, as seen in Figure 10.20. The finding is characteristically benign in appearance by mammographic imaging and not so obviously benign by DCE breast MRI. The case in Figure 10.20 illustrates the need for mammographic correlation when interpreting breast MRI.

Explantation

Silicone gel–filled implant removal was common in the 1990s because of concerns about systemic symptoms and has remained an important procedure for implant rupture, contractures, or local symptoms. Typically, explantation involves removal of the entire implant, including the capsule. However, if there has been prior rupture, some of the shell can be fragmented and left behind. Additionally, in silicone implant rupture, silicone gel can migrate elsewhere in the breast or axilla.[32] Using specific MRI sequences, silicone can be distinguished from other common postsurgical changes such as fibrosis, hematoma, seroma, or tumor. On T1-weighted fat-suppressed images, silicone appears hypointense, or black, compared with the enhancement of surrounding breast tissue. Cysts or fluid will also have this signal characteristic. However, a T2-weighted water-suppression sequence can easily differentiate these two because the cyst or water will become dark and the silicone will remain bright.[32] As with other breast surgical procedures, MRI findings also include skin thickening at the incision site, magnetic susceptibility, fat necrosis, fibrosis, or hematoma or seroma. Figure 10.21 shows examples of the varied appearance of explantation in two patients, one with residual seroma and the second with a scar characteristically located in the prepectoral region.

Male Breast

Occasionally, the male breast is evaluated and may have postsurgical changes. Most commonly, the postsurgical changes are secondary to removal of excess breast tissue for gynecomastia, as seen in Figure 10.22. Although there is less breast tissue in men than in women, the postsurgical

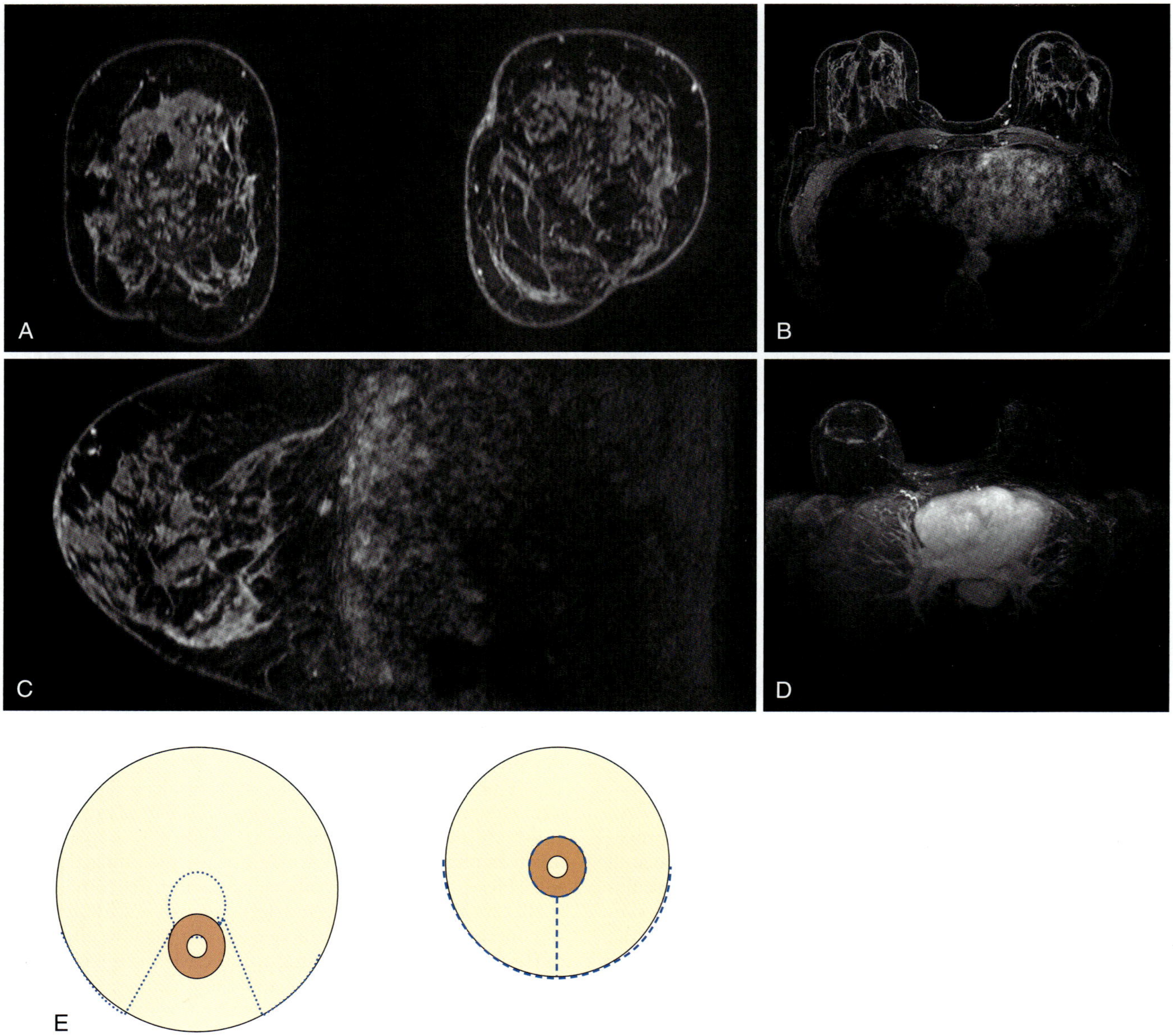

FIGURE 10.18 Coronal **(A)**, axial **(B)** and sagittal **(C)** postcontrast MRI images of a patient after reduction mammoplasty. MIP image **(D)** of a different patient demonstrates minimal enhancement of the scar in a circumareolar distribution. Postreduction scarring follows the pattern of circumareolar, horizontal, and sagittal incisions to the inframammary fold that is shown on **(E)**.

changes are the same, including skin thickening, fibrosis, magnetic susceptibility, and fat necrosis.

Regional Surgical Procedures

Extramammary surgical changes are occasionally encountered. These are significant because related artifacts may obscure regions of interest within the breast. In the majority of cases, these extramammary findings are incidental. Depending on the imaging protocol being used, portions of the chest, upper extremity, and upper abdomen may be included in the images, and therefore regional surgical procedure changes may be observed in breast MRI. Figure 10.23 demonstrates some of the more common extramammary surgical changes from sternotomy wires, port placement, and axillary lymph node dissection.

Conclusion

Breast MRI is frequently used for pretreatment evaluation of patients with a new diagnosis of breast cancer, for additional evaluation of clinical or imaging findings, and for breast cancer screening in patients at high risk of developing breast cancer. Many of these patients have had previous breast interventions, and it is important for radiologists to be aware of the related morphologic and kinetic MRI findings. Overall, breast MRI postoperative findings have similar morphologic appearances to those seen with mammography and ultrasound. However, the improved spatial resolution, contrast enhancement kinetics, and signal intensity of some of the postsurgical changes are features specific to breast MRI, making it a valuable adjunct in the evaluation of the postsurgical breast.

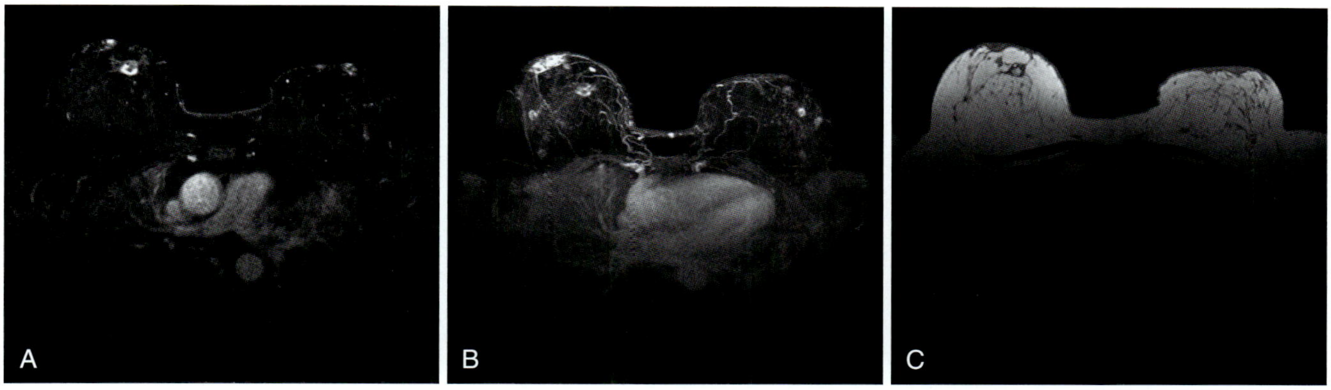

FIGURE 10.19 The MRI appearance of fat necrosis is shown in a DCE breast MRI subtracted image (**A**), MIP image (**B**), and T1-weighted non–fat-saturated image (**C**). The postcontrast images demonstrate multiple ring enhancing lesions in both breasts in a patient who had undergone bilateral reductions 5 months previously. The non–fat-saturated T1-weighted image identifies the presence of fat within the lesions, consistent with fat necrosis.

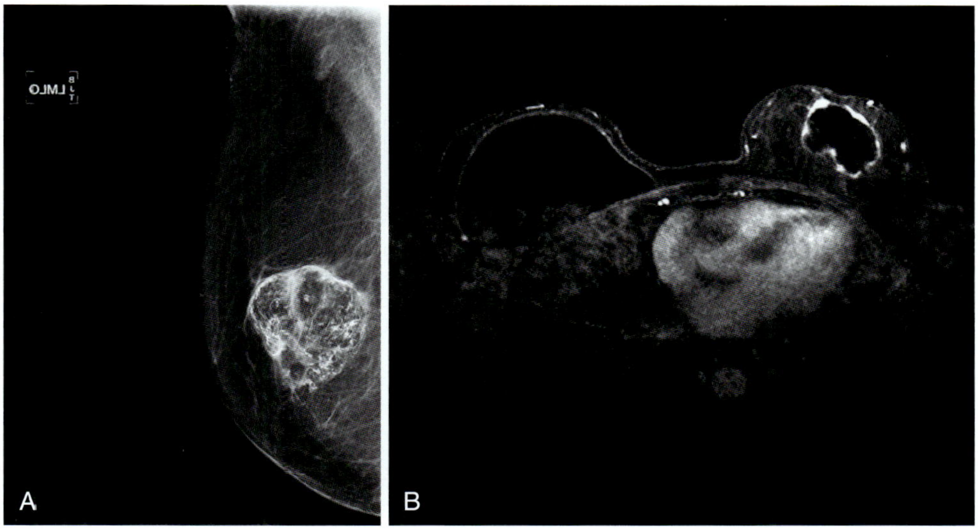

FIGURE 10.20 Exuberant fat necrosis is shown in images of a patient with a previous mastectomy and implant reconstruction on the right and a reduction mammoplasty for symmetry on the left. Mammogram (**A**) and DCE breast MRI subtracted image (**B**). Fat necrosis is easily recognized mammographically because of the bizarre eggshell calcifications, exemplifying the importance of mammographic correlation at the time of breast MRI interpretation.

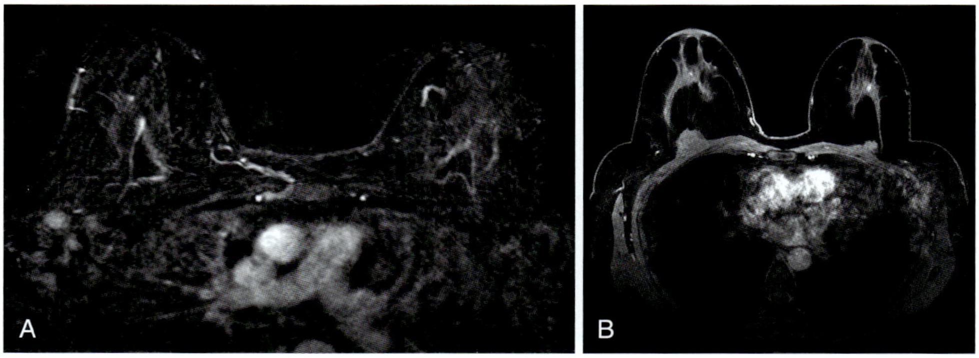

FIGURE 10.21 Explantation changes in two patients. **A**, Subtracted axial MR image of a patient with previous removal of breast implants, now demonstrating residual seromas at the site. **B**, Nonenhancing masses abutting the pectoralis muscles are shown representing scarring at the explantation site on this MRI scan of a second patient.

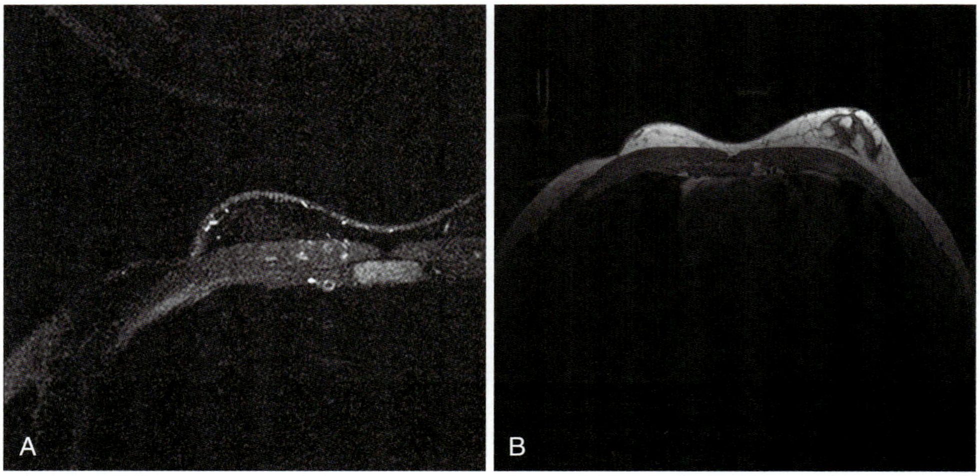

FIGURE 10.22 Postsurgical changes in a male patient undergoing DCE breast MRI. **A,** T2-weighted image. **B,** T1-weighted non–fat-saturated MRI scans of a man with a remote history of cosmetic surgery to remove excess right breast tissue (gynecomastia), demonstrating resultant skin retraction. The patient has since developed gynecomastia in the left breast.

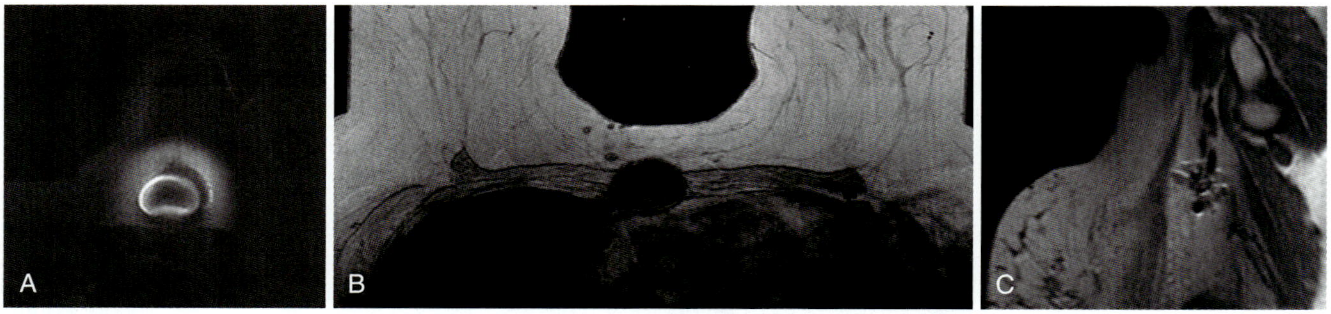

FIGURE 10.23 Incidentally noted extramammary surgical changes identified at the time of DCE breast MRI. **A,** Implantable port artifact is often seen in the superior chest in patients receiving chemotherapy or needing chronic intravenous medications or total parenteral nutrition. **B,** T1-weighted non–fat-saturated images demonstrating a "blooming" artifact from sternotomy wires. Depending on the body habitus of the patient, the artifact can obscure portions of the medial breast. **C,** Sagittal T1-weighted non–fat-saturated image of the axilla shows susceptibility artifact at the site of surgical nodal dissection.

References

1. Sickles EA, Herzaog KA: Mammography of the postsurgical breast, *Am J Radiol* 136:585–588, 1980.
2. Sickles EA, Herzaog KA: Intramammary scar tissue: a mimic of the mammographic appearance of carcinoma, *Am J Radiol* 135:349–352, 1980.
3. Lamm RL, Jackman RJ: Mammographic abnormalities caused by percutaneous stereotactic biopsy of histologically benign lesions evident on follow-up mammograms, *Am J Radiol* 174: 753–756, 2000.
4. Krishnamurthy R, et al: Mammographic findings after breast conservation therapy, *Radiographics* 19:S53–S62, 1999.
5. Dershaw DD: Mammography in patients with breast cancer treated by breast conservation (lumpectomy with or without radiation), *Am J Radiol* 164:309–316, 1995.
6. Balu-Maestro C, Bruneton JN, Geofray A, et al: Ultrasonographic posttreatment follow-up of breast cancer patients, *J Ultrasound Med* 10(1):1–7, 1991.
7. Whitehouse G, Moore NR: MR Imaging of the breast after surgery for breast cancer, *MRI Clin North Am* 2(4):591–603, 1994.
8. Devon RK, et al: Breast reconstruction with a transverse rectus abdominis myocutaneous flap: spectrum of normal and abnormal MR imaging findings, *Radiographics* 24:1287–1299, 2004.
9. Ojeda-Fournier H, Choe KA, Mahoney MC: Recognizing and interpreting artifacts and pitfalls in MR imaging of the breast, *Radiographics* 27:S147–164, 2007.
10. American College of Radiology: *ACR Practice guidelines®: The Performance Of Contrast- Enhanced Magnetic Resonance Imaging (MRI) Of The Breast*. Available at http://www.acr.org/~/media/ACR/Documents/PGTS/guidelines/MRI_Breast.pdf. Accessed December 2012.
11. Poplack SP, Weiss JE, Titus-Ernstoff L, et al: Screening mammography: costs and use of screening-related services, *Radiology* 234(1): 79–85, 2005.
12. Liberman L: Percutaneous imaging-guided core breast biopsy, *AJR Am J Roentgenol* 174(5):1191–1199, 2000.
13. Veronesi U, Saccozzi R, Del Vecchio M, et al: Comparing radical mastectomy with quadrantectomy, axillary dissection, and radiotherapy in patients with small cancers of the breast, *N Engl J Med* 305(1):6–11, 1981.
14. Frei KA, Kinkel K, Bonel HM, et al: MR imaging of the breast in patients with positive margins after lumpectomy, *AJR Am J Roentgenol* 175(6):1577–1584, 2000.
15. Daly CP, Jaeger B, Sill DS: Variable appearances of fat necrosis on breast MRI, *AJR Am J Roentgenol* 191:1374–1380, 2008.
16. Hogge JP, Robinson RE, Magnant CM, et al: The mammographic spectrum of fat necrosis of the breast, *Radiographics* 15(6):1347–1356, 1995.
17. Taboada JL, Stephens TN, Krishnamurthy S, Brandt KR, Whitman GJ: The many faces of fat necrosis in the breast, *Am J Radiol* 192: 815–825, 2009.
18. Bassett L, Gold R, Cove H: Mammographic spectrum of traumatic fat necrosis: the fallibility of "pathognomonic" signs of carcinoma, *AJR Am J Roentgenol* 130:119–122, 1978.
19. Li J, Dershaw DD, Lee CF, et al: Breast MRI after conservation therapy: usual findings in routine follow-up examinations, *AJR Am J Roentgenol* 195(3):799–807, 2010.
20. Gold RH, Montgomery CK, Minagi H, et al: The significance of mammary skin thickening in disorders other than primary carcinoma: a roentgenologic-pathologic correlation, *AJR Am J Roentgenol* 112:613–621, 1971.

21. Willson SA, Adam EJ, Tucker AK: Patterns of breast skin thickness in normal mammograms, *Clin Radiol* 33:691–693, 1982.
22. Ojeda-Fournier H, et al: Accelerated partial breast irradiation and post-treatment imaging evaluation, *Radiographics* 31:1701–1716, 2011.
23. Dao TH, Rahmouni A, Campana F, et al: Tumor recurrence versus fibrosis in the irradiated breast: differentiation with dynamic gadolinium-enhanced MR imaging, *Radiology* 187:751–755, 1993.
24. Lewis-Jones HG, Whitehouse GH, Leinster SJ: The role of magnetic resonance imaging in the assessment of local recurrent breast carcinoma, *Clin Radiol* 43:197–204, 1991.
25. Rieber A, Schramm K, Helms G, et al: Breast-conserving surgery and autogenous tissue reconstruction in patients with breast cancer: efficacy of MRI of the breast in the detection of recurrent disease, *Eur Radiol* 13(4):780–787, 2003.
26. Morakkabati N, Leutner CC, Schmiedel A, et al: Breast MR imaging during or soon after radiation therapy, *Radiology* 229:893–901, 2003.
27. Tran Cao HS, Tokin C, Konop J, et al: A preliminary report on the clinical experience with AlloDerm in breast reconstruction and its radiologic appearance, *Am Surgeon* 76:1123–1126, 2010.
28. Langstein HN, Cheng MH, Singletary SE, et al: Breast cancer recurrence after immediate reconstruction: patterns and significance, *Plastic Reconstr Surg* 111:712–720, 2003.
29. Kang BJ, Jung JI, Park C, et al: Breast MRI findings after modified radical mastectomy and transverse rectus abdominis myocutaneous flap in patients with breast cancer, *J Magne Reson Imaging* 21:784–791, 2005.
30. Ainslie NB, Ojeda-Fournier H: Creating a realistic breast: the nipple-areola reconstruction, *Plastic Surg Nurs* 16:156–166, 1996.
31. Schusterman MA: The free TRAM flap, *Clin Plast Surg* 25:191–195, 1998.
32. Ahn CY, Shaw WW, Narayanan K, et al: Residual silicone detection using MRI following previous breast implant removal: Case reports, *Aestheti Plastic Surg* 19(4):361–367, 1995.

CHAPTER 11

MRI for Breast Implant Evaluation

Anne E. Kleimeyer
Mary C. Mahoney

More than 2 million women in the United States have undergone breast implantation since the 1960s, either for cosmetic augmentation or breast reconstruction. During this time, both the silicone controversy and the known complications of breast augmentation have necessitated an accurate imaging modality to evaluate breast implants. Magnetic resonance imaging (MRI) has become the accepted standard for the evaluation of implant integrity. In this chapter, we will discuss the history of breast augmentation and the types of implants that can be encountered in daily practice. The advantages of MRI over both mammography and sonography in evaluating implant rupture will also be addressed.

History of Breast Implantation

The first breast augmentation procedure was performed in 1895 by Czerny. The breast was reconstructed with autologous fat implantation, after the excision of a large fibroadenoma.[1,2] Throughout the remainder of the 1800s, a variety of materials were injected into the breast, including mineral oil, fat and Vaseline. In the early 1900s, paraffin injections were performed for breast reconstruction. However, this practice was discontinued by the early 1920s secondary to both local and lethal complications, including breast lumps, skin necrosis, lung emboli, and brain emboli.[3] Other materials, such as glass balls and ivory, have been inserted into the breast for reconstruction.[3]

Silicone was developed in the 1930s. The material was soon considered ideal for breast augmentation for two reasons. Silicone could be easily manufactured in a variety of sizes and shapes, and silicone was the first material to have a "normal" feel once inserted into the breast. The injection of liquid silicone into the breast was first performed in Japan, reportedly in the late 1940s.[4] In the United States in the 1950s and 1960s, liquid silicone was directly injected into the breast parenchyma for augmentation. The main problem encountered by use of free silicone was the tendency of the silicone to migrate a far distance from the site of the injection. "Adulterated" silicones were then created to keep the silicone from migrating away from the injection site. These adulterated silicone substances contained fibrosing agents such as vegetable oil or fatty acids. The free injections of adulterated silicones resulted in a silicone-induced mastopathy in many women. The mastopathy included lymphadenopathy, granulomatous masses, fibrosis, skin retraction, nipple inversion, and infections. The practice of direct silicone injections was prohibited by the U.S. Food and Drug Administration (FDA) in the 1970s.

The first silicone gel-filled implant was inserted into the breast by Dr. Thomas Cronin at Baylor University in 1962. The creation of the silicone gel prosthesis revolutionized plastic surgery of the breast. The first silicone implants were produced commercially by Dow Corning Corp. starting in October 1963.[3] The early silicone implants were made of a silicone polymer capsule and a liquid silicone gel. These early-generation implants were prone to rupture, predominantly as a result of the thinner shells and less-viscous silicone gel used at the time. Since the 1980s, silicone implants have contained a more viscous or adhesive gel, which is designed not to leak, even if the outer shell is breached.[5]

The use of silicone breast implants has been a controversial and debated topic since the beginning of their use in the 1960s. Most of the controversy has centered on the suggested association of silicone implants with connective tissue disorders and malignant diseases of the breast.[6-8] As a response to the concern over silicone breast implants and their association with systemic disease, the FDA imposed a moratorium on silicone gel implants in 1992.

In 1999, a formal report was published by the Institute of Medicine: "Safety of Silicone Breast Implants." The report concluded that the local complications of silicone implant rupture were frequent. However, these complications were difficult to diagnose because of the large variety of implant types and styles available on the market. The report also came to two separate conclusions, assuring patients of the safety of silicone implants. First, the report asserted that there was no increase in either primary or recurrent breast cancer in women with silicone implants. Second, it asserted that there was no higher risk of malignancy, connective tissue disorders, or neurologic diseases in women with implants than in women without implants.[9] In a slow response to this report, the FDA re-approved silicone gel implants in 2006, with some mild limitations. Silicone devices are permitted for all women undergoing breast reconstruction following breast cancer, trauma to the breast, or developmental disorders involving the chest wall. However, silicone implants

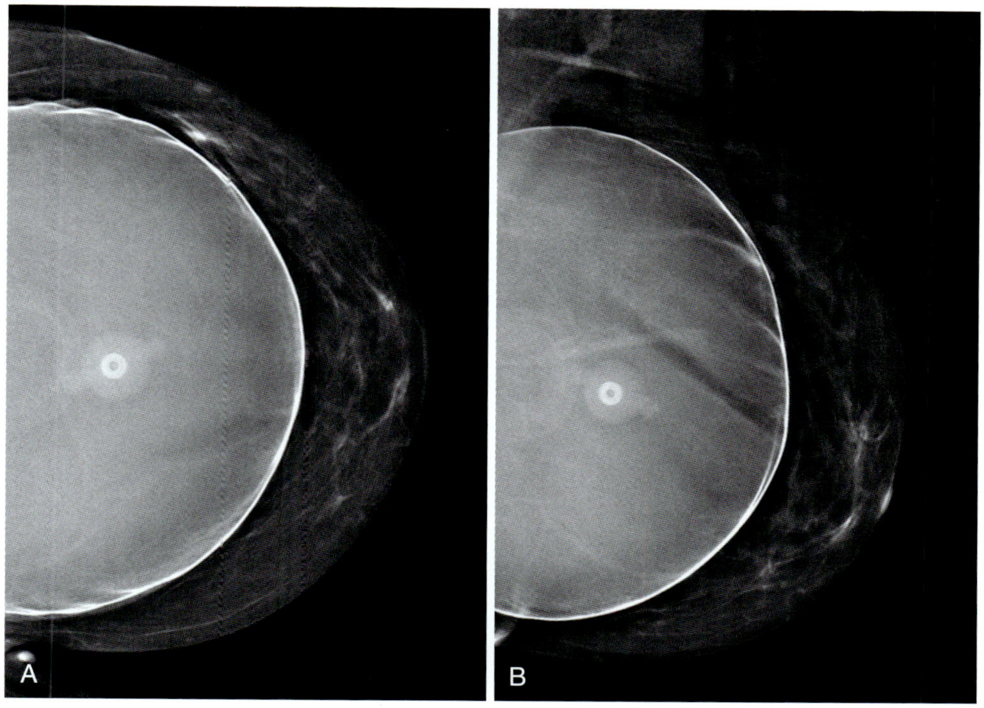

FIGURE 11.1 Mammogram of a saline implant showing valve. (A) Standard craniocaudal (CC) and (B) mediolateral oblique (MLO) views of the breast demonstrate an intact subpectoral saline implant with visualization of a fill valve.

are not available for women younger than age 22 years for purely cosmetic use.

The FDA also made recommendations to guide imaging practices. The FDA suggests a baseline breast MRI to evaluate for implant integrity 3 years after the placement of silicone implants and then every 2 years thereafter, to evaluate for rupture in asymptomatic women.

Implant Basics

A wide variety of implants are available to the American consumer, including silicone and saline implants and numerous varieties that contain a combination of both materials. To better evaluate for the complication of rupture, familiarity with the types of implants is necessary for the interpreting radiologist. The types of implants, the location of implants, and the known complications of implant rupture are discussed later. For a thorough review of breast implants, Middleton and McNamara[3] created a comprehensive breast implant classification scheme, based on historical and MRI considerations.

A saline implant is constructed with an elastomer shell filled with saline. The implant can contain a variable amount of saline, which can be adjusted via a fill valve. Often, the valves used to adjust saline volume are mammographically visible and frequently palpable on physical examination (Figure 11.1). A saline implant rupture is a clinical diagnosis with rapid implant decompression when the elastomer shell develops a tear (Figure 11.2). Hence there are few indications for MRI evaluation of a patient with saline implants. If the patient has a history of a prior silicone implant or free silicone injections, MRI may be useful to determine if any free silicone remains. If MRI is performed, it is important to note that the presence of fluid outside the shell is not specific for rupture in patients with saline implants. Normal migration of saline or reactive serous fluid can develop around the saline implant.[10]

A variety of silicone implants can be encountered with MRI scans, including single-lumen, double-lumen, and reverse double-lumen implants. The standard single-lumen silicone implant has an outer silicone elastomer shell and contains homogeneous high signal intensity silicone on T2 images (Figure 11.3). A typical double-lumen implant contains two elastomer shells, with silicone in the inner gel space and saline in the outer lumen. The amount of saline in the outer lumen can either be a fixed amount or variable, depending on the manufacturer. Double-lumen implants were created to reduce silicone gel bleeding and associated capsular contracture (Figure 11.4).

A reverse double-lumen implant contains a variable amount of saline in the inner lumen and a fixed amount of silicone in the outer lumen. The reverse double lumen implant is frequently seen in the setting of breast reconstruction. The benefit of this implant is a more natural feel because the silicone component is located on the outside.[10] In the Middleton and McNamara series,[3] only 11% of the implants were of the standard double-lumen variety and fewer than 1% were reverse double-lumen implants.

Because of the bicompartmental nature of dual-lumen implants, failure of the inner elastomer shell can have a unique outcome not visualized with single-lumen silicone implants. Failure of the inner shell leads to intermixing of the saline and silicone, a type of intracapsular rupture easily identified with MRI. Failure of the inner elastomer shell has been termed an *internal rupture*.[10] The mixture of the silicone and saline contents has also been described as the *salad oil* sign on breast MRI because of the appearance of large globules of silicone intermixed with saline (Figures 11.5 and 11.6).

Silicone implants can have a smooth or textured surface to the elastomer shell. The textured surface was developed to decrease the rate of capsular contracture. Some implants also have a coating of polyurethane (PTU) over the surface

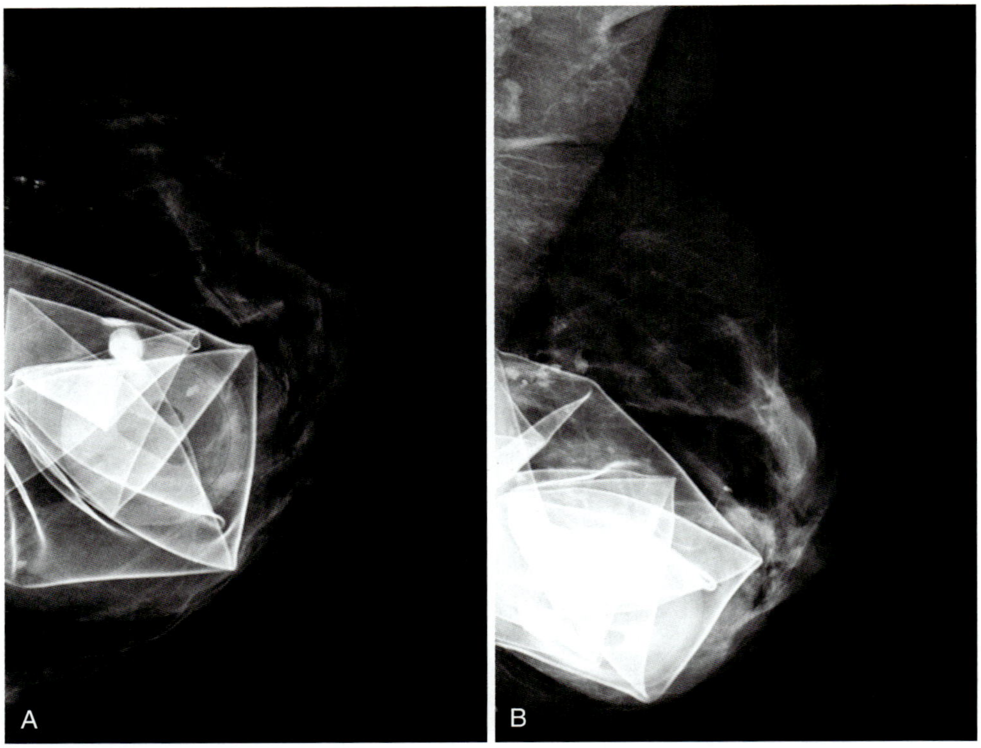

FIGURE 11.2 Mammogram of a collapsed saline implant. **(A)** Standard CC and **(B)** MLO views of the breast demonstrate a collapsed subglandular saline implant.

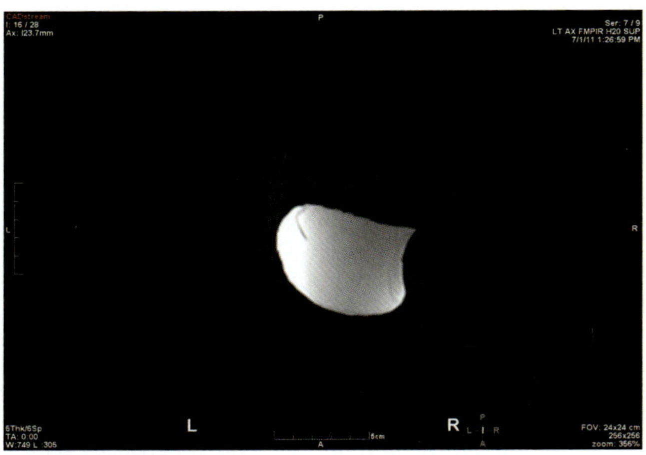

FIGURE 11.3 MRI of standard silicone implant. Axial, subglandular, prepectoral, fat- and water-suppressed image of the left breast demonstrates an intact silicone implant.

of the silicone envelope. This PTU layer serves a similar purpose as a textured implant, decreasing the rate of capsular contracture. Both the textured and PTU-covered implants commonly have a small to moderate amount of serous reactive fluid surrounding the implants. If pronounced, the reactive fluid surrounding a single-lumen device can mimic an intact double-lumen implant.[11] The presence of this extracapsular fluid on MR imaging has been described as a *picture frame* appearance.[3]

Additional, rarer types of implant devices are occasionally seen with implant-integrity breast MRI. These types of implants account for fewer than 1% of breast implants. A silicone gel/gel double-lumen implant has been commercially available since the 1980s. The inner lumen is usually overfilled with silicone gel and therefore holds a more spherical shape. The outer lumen is usually underfilled to achieve a more reasonable cosmetic outcome. Triple-lumen implants are also available, containing an overfilled silicone gel inner layer, an underfilled silicone gel middle layer, and an outer layer of saline (Figure 11.7). Soft pectus implants are made of a solid silicone elastomer and are dark on all MRI sequences. These pectus implants were developed to cosmetically correct either an acquired or congenital absence of the pectoralis muscle.[3] Finally, "stacked" implants have been used for the purpose of breast reconstruction. This technique utilizes more than one implant per breast.

Breast implants are placed in either a subglandular or subpectoral location. The subglandular location places the implant between the patient's fibroglandular breast tissue and the pectoralis major muscle. With both mammography and breast MRI, the pectoralis muscle is seen diving behind the implant when the implant is placed in a subglandular location (Figure 11.8). The subpectoral location places the implant between the pectoralis major and minor muscles (Figure 11.9). The choice of a subpectoral versus subglandular location greatly varies from patient to patient, and the decision is often based on the surgeon's preference. The surgical insertion of a subpectoral implant is technically more difficult. However, a subpectoral implant allows for better visualization of native breast tissue on mammography, has a lower incidence of capsular contracture, and has been associated with reduced surgical scarring.[4]

Implants can be placed by an inframammary, periareolar, or axillary approach. The inframammary approach provides the easiest surgical access but does result in a scar along the inframammary fold. The periareolar semicircular incision

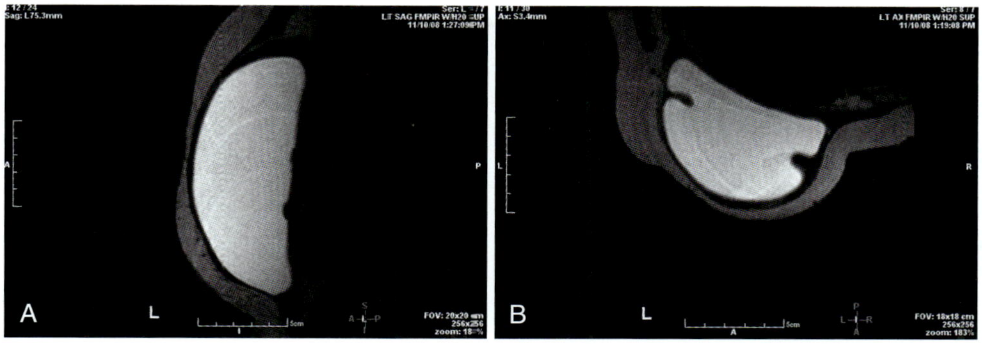

FIGURE 11.4 MRI of double lumen implant. **A,** Standard dual-lumen implant. MRI sagittal short tau inversion recovery (STIR) image with water suppression demonstrates an intact subpectoral dual-lumen implant with silicone in the inner chamber and saline in the outer chamber. **B,** A standard dual-lumen implant. MRI axial STIR images with water and fat suppression demonstrates an intact subpectoral dual-lumen implant with silicone in the inner chamber and saline in the outer chamber.

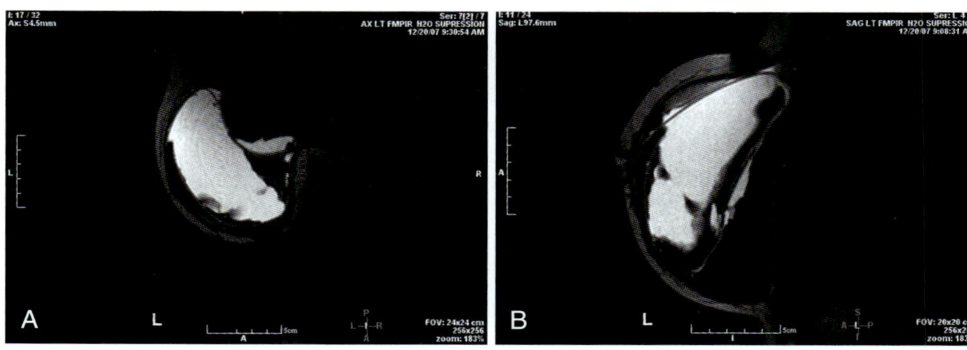

FIGURE 11.5 MRI of double-lumen implant with internal rupture. **(A)** Axial and **(B)** sagittal MRI STIR images with water suppression demonstrate a standard dual-lumen implant with failure of the inner lumen or *internal rupture.* There is mixing of the inner-lumen silicone compartment and the outer-lumen saline compartment, described as the salad oil sign.

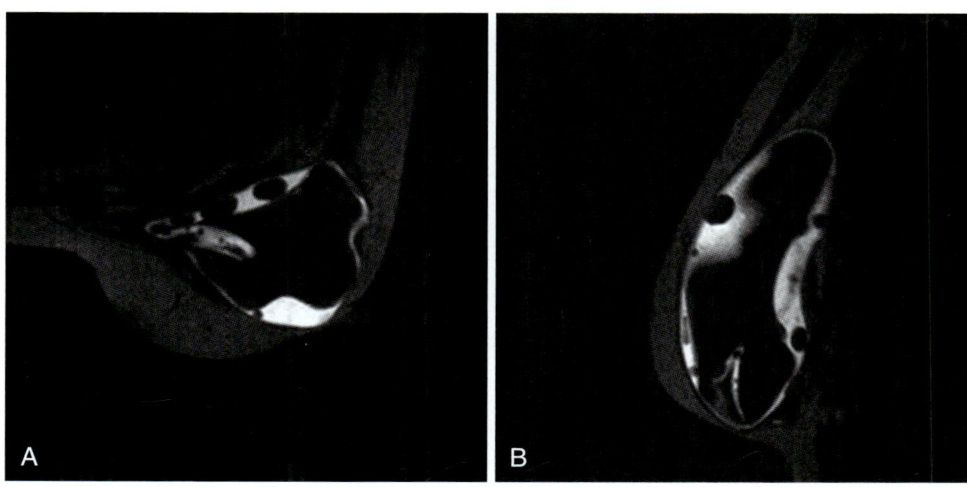

FIGURE 11.6 Reverse double-lumen implant with internal rupture. **(A)** Axial and **(B)** sagittal MRI STIR images of the breast with water suppression demonstrate a reverse dual-lumen implant with an outer silicone lumen and an inner saline lumen. There has been failure of the inner lumen with mixing of both the saline and silicone, resulting in the salad oil sign. *(Courtesy of Biren A. Shah, MD, Henry Ford Health Systems, Detroit, MI, and Shreya M. Sharman, B.S., University of Michigan, Ann Arbor.)*

causes the least amount of scarring, but there is a risk of decreased nipple sensation. The axillary approach causes minimal scarring but is technically more difficult.[1]

The risk of rupture of a silicone-containing implant is directly related to the age of the implant and placement of the implant behind the pectoralis muscle.[12,13] The majority of ruptures have no known traumatic origin, and implant rupture increases in incidence with time.[14,15] The exact incidence of breast implant rupture is unknown. Silicone implant ruptures have been linked to breast pain, paresthesias, asymmetric swelling, and breast contracture. In symptomatic women, with either breast pain or contracture, the incidence of rupture is 15% to 33%.[16] In most cases, however, implant rupture goes unnoticed by the patient, with no changes to the shape or feeling of the breast.[17] The frequency of rupture in asymptomatic women has been reported up to 6%.[10]

Magnetic Resonance Imaging of the Implanted Breast

Breast MRI is the modality of choice for the evaluation of silicone implant rupture. MRI conveys the highest sensitivity and specificity for silicone implant rupture.[16-19] In 2005, Holmich and coworkers[17] calculated an accuracy of 92%,

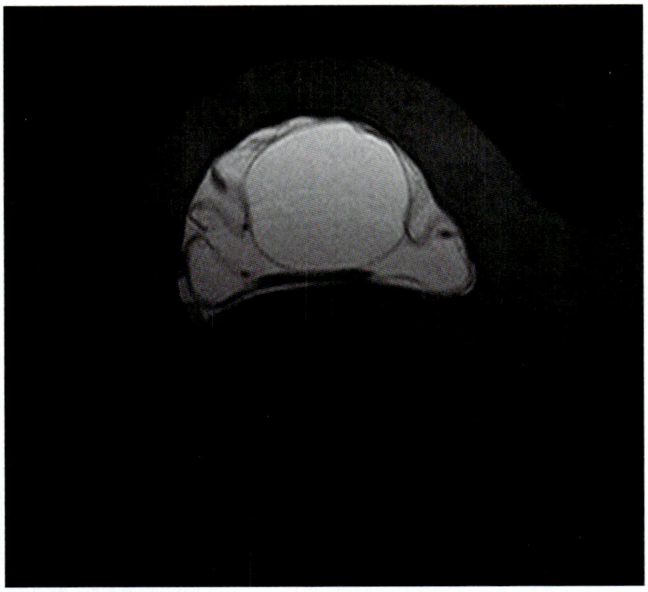

FIGURE 11.7 MRI scan of a triple-lumen implant. Axial T2-weighted image of the breast with fat and water suppression demonstrates an overfilled silicone inner lumen, a collapsed silicone middle lumen, and an intact small outer saline lumen. *(Courtesy of Haydee Fournier Ojeda, MD, University of California, San Diego.)*

a sensitivity of 89%, and a specificity of 97% for implant rupture detection in a population of 118 implants, after comparing with findings at explantation. Silicone has a unique magnetic resonance frequency that allows for silicone-selective sequences to be performed. It is this selective frequency that accounts for the high accuracy and specificity seen with implant-integrity breast MRI. According to Monticciolo and colleagues,[20] the creation of silicone-selective pulse sequences has contributed to the use of MR for detection of implant rupture and subsequent silicone leakage.

Breast MRI also has additional advantages over both mammography and sonography, including the ability to image with multiplanar capability and the lack of ionizing radiation conveyed to the patient. In the setting of an extracapsular rupture, MRI gives a detailed account of silicone migration and the relationship to vital structures, including axillary lymph nodes and the brachial plexus. However, breast MRI has several limitations. MRI is an expensive imaging modality, with a cost several times greater than either mammography or ultrasound. Also, the use of MRI is not available for patients with pacemakers, certain aneurysm clips, foreign bodies in sensitive locations, and for patients limited by claustrophobia or body habitus.

Adequate MRI of the breast requires both specific sequences and dedicated breast imaging equipment to evaluate for implant rupture. A 1.5 Tesla (T) magnet strength or greater is preferred, which allows for detection of more

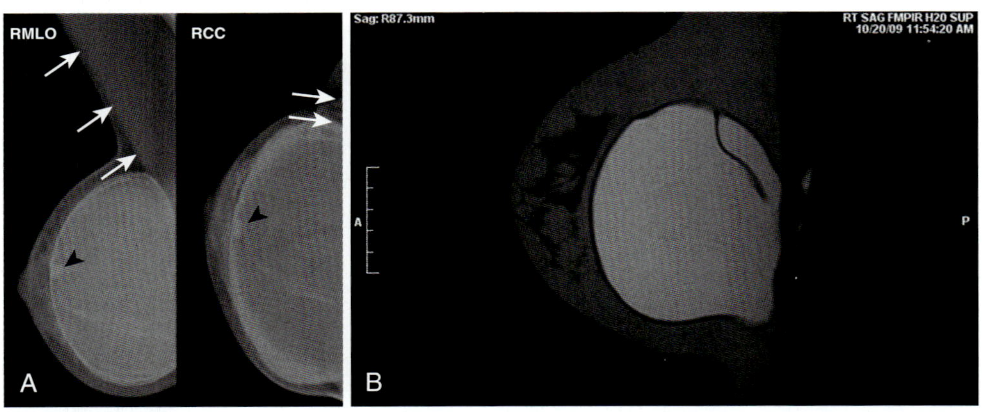

FIGURE 11.8 **(A)** Mammogram and **(B)** sagittal MRI scans demonstrate a silicone implant in a subglandular location. The pectoralis major muscle is seen diving behind the implant *(arrows)*.

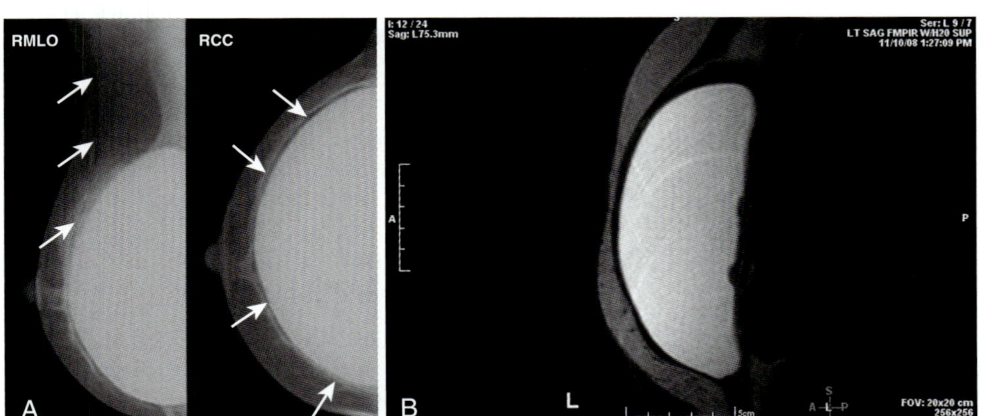

FIGURE 11.9 **(A)** Mammogram and **(B)** sagittal MRI scans demonstrate a silicone implant located behind the pectoralis major muscle *(arrows)*.

subtle signs of intracapsular or extracapsular rupture.[19] Also, the use of a standard body coil does not provide adequate resolution in breast imaging. A dedicated magnetic resonance breast coil is needed for implant-integrity breast imaging. The use of a dedicated breast surface coil improves the accuracy of breast MRI in diagnosing implant rupture.[19,21] For diagnosing extracapsular rupture, T2-weighted images with both chemical fat suppression and water suppression should be obtained. This sequence allows for the greatest contrast difference between silicone and the surrounding breast tissue. Extracapsular rupture is not well depicted on fast spin echo T1-weighted images.

MRI of the breast can also be used as a problem-solving tool in patients who plan to undergo revision implant surgery. Often, patients who need a revision of their silicone implants have no specific information about their current implant size, making surgical planning difficult. Clinical estimates of implant volumes can be widely inaccurate, especially if the implants have ruptured or are severely contracted. A calculation of silicone breast implant volume can be performed using breast MRI and a commercially available computer-aided detection (CAD) system with sufficiently accurate results.[22] Calculating accurate implant volume may have a clinical benefit in planning implant revision surgery.

MRI of the breast is also considered the modality of choice for detecting breast cancer in patients who have undergone free silicone injections.[23] In the 1960s and 1970s, free silicone injections were less costly than implants and therefore appealed to women who were unaware of the risks and complications. The injected free silicone is randomly distributed in the breast and limits both the mammographic and sonographic evaluation for breast cancer (Figure 11.10). In the setting of silicone-induced mastopathy, fibrous silicone breast masses are difficult to distinguish from a breast carcinoma. Therefore a combined breast MRI technique using both contrast-enhanced sequences and the T2-weighted sequence with fat and water suppression can be helpful in identifying malignancy in patients with free silicone injections (Figure 11.11).

Finally, MR imaging of the breast using dynamic contrast-enhanced sequences can play an important role in diagnosing malignancies in women with implants. In 1992, Silverstein and coworkers[24] observed a delay in breast cancer diagnosis in patients who had undergone breast implant surgery. However, a 1995 metaanalysis study published in the *New England Journal of Medicine* concluded that there was no significant difference in breast cancer survival rates between women with or without implants. The study also concluded that the distribution of cancers, by stage, in women with breast implants is similar to that of general screened populations.[25] Hence contrast-enhanced imaging of the breast in implanted women should be used as a problem-solving tool, rather than as a screening modality (Figure 11.12).

Implant Complications

The known complications of silicone gel-filled implants include intracapsular rupture, extracapsular rupture, and capsular contracture. Although capsular contracture is predominantly a clinical diagnosis, MRI is the modality of choice to both identify and characterize intracapsular and extracapsular rupture.

Intracapsular rupture is the most common type of rupture, accounting for approximately 80% to 90% of all silicone implant ruptures.[19] In the majority of patients, a fibrous capsule forms as a normal foreign body response around the implant. This fibrous capsule is low signal on all MRI sequences. An intracapsular rupture is a tear or rupture

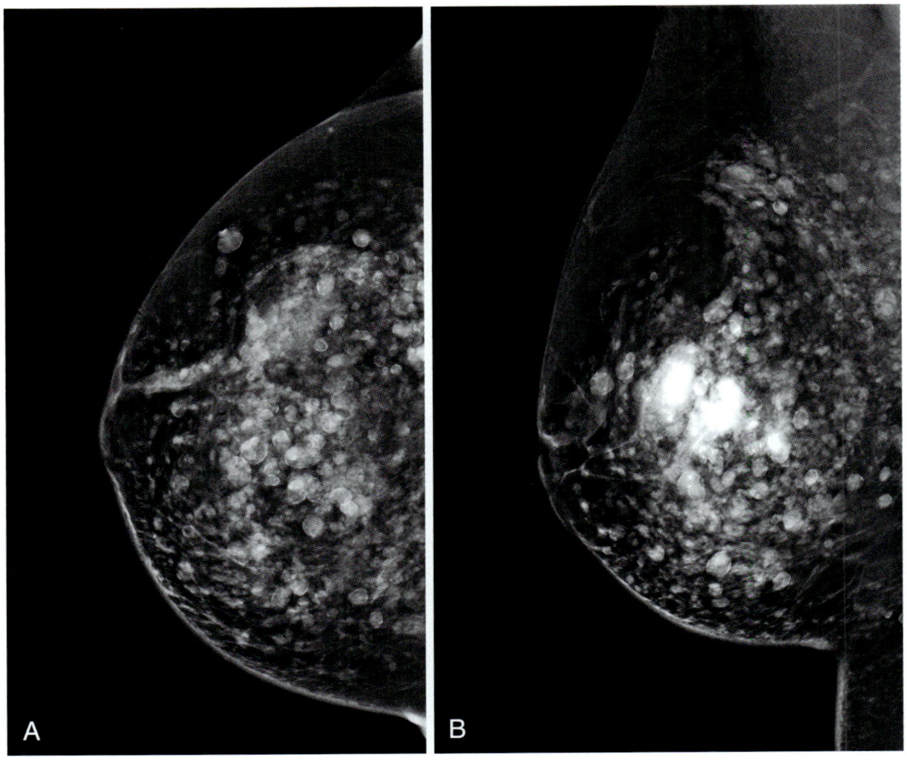

FIGURE 11.10 Mammogram of free silicone injections. **(A)** CC and **(B)** MLO views demonstrate multiple high-density areas throughout the breast representing free silicone injected into the breast.

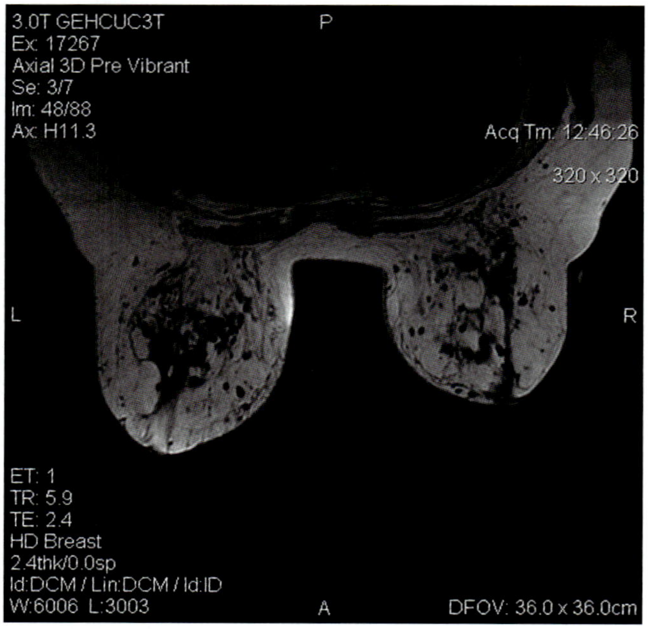

FIGURE 11.11 MRI scan of free silicone injections. Axial precontrast T1-weighted MRI scan demonstrates multiple, round, low-signal masses corresponding to silicone globules.

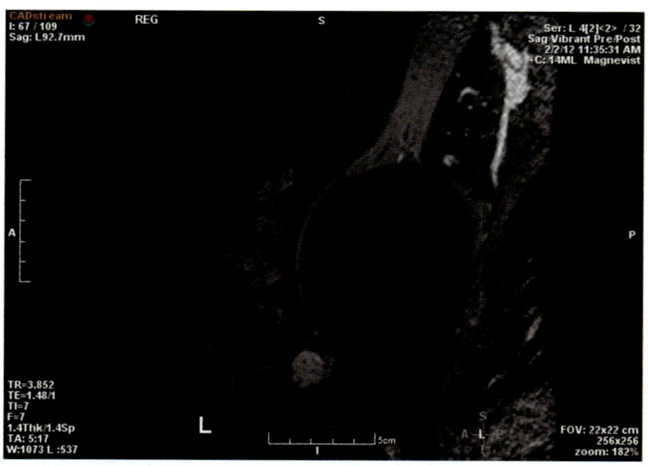

FIGURE 11.12 MRI scan of implant and cancer. Sagittal T1-weighted, fat-suppressed, postcontrast image of the left breast demonstrates a subpectoral implant and irregularly shaped and marginated, enhancing mass proved on biopsy to represent poorly differentiated ductal carcinoma.

of the implant elastomer shell with subsequent silicone leakage that does not extend beyond the fibrous capsule. The silicone is free within the fibrous capsule and no longer contained by the elastomer shell of the implant. An isolated intracapsular rupture cannot be identified mammographically because the intact fibrous capsule maintains the normal shape of the implant on a mammogram.

The *linguini* sign is the most specific MRI finding for the diagnosis of silicone intracapsular rupture.[16,19] The linguini sign is the presence of multiple curvilinear low signal lines floating within the silicone gel, representing the complete collapse of the elastomer implant shell (Figure 11.13). The linguini sign was first coined by Gorczyca and colleagues[26] in a *Radiology* article from 1992. The linguini sign alone is 80% sensitive and 93% specific for the presence of intracapsular rupture.[14]

An early variant of the linguini sign is the *subcapsular* sign. The subcapsular sign is a hypointense line that runs almost parallel to the fibrous capsule, with the beginning and end of the line being followed to the surface of the implant (Figure 11.14). In a 2005 study performed by Holmich and coworkers,[17] the subcapsular line finding was found to be another specific sign of intracapsular rupture.

There are additional signs of intracapsular rupture that are much less specific and can be subtle on magnetic resonance imaging. These signs include both the *keyhole* sign and the *inverted teardrop* or *noose* sign. The keyhole sign is a local invagination of the silicone elastomer shell in which the two sides of the shell do not touch (Figure 11.15). High-signal silicone is seen along the outside of the invaginated shell, suggesting a localized intracapsular rupture. The inverted teardrop or noose sign occurs when the silicone elastomer shell invaginates and the two sides of the membrane oppose one another (Figure 11.16). The implications of a teardrop sign are the same as a keyhole sign, suggesting a localized intracapsular rupture. However, neither the presence of a keyhole or inverted teardrop sign is specific for intracapsular rupture. As much as 50% of the time, these localized findings seen on MRI will be normal at explantation.[12] However, at the same time, 52% of ruptured implants will show only these subtle findings at the time of MR examination.[27]

The phenomena of either a keyhole sign or an inverted teardrop sign has been termed an *uncollapsed silicone implant rupture*. This is considered a type of intracapsular rupture in which there is a localized tear of the implant shell, but the shell collapses only partially. This finding is thought to be common in the third-generation implants that have been manufactured from the 1980s forward. These

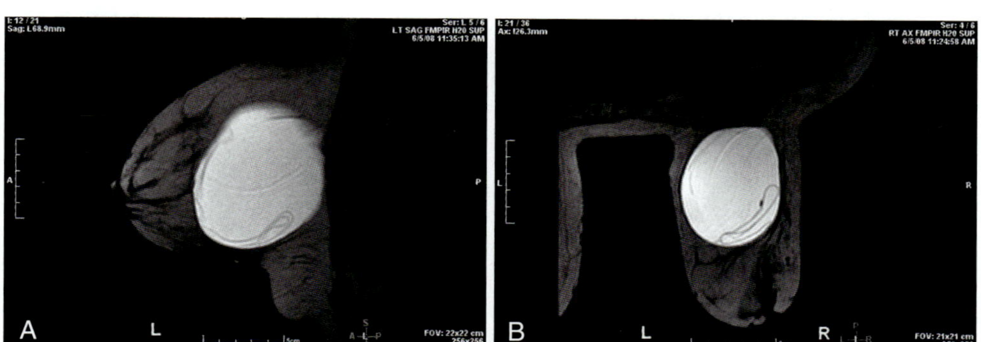

FIGURE 11.13 MRI scan demonstrates the linguini sign. **(A)** Sagittal and **(B)** axial fast spin echo STIR images with water suppression demonstrate a single-lumen subglandular implant with collapse of the elastomer shell, or linguini sign.

implants contain both a thick multilayer elastomer shell and more viscous internal silicone gel. In the event of a rupture these attributes keep the elastomer shell from completely collapsing within the implant and creating the linguini sign.[18]

A gel bleed is the microscopic diffusion of silicone gel through an intact elastomer implant shell. The majority of gel bleeds cannot be detected by MR imaging. When a gel bleed is extensive, either an inverted teardrop or keyhole sign can form. Therefore an uncollapsed implant rupture can have an identical appearance to a large gel bleed. This helps to explain why 50% of the time, the localized MR findings of intracapsular rupture can be normal at explantation. Gel bleeds remain a controversial entity; some feel that the diffusion represents the natural history of silicone implants, and others feel that a gel bleed is a sign of a microscopic tear of the implant shell and impending intracapsular rupture.[16]

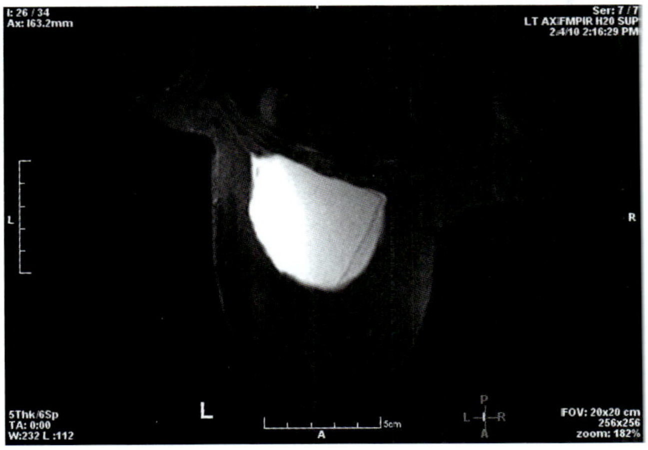

FIGURE 11.14 MRI scan of subcapsular sign. Axial STIR image with water suppression demonstrates a single-lumen silicone implant with an isolated subcapsular line sign along the medial side of the left breast. The subcapsular line is another specific sign of intracapsular rupture.

There are normal postoperative variants of a silicone implant that can mimic the presence of an intracapsular rupture. A radial fold is a normal infolding of the implant (Figure 11.17). Radial folds can be seen as curvilinear lines along the periphery of the implant. A radial fold should always abut the periphery of the implant and should span the entire substance of the gel only at the periphery.[10] Complex or atypical radial folds can be mistaken for an intracapsular rupture. The use of orthogonal imaging can be helpful in differentiating the two entities.

After placement of silicone implants, it is a common practice to inject saline or saline mixed with antibiotics and steroids into the breast prostheses. This practice is used to affect symmetry of the breasts and to decrease the rate of capsular contracture. Therefore small amounts of water signal can be a normal finding in an intact silicone implant, not a sign of intracapsular rupture.[10] However, this appearance of an injected implant can look identical to a double lumen silicone and saline implant with failure of the inner lumen shell.

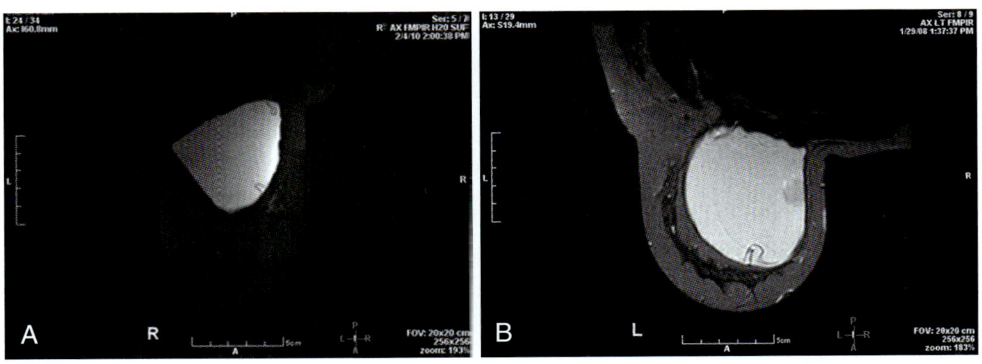

FIGURE 11.15 MRI scan showing the keyhole sign. **A,** Axial STIR image with water suppression demonstrates a keyhole sign along the anterior lateral margin of the right implant. **B,** An axial STIR image of the left breast also has a "keyhole" sign along the anterior margin.

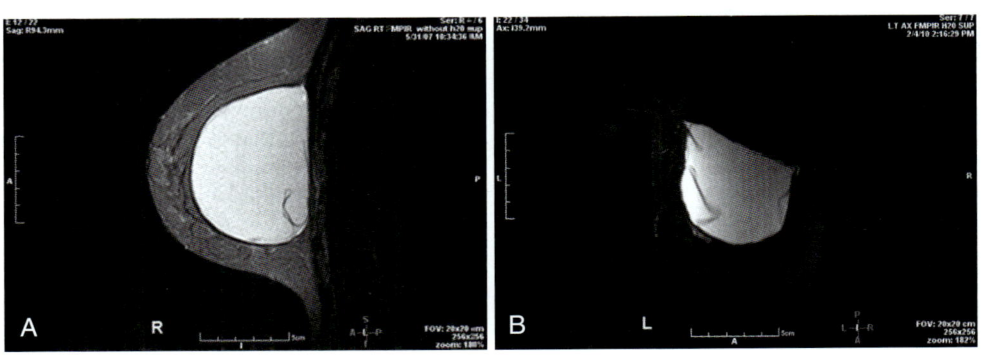

FIGURE 11.16 MRI scan showing an inverted teardrop or noose sign. **A,** A sagittal T2-weighted image of a subglandular implant demonstrating an "inverted teardrop" sign. **B,** A T2-weighted fast spin echo axial image with both water and fat suppression that demonstrates two inverted teardrop signs along the anterior and posterior lateral margins of the left implant. An additional subcapsular sign is seen along the medial margin.

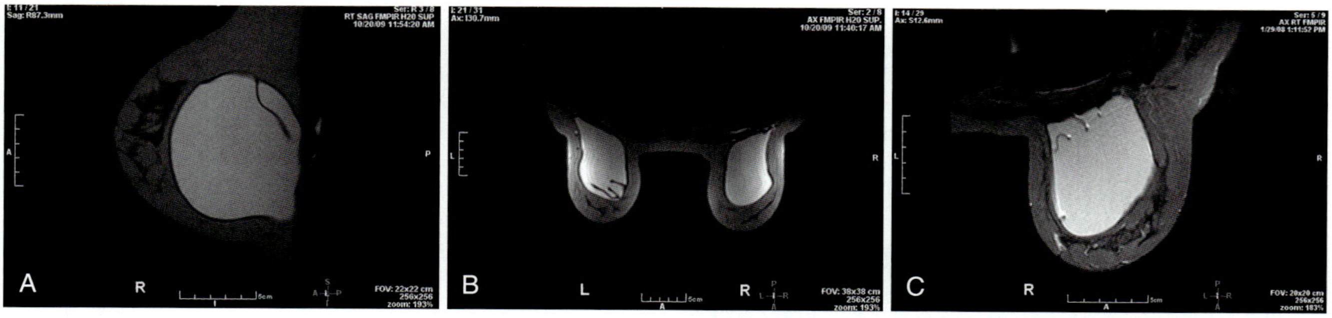

FIGURE 11.17 MRI scan showing a radial fold. **A,** Sagittal T2-weighted water- and fat-suppressed image of the right breast with a single radial fold along the superior margin of the subglandular silicone implant. **B,** Axial images of both breasts with multiple radial folds seen anteriorly on the left. **C,** A T2-weighted axial fast spin echo image with fat suppression only. This image demonstrates multiple radial folds along the posterior medial margin of the right breast.

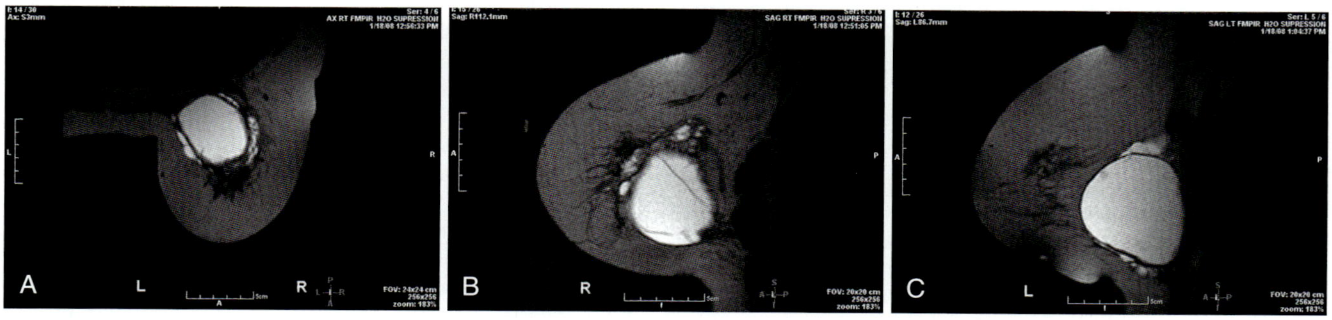

FIGURE 11.18 MRI scan showing extracapsular rupture. **(A)** Axial and **(B and C)** sagittal T2-weighted fast spin echo images with fat and water suppression demonstrate bilateral extracapsular ruptures. Multiple high-signal masses of extracapsular silicone are seen extending along the periphery of both implants.

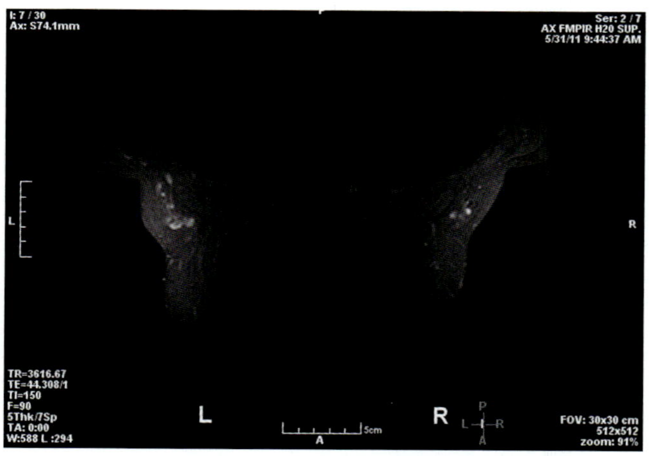

FIGURE 11.19 MRI scan showing silicone migration. An axial T2-weighted fast spin echo image with water and fat suppression of both axillae demonstrates multiple high-signal lymph nodes. Silicone from an extracapsular rupture has been taken up by the lymphatic system, resulting in silicone migration and silicone lymphadenopathy.

An extracapsular rupture is a breach of both the elastomer shell of the implant and the surrounding fibrous capsule (Figure 11.18). This results in a macroscopic leakage of silicone through the fibrous capsule and into the surrounding tissues of the breast. On T2-weighted fat- and water-suppressed MRI scans, this extracapsular rupture is frequently seen as one, or often more, high-signal round or oval masses, adjacent to or extending away from the implant. An intracapsular rupture must be present in the setting of an extracapsular rupture. The prevalence of extracapsular spread of silicone has been reported as 11% to 23% in studies of surgically removed implants.[27,28]

When silicone gel extends beyond the fibrous capsule, a granulomatous reaction and scar formation usually develop. A siliconoma is a masslike focal collection of histiocytes and foreign body giant cells surrounded by and engulfing silicone. The formation of a siliconoma is the body's natural response to help wall off the foreign substance. These siliconomas result in palpable and sometimes painful masses in the breast. Silicone lymphadenopathy is also a common finding in the setting of an extracapsular rupture. Silicone can be taken up by the lymphatic system and migrate to the axilla. Silicone migration into the axilla can then involve the brachial plexus, resulting in varying neuropathies.

Silicone migrations to the lymph nodes, arms, subcutaneous tissues of the abdominal wall, and to the inguinal canals have also been reported (Figure 11.19).[27] Fistulous drainage of the siliconoma and formation of skins ulcers are also known complications of extracapsular rupture.[27] The local complications of free silicone from extracapsular rupture are the same adverse effects as are seen with direct silicone injection. The surgery performed to remove extracapsular silicone can be technically difficult. Often multiple surgeries are required to remove the full extent of the silicone.[21]

With implant-integrity MRI of the breast, false-positive diagnoses of extracapsular rupture can occur. A detailed

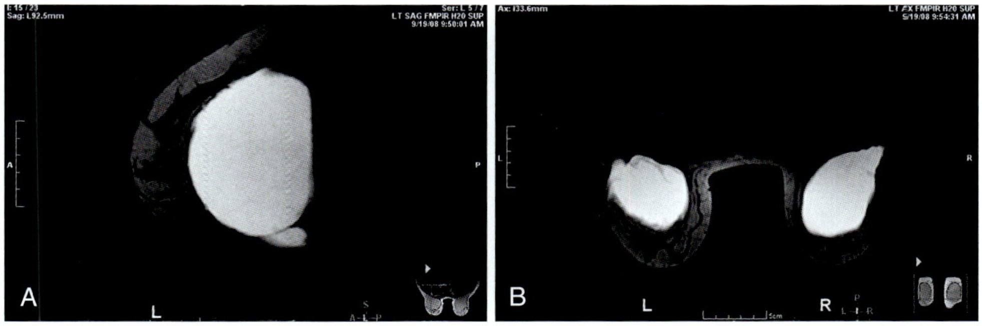

FIGURE 11.20 MRI scan shows a bulge, not a rupture. **(A)** Sagittal and **(B)** axial T2-weighted fast spin each image with both fat and water suppression, demonstrating a focal bulge of the inferior, lateral, and posterior left subglandular implant. On the sagittal image, the focal bulge of the implant mimics an extracapsular rupture.

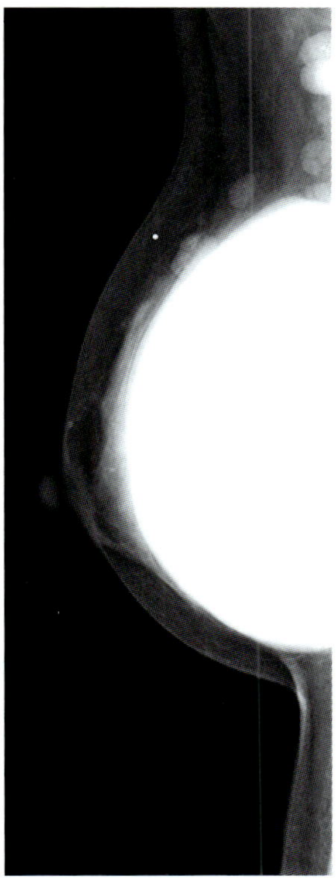

FIGURE 11.21 Mammogram of extracapsular rupture. MLO view of the right breast demonstrates a subpectoral silicone implant. A BB overlies the superior breast, marking the site of a palpable lump. There are multiple high-density masses in the superior breast and axilla, evidence of an extracapsular rupture and silicone lymphadenopathy.

clinical history should be obtained prior to interpreting implant studies. For a subset of patients, there may be a clinical history of previous extracapsular implant rupture or of free silicone injections into the breast. Thus the presence of extracapsular silicone on an implant-integrity MRI scan may not always indicate an acute rupture. Also, a focal bulge of the fibrous capsule can be problematic when interpreting an implant-integrity breast MRI. The bulge can be difficult to distinguish from a true extracapsular rupture (Figure 11.20).[12,21] Finally, fluid collections surrounding the implant should not be considered a sign of extracapsular rupture. The textured surface or PTU-covered silicone implants are commonly associated with reactive fluid collections around the implant. On a T2-weighted sequence with fat and water suppression, these peri-implant fluid collections should remain low in signal and therefore not mimic an extracapsular rupture.

Capsular contracture is the most common long-term complication of breast implants. A fibrous capsule is the body's normal response to the placement of a breast implant, and this fibrous capsule occurs around all implants to a varying degree. If this capsule becomes thickened, the capsule can begin to strangulate the implant. This can result in an alteration of the breast shape and a stiffening of the breast that no longer feels natural to the patient. Capsular contracture can also result in profound discomfort in the breast.

Capsular contracture is more frequently seen in patients with either smooth-surfaced implants or with subglandular implants. According to Morgan and colleagues,[10] capsular contracture occurs in up to 10% to 25% of patients who have received smooth-surfaced silicone prostheses. The intended purpose of both the textured surface and the PTU coating on more recent implant designs has been to promote tissue ingrowth and to reduce capsular contracture.[3] The breast contracture can occur any time after the placement of the implants but most commonly occurs within the first few postoperative months.[1]

Capsular contracture is predominantly a clinical diagnosis, with the palpation of a spherical, firm, or distorted breast. Radiographic findings are rarely present. On breast MRI, a focal asymmetric serrated appearance to the fibrous capsule has been described as a typical finding in capsular contracture.[10] Also, a transverse diameter of the breast that measures less than 2 times the anterior to posterior depth of the implant corresponds to clinically evident contracture.[10]

The treatment of capsular contracture consists of either a closed or open capsulotomy.[29] The closed capsulotomy consists of physical compression of the breast to break the capsule and soften the feel of the implant. An open capsulotomy involves surgical removal of the fibrous capsule.

Mammographic and Sonographic Evaluation of Implants

Although implant-integrity breast MRI is the imaging modality of choice for the diagnosis of silicone implant rupture, both mammography and ultrasound are additional tools that can be used by the radiologist. Both mammography and ultrasound can be diagnostic for silicone implant rupture, although the sensitivity of these two modalities does not approach that of breast MRI.

Mammography can accurately depict extracapsular silicone that has been extruded into the breast tissue adjacent

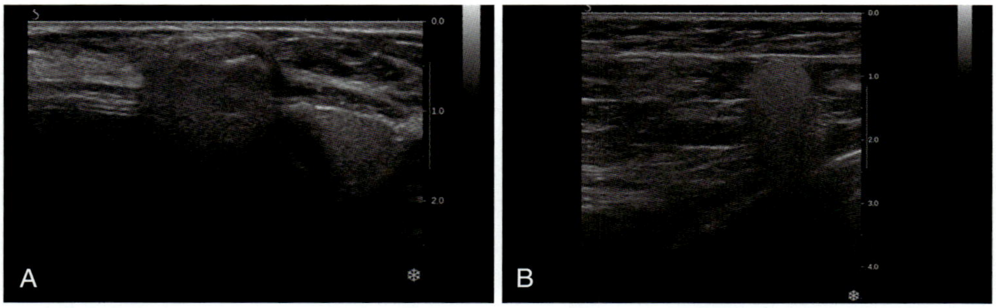

FIGURE 11.22 Ultrasound image shows the snowstorm sign. **A** and **B**, Echogenic masses along the periphery of the implant with sharp anterior and fading posterior margins consistent with the snowstorm sign.

to the implant (Figure 11.21). On a mammogram, extracapsular silicone appears as lobular or spherical dense areas of opacity that are immediately adjacent to the implant or separate from it. An additional sign of implant rupture includes a new asymmetry in either the size or shape of the implant. A new focal herniation or bulge of the implant is also concerning for rupture. Before the diagnosis of rupture is made, a review of the patient's pertinent clinical history is recommended. The patient may have a history of a prior ruptured implant with subsequent revision or a history of free silicone injections. Both of these events could be mistaken for a rupture of the current implant.

There are advantages in using mammography over other modalities in the diagnosis of implant rupture. Mammography is inexpensive, with the cost of a mammogram being at least 3 times less than a breast MRI. Also, women older than the age of 40 years typically already undergo yearly mammography.

However, there are significant limitations to mammography. Dense silicone is not easily penetrated by x-ray, and therefore intracapsular rupture cannot be diagnosed with a mammogram. Mammography also has a limited field of view, with only the breast tissue immediately adjacent to the implant being imaged. An extracapsular rupture with migration to the axilla may be missed with mammography, as well as an extracapsular rupture that is located posterior to the implant. Finally, a focal bulge of the fibrous capsule can be difficult to differentiate from extruded extracapsular silicone.

Ultrasound can also be a valuable imaging tool in detecting a ruptured silicone implant. Ultrasound can detect implant rupture with a sensitivity ranging from 50% to 77%, and a specificity ranging from 55% to 84%.[30,31] Ultrasonography is extremely operator-dependent, and the large range of sensitivities and specificities may reflect differences in operator experience and the type of equipment used. Ultrasonographic signs of implant rupture include both the *stepladder* and the *snowstorm* signs.

The stepladder sign is used to identify an intracapsular rupture. The stepladder sign is a series of echogenic straight or curvilinear lines that traverse the interior of the implant. These lines represent the collapsed elastomer shell of the implant. The stepladder sign is analogous to the linguini sign seen on MRI of the breast.

The snowstorm sign is used to identity an extracapsular rupture on ultrasound. The snowstorm appearance is a highly echogenic pattern of scattered and reverberating echoes seen along the periphery of the implant (Figure 11.22). These echogenic nodules have a well-defined anterior margin and a loss of the circumscribed margin posteriorly. These echogenic nodules are synonymous with silicone granulomas, causing an abnormal dispersion of the ultrasound beam. The same appearance occurs in the axilla in cases of silicone migration to axillary lymph nodes.

An advantage of ultrasound is that the cost is relatively low compared with MRI of the breast. Ultrasound is also a useful tool in patients who are unable to undergo MRI because of claustrophobia, body habitus, or other contraindications. Finally, ultrasound is similar to MRI in that the patient is not exposed to ionizing radiation.

The limitations of ultrasonography for evaluating implant rupture cannot be ignored. Because of silicone's ability to markedly attenuate the ultrasound beam, evaluation of the back wall of an implant and the tissues posterior to the implant is limited. Also, normal reverberation artifact from the implant can be confused with the stepladder sign and intracapsular rupture. Similar to what happens with mammography and MRI, a prior history of either silicone injections or previous extracapsular rupture can be mistaken for a current implant rupture. Echogenic noise from a remote silicone rupture can make accurate evaluation of the current implant impossible.

Conclusion

MRI is the procedure of choice for evaluation of silicone breast implant integrity. Familiarity with the types of implants available, the various surgical procedures for placement, and the patient's prior breast history are critical for accurate assessment.

References

1. Yang N, Muradali D: The augmented breast: a pictorial review of the abnormal and unusual, *AJR Am J Roentgenol* 196:W451–W460, 2011.
2. Spear SL, Parikh PM Goldstein JA: History of breast implants and the Food and Drug Administration, *Clin Plast Surg* 36:15–21, 2009.
3. Middleton MS, McNamara MP: Breast implant classification with MR imaging correlation, *Radiographics* 20:e1–e2, 2000.
4. Bassett LW, Mahoney MC, Apple SK, D'Orsi CJ: *Breast imaging*, Philadelphia, PA, 2011, Elsevier Inc.
5. Glynn C, Litherland J: Imaging breast augmentation and reconstruction: pictorial review, *Br J Radiol* 81:587–595, 2008.
6. Hennekens CH, Lee IM, Cook NR, et al: Self-reported breast implants and connective-tissue diseases in female health professionals. A retrospective cohort study *JAMA* 275:616–621, 1996.
7. Solomon G: A clinical and laboratory profile of symptomatic women with breast implants, *Semin Arthritis Rheum* 24:29–37, 1994.
8. Gabriel SE, O'Fallon WM, Kurland LT, et al: Risk of connective-tissue diseases and other disorders after breast implantation, *N Engl J Med* 330:1697–1702, 1994.
9. Bondurant S, Ernster V, Herdman R, editors: *Safety of silicone breast implants. Institute of Medicine (US) Committee on the Safety of Silicone Breast Implants*, Washington, 1999, National Academies Press.
10. Morgan DE, Kenney PJ, et al: MR imaging of breast implants and their complications, *AJR Am J Roentgenol* 167:1271–1275, 1996.
11. Berg WA, Anderson ND, Zerhouni EA, et al: MR imaging of the breast in patients with silicone breast implants: normal postoperative variants and diagnostic pitfall, *AJR Am J Roentgenol* 163:575–578, 1994.
12. Berg WA, Nguyen TK, Middleton MS, et al: MR imaging of extracapsular silicone from breast implants: diagnostic pitfalls, *AJR Am J Roentgenol* 178:465–472, 2002.
13. Brown SL, Middleton MS, Berg WA, et al: Prevalence of rupture of silicone gel breast implants revealed on MR imaging in a population of women in Birmingham, Alabama, *AJR Am J Roentgenol* 175:1057–1064, 2000.
14. Herborn CU, Marincek B, Erfmann D, et al: Breast augmentation and reconstructive surgery: MR imaging of implant rupture and malignancy, *Eur Radiol* 12:2198–2206, 2002.
15. De Camara DL, Sheridan JM, Kammer BA: Ruptures and aging of silicone gel breast implants, *Plast Reconstr Surg* 91:828–834, 1993.
16. Paetau AA, McLaughlin SA, McNeil RB, et al: Capsular contracture and possible implant rupture: Is magnetic resonance imaging useful? *Plast Reconstr Surg* 125:830–835, 2010.
17. Holmich LR, Vejborg I, Conrad C, et al: The diagnoses of breast implant rupture: MRI findings compared with findings at explantation, *J Radiol Online* 53:2123–2225, 2005.
18. Gorcyzca DP: MR imaging of breast implants, *Magn Reson Imaging Clin North Am* 2:659, 1994.
19. Gorcyzca DP, Gorczyzca SM, Gorczyca KL: The diagnosis of silicone breast implant rupture, *Plast Recosntr Surg* 120(Suppl 1):S49, 2007.
20. Monticciolo DL, Nelson RC, Dixon WT, et al: MR detection of leakage from silicone breast implants: value of a silicone-selective pulse sequence, *AJR Am J Roentgenol* 163:51–56, 1994.
21. Berg WA, Caskey CI, Hamper UM, et al: Diagnosing breast implant rupture with MR imaging, US and mammography, *Radiographics* 13:1323–1336, 1993.
22. Rudolph R, Forcier N: Calculation of silicone breast implant volumes using breast magnetic resonance imaging, *Aesthetic Surg J* 29:310–313, 2009.
23. Po J, Margolis DJ, Cunningham CH, et al: Water-selective spectral-spatial contrast-enhanced breast MRI for cancer detection in patients with extracapsular and injected free silicone, *Magn Reson Imaging* 24:1363–1367, 2006.
24. Silverstein MJ, Handel N, Gamagami P, et al: Breast cancer diagnosis and prognosis in women following augmentation with silicone gel-filled prostheses, *Eur J Cancer* 28:635–640, 1992.
25. Bryant H, Brasher P: Breast implants and breast cancer: reanalysis of a linkage study, *N Engl J Med* 332:1535–1539, 1995.
26. Gorczyca DP, Sinha S, Ahn CY, et al: Silicone breast implants in vivo: MR imaging, *Radiology* 185:407–410, 1992.
27. Caskey CI, Berg WA, Hamper VM, et al: Imaging spectrum of extracapsular silicone: correlation of US, MR imaging, mammographic and histo-pathologic findings, *Radiographics* 19:S39–S51, 1999.
28. Brown SL, Silverman BG, Berg WA: Rupture of silicone-gel breast implants: causes, sequelae, and diagnosis, *Lancet* 350:1531–1537, 1997.
29. Cardenosa G: *Breast imaging companion*, ed 3, Philadelphia, 2008, Lippincott Williams &Wilkins, p 462.
30. Venta LA, Salomon CG, Flisak ME, et al: Sonographic signs of breast implant rupture, *AJR Am J Roentgenol* 166:1413–1419, 1996.
31. Caskey CI, Berg WA, Anderson ND, et al: Breast implant rupture: diagnosis with US, *Radiology* 190:819–823, 1994.

CHAPTER 12

MRI-Guided Breast Biopsy

Carol H. Lee

When a suspicious finding is seen on a breast magnetic resonance imaging (MRI) examination and other imaging and clinical examinations are negative, the only way to perform a biopsy of the lesion is by using MRI guidance. All facilities that perform breast MRI should have the ability to perform MRI-guided biopsy. If it is not offered, patients must go elsewhere for the procedure, adding time, inconvenience, and cost to the process.

The American College of Radiology breast MRI accreditation program requires that facilities have MRI biopsy capability or have a formal relationship with another facility that will accept their patients for biopsy without repeating the examination.[1] Not only is offering MRI-guided biopsy good medical practice that benefits patients more and more insurers are demanding accreditation of facilities in various modalities, including breast MRI, in order to receive reimbursement.

The steps in performing MRI-guided biopsy are similar to stereotactic breast biopsy, but there are factors and challenges that are unique to this procedure, including limited time of lesion visibility and lack of confirmation of lesion sampling. Despite this, experience with MRI-guided core biopsy has shown that this technique is effective[2-6] with a high technical success rate. Lehman and colleagues[4] reported successful tissue retrieval in 100% of 35 lesions. Liberman and coworkers[5] were able to retrieve tissue in 95 (97%) of 98 biopsies, and Perlet and colleagues[6] reported that 517 (96%) of 538 biopsies in their series could be completed.

The positive predictive value (PPV) of MRI-guided biopsies has been reported to be 18% to 61%, with most studies reporting a PPV of about 25% to 40%.[2-7] The variation is likely caused by differences in patient populations and in interpretive criteria. It has been shown that the positive biopsy rate is higher for abnormalities found on diagnostic MRI than on screening studies and is highest for lesions found in the ipsilateral breast of women with a new diagnosis of breast cancer.[8,9]

Patient and Lesion Selection

There are safety considerations in performing breast MRI, and some patients are not candidates for this examination. However, patients in whom MRI-guided biopsy is being considered have already had an MRI that identified the suspicious abnormality, making it less likely that safety is a contraindication. Aside from safety considerations, patient factors that are relative contraindications to MRI-guided biopsy are very few and are largely limited to bleeding diatheses.

In terms of lesion selection, when a suspicious abnormality is seen on MRI and biopsy is recommended, the most recent mammogram should be reviewed to determine whether there is a corresponding abnormality that might guide excision. Targeted ultrasound should also be considered, especially for enhancing masses because biopsy under ultrasound guidance is faster, easier, and less expensive than MRI-guided procedures. Abe and coworkers[10] reported finding a sonographic correlate in 57% (115/202) of suspicious MRI lesions for which targeted ultrasound was done, and Meissnitzer and colleagues[11] reported finding a sonographic correlate in 56% (290/519). However, the Meissnitzer group also reported that on follow-up of 80 cases, the ultrasound finding was not the same as the MRI finding in 10 lesions (12.5%), 5 of which had been benign on ultrasound but actually proved to be malignant on MRI-guided biopsy. Therefore, whenever an ultrasound correlate is thought to be found for a suspicious MRI lesion and the biopsy results are benign and concordant, follow-up MRI should be done to be certain that the lesions are the same (Figure 12.1).

When there is no sonographic or mammographic correlate and MRI-guided biopsy is necessary, it should be recognized that there are lesions that are not amenable to MRI-guided core biopsy. These include those that are very posterior in the breast, very superficial, close to the nipple, lesions in breasts that are very thin, and some lesions in women with implants. For suspicious lesions that are seen only on MRI for which tissue diagnosis is desired and for which MRI-guided core biopsy is not technically feasible because of lesion location or the size of the breast, MRI-guided wire localization with an MRI-compatible wire can be performed. These wires are virtually identical in design to conventional localizing wires that are placed under mammographic or ultrasound guidance, but they are thinner and tend to be more prone to transection in the operating room.[12]

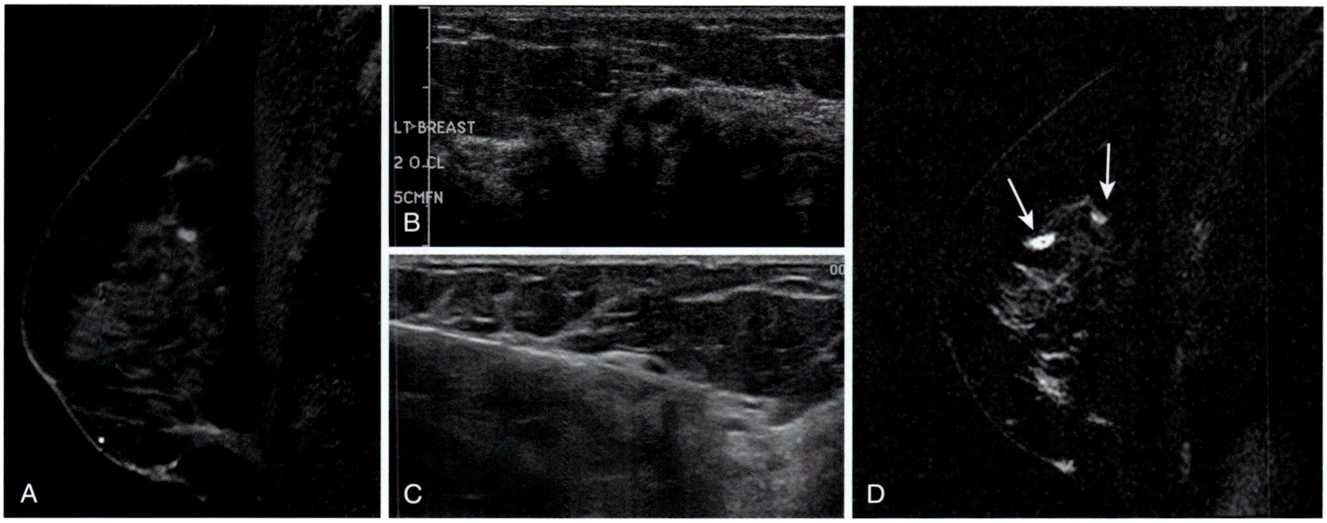

FIGURE 12.1 Mistaken sonographic correlate to MRI lesion. **A,** Sagittal T1 postcontrast subtraction MRI scan of a 48-year-old woman with newly diagnosed invasive lobular carcinoma left breast (not shown) has an enhancing mass in a different quadrant of the left breast. **B,** Image from a targeted ultrasound shows a mass of similar size and shape to the MRI finding thought to represent the sonographic correlate. **C,** Ultrasound-guided biopsy was done and yielded fibroadenoma, which was thought to be concordant. **D,** T2-weighted postbiopsy MRI scan shows the postbiopsy change (*arrow*) separate from enhancing mass (*arrowhead*). MRI-guided biopsy was done and showed invasive lobular carcinoma.

Patient Preparation Before the Procedure

Anticoagulation with warfarin (Coumadin) is usually reversed before performing core biopsy procedures. In some women, however, the medical risks of reversing anticoagulation may be so great as to require bridge therapy with low-molecular-weight heparin to safely prevent thrombotic or embolic events. Communication and cooperation between the radiologist who is recommending and/or performing the biopsy and the referring clinician are especially crucial in these patients.

Aspirin and nonsteroidal anti-inflammatory agents such as ibuprofen can also be associated with prolonged bleeding and are often stopped for 5 to 7 days before the biopsy. Melotti and Berg[13] reviewed their experience with performing core biopsies on women on anticoagulation and reported that 3 (38%) of 8 patients on anticoagulation developed hematomas larger than 1 cm compared with 13 (8%) of 171 women who were not anticoagulated. However, none of the patients on either warfarin or aspirin who underwent stereotactic core biopsy with an 11-gauge needle required surgical intervention to stop bleeding or to evacuate a hematoma. They concluded that core biopsy in women on anticoagulation or aspirin therapy can be performed without stopping the medication if there are compelling reasons to do so, such as a patient's inability to come back for the procedure at another time or possible noncompliance with a recommendation for biopsy if performed at a later date. Similar results were reported by Somerville and coworkers,[14] who compared 200 women on anticoagulation with 855 women who were not and who underwent biopsy with 14-gauge or larger needles. There were significantly more bruises among women on anticoagulation but no significant difference in hematoma formation between the two groups, and none of the patients required surgical intervention. The numbers in these studies are small, however, with only 8 anticoagulated patients undergoing biopsy with an 11-gauge vacuum device in the report by Melotti and Berg and a total of 16 patients on warfarin in the report by Somerville and coworkers.[13,14] Melotti and Berg report that they still reverse anticoagulation or withhold aspirin for 7 days in most cases, and Somerville and coworkers give the patients the option of stopping anticoagulation medications or proceeding with the biopsy.[13,14] If a patient on warfarin elects not to stop anticoagulation, they recommend that the international normalized ratio be checked to be certain the patient is not above the therapeutic range.

With regard to prophylactic antibiotics, there is no evidence that these are indicated prior to MRI-guided core biopsy.

Informed Consent

As with any interventional procedure, informed consent should be obtained after the risks and benefits are explained to the patient. There are little data on the incidence of complications associated with MRI-guided biopsies. There is information, however, on other core biopsy procedures, namely those done with stereotactic and ultrasound guidance, showing a low incidence of complications.[15,16] Serious complications from vacuum-assisted core biopsies are infrequent, reported in about 1% of cases.[15,16] Infection after core biopsy is another uncommon occurrence.[15]

Besides potential complications, a discussion of the need for clip placement, as well as the need for follow-up MRI if the results of the biopsy prove to be benign, is sometimes included. Additionally, it is often a good idea to formulate a plan before the biopsy for conveying results to the patient, including when pathology results can be expected, who will convey them, and how this will be done (either in person or by telephone).

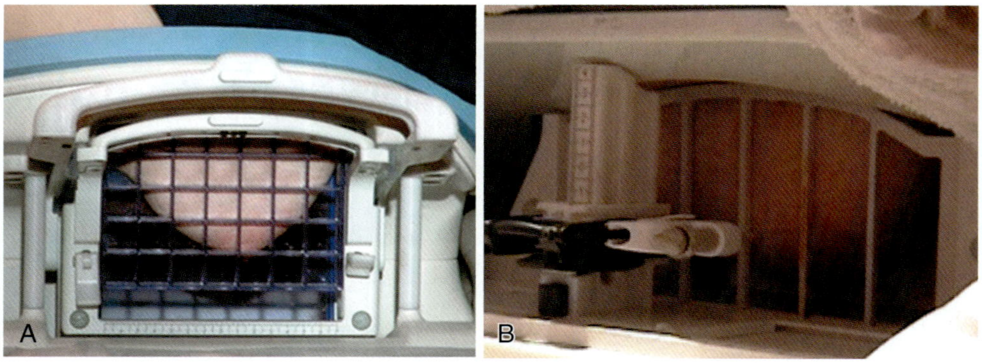

FIGURE 12.2 Targeting devices. **A,** Grid device. **B,** Pillar-and-post device.

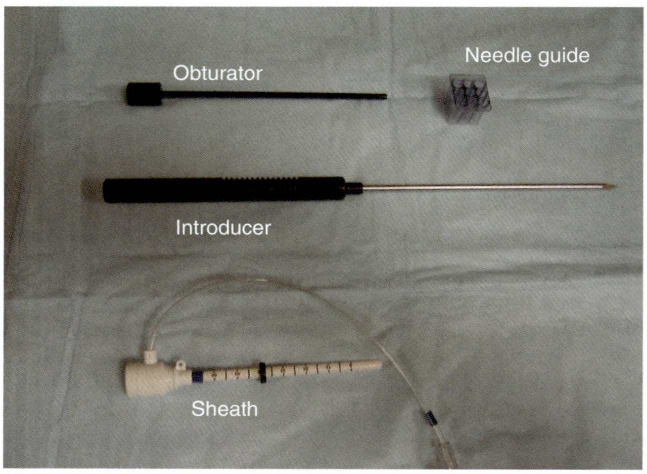

FIGURE 12.3 An introducer set.

Equipment Selection

Magnet Strength

Equipment is available for performing MRI-guided core biopsies on both 1.5 and 3.0 Tesla (T) magnets. There is no evidence that doing the biopsy on a machine with a different field strength from that in which the diagnostic study was done poses any problems. For example, a biopsy can be done on a 1.5 T scanner after a diagnostic study is done on a 3.0 T magnet, and vice versa.

Targeting Equipment

A variety of different devices that add onto the breast coil are available that allow for targeting of the enhancing lesion. These devices use either a grid compression plate or a pillar-and-post apparatus (Figure 12.2). All allow approach from the lateral aspect of the breast, and many also allow medial access. Newer coils are being developed that will enable approach from other directions.

Vacuum-Assisted Devices

A number of different devices are used for vacuum-assisted MRI core biopsies ranging from 7- to 11-gauge needles. Vacuum-assisted core biopsy with needles that are 11 gauge or larger have been shown to result in more accurate results than 14 gauge automated core biopsies.[17] All have basically the same design, with a plastic sheath that allows the calculated depth of the lesion to be set. A sharp introducer is placed through the sheath and allows the sheath to be positioned in the breast. There is a plastic obturator that is then placed to allow scanning to confirm accurate positioning of the sheath. Finally, the sampling device is placed through the sheath, and tissue samples are obtained. An example of an introducer set is shown in Figure 12.3. Some of the vacuum-assisted devices have a self-contained vacuum, but most have a console that provides the suction and remains outside of the magnet room, connected to the needle by long tubing. With some of the vacuum-assisted devices, the cores are collected automatically in a chamber, and with others the cores are retrieved manually with each pass. Following the procedure, a variety of MRI-compatible clips are available that can be placed at the biopsy site.

Biopsy Technique

Before an MRI-guided biopsy is performed, the diagnostic study that prompted the biopsy recommendation should be thoroughly reviewed and the approach planned. This is particularly important for MRI-guided procedures because of limited time of lesion visibility owing to washout of contrast and enhancement of the surrounding normal parenchyma over time. The reported average time to perform a vacuum-assisted core biopsy of a single lesion under MRI ranges from 35 to 58 minutes.[2,18,19] Scheduling one or one-and-a-half hours of magnet time is usually sufficient. Multiple and bilateral lesions will, of course, require more time. Lehman and coworkers[18] reported that the mean time for biopsy of multiple lesions in one breast was 59 minutes and for bilateral lesions was 64 minutes, compared with a mean of 38 minutes for a single lesion. Similarly, Liberman and colleagues[2] reported a mean time of 35 minutes for a single lesion and 65 minutes for two lesions.

Biopsy coils generally allow approach from either the lateral or medial surface, and the approach that represents the shortest distance to the lesion should be chosen. In general, a sagittal sequence is used to determine which opening in the grid is to be used. It is useful for facilities that acquire primary diagnostic images axially either to obtain a sagittal sequence as the last postcontrast series or to acquire images with isotropic voxels that allow subsequent reformatting in any plane without substantial loss of resolution. Some biopsy coils allow a fenestrated grid to be placed laterally and medially at the same time. This is advantageous when the lesion is close to the midline and allows more flexibility of approach. Care should be taken, however, not to confuse the medial and lateral aspects of the breast on the subsequent images. One way of ensuring easy differentiation is to place one fiducial on one side and two on the other, or to place the fiducial marker on the superior aspect of the breast on one surface and inferiorly on the other.

Multiple Lesions

Multiple lesions in one breast can often be biopsied during the same session. Coils that allow both a lateral and medial approach at the same time can be used if the lesions are on opposite sides of the breast. Bilateral lesions can also be successfully biopsied during the same session if the lesions are accessible from the lateral approach in each breast. If not, they will likely need to be sampled on different days.

Patient Positioning

As with diagnostic MRI, the intravenous line should be placed before the patient is put in the magnet and the patient should be positioned in the breast coil by either an experienced technologist or by the physician who is doing the procedure. Often, facilities that are just starting to perform MRI-guided biopsies will have mammography technologists who are experienced in positioning for stereotactic biopsies position the patient's breast in the coil, because the techniques are similar. The breast tissue should be pulled into the coil to maximize the amount of tissue visualized, and then compression can be applied. The compression should be firm enough to ensure that the lesion does not move, but not so much as to compromise enhancement. Time and care should be taken to maximize patient comfort to minimize patient movement during the procedure.

Contrast Administration

Most abnormalities that are undergoing MRI-guided biopsy are not seen without the administration of intravenous contrast. Power injection is not necessary because kinetics will not be assessed. However, giving a contrast agent without having to move the patient out of the magnet—either with a power injector that is connected to the IV line beforehand or hand injecting through connecting tubing—is desirable to minimize the possibility of patient motion.

Targeting

All of the commercially available computer-aided detection (CAD) products have biopsy-targeting software that can be used to target lesions. These programs usually require use of a particular fiducial marker and can automatically calculate lesion location in relation to the position of the fiducial marker from either an axial or a sagittal sequence (Figure 12.4). However, biopsies can be quickly and successfully performed without these programs, and computer malfunction or software problems can occur. Therefore knowledge of the procedure of manual lesion targeting without computerized software is essential. Targeting is slightly different between a grid compression device and the pillar-and-post method. There are advantages and disadvantages to each. Targeting with the grid device is often simpler and faster.

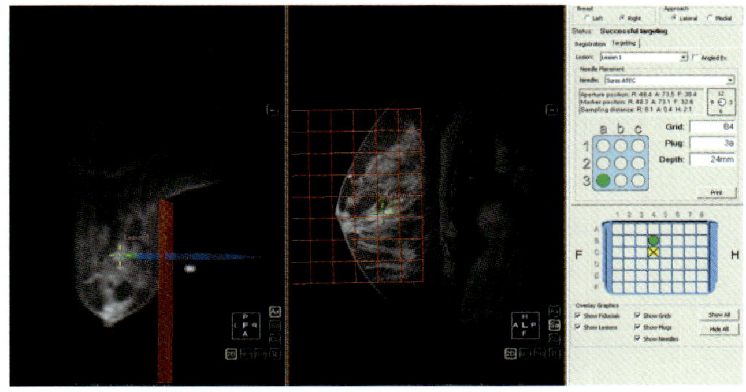

FIGURE 12.4 Automated targeting software. A cursor is placed over the lesion on the MR image, and the appropriate grid and needle opening are indicated. The depth of the lesion is also determined and displayed.

The pillar-and-post technique allows angulation of the needle to access lesions close to the chest wall, and the needle entrance site in the skin is more readily visualized.

Targeting with a Grid Device

To locate an enhancing lesion in the breast, a fiducial marker needs to be placed and included on the images. Several options exist for fiducial markers, including simple vitamin E capsules. Some of the biopsy grids have built-in markers. If a marker is placed manually, it can be put either in the grid opening that is likely to be directly over the lesion as determined by the diagnostic study or in a grid opening that is not likely to be over the lesion, so that the fiducial does not have to be moved prior to placing the needle.

For the manual grid technique, a sagittal sequence is needed, either acquired directly or reformatted with high enough resolution to visualize the lesion. A precontrast T1-weighted sequence is usually obtained to ensure that technical factors such as positioning and fat suppression are adequate and that the fiducial is seen. Additionally, in occasional cases subtraction images help clinicians visualize the enhancing lesion, and having a precontrast sequence allows for subtraction to be performed. Once the lesion is identified, the appropriate grid opening and appropriate hole in the needle guide are identified by determining the relative position of the lesion to the fiducial marker. This determines the *x* and *y* coordinates of the lesion. The lesion depth, the z coordinate, is easily determined by counting the number of slices between the skin surface and the center of the lesion. The number of slices is then multiplied by the slice thickness to obtain the depth (Figure 12.5).

Because the orientation of the image on the imaging monitor is different from the orientation of the patient on the scan table, it is relatively easy to choose the incorrect grid opening. To avoid this mistake, diagrams of the grid can be used to mark the location of the fiducial and the lesion (Figure 12.6). The diagram can then be brought into the magnet room and turned to orient it in the same position as the patient.

Targeting with a Pillar-and-Post Device

Manual targeting when using a pillar-and-post device can be done with either an axial or a sagittal sequence. Once the patient is positioned, compression is applied and the pillar is set to zero for both the *x* and y axes. Again, a fiducial marker

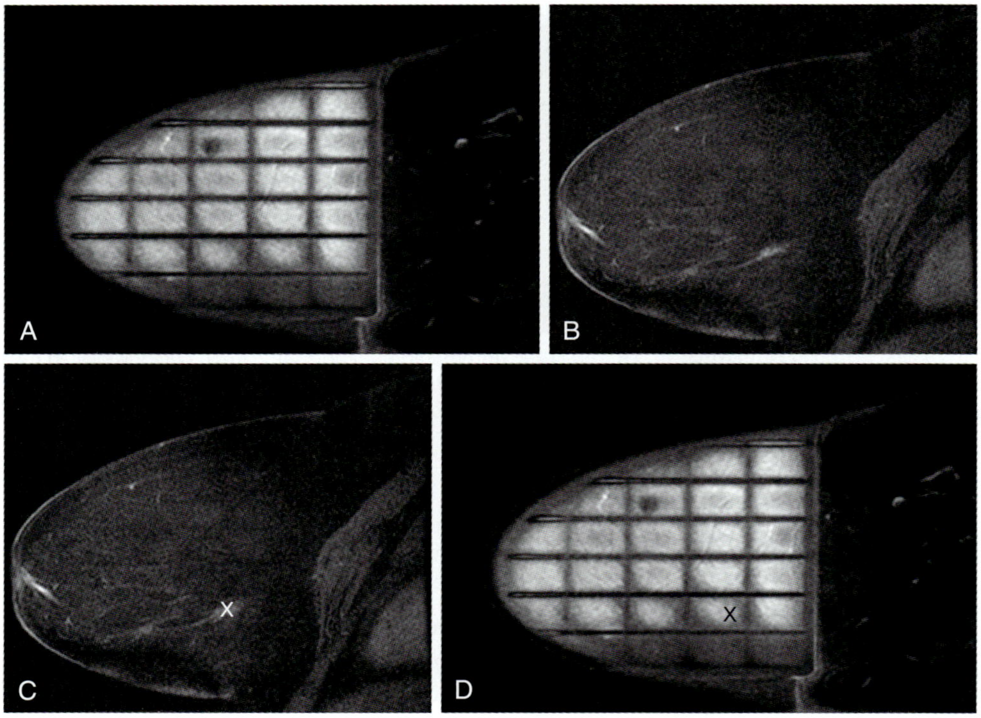

FIGURE 12.5 Targeting with a grid device seen on MRI images. **A,** Patient is positioned in grid device, a fiducial marker is placed, and the patient is scanned. The image number indicating the location of the skin surface is noted. **B,** The lesion is identified and the image number showing the center of the lesion is noted. **C,** A cursor is placed over the lesion. **D,** With the cursor kept in place, the image is scrolled to show the grid. The position of the cursor indicates the appropriate grid and needle opening to use. The number of slices between the skin surface and the lesion multiplied by the slice thickness indicates the depth of the lesion.

is placed and included in the precontrast scan. Contrast is administered, and an image sequence, usually in the axial plane, is obtained. The position of the fiducial is marked on the slice on which it is seen, and a reference line is placed on the workstation across the breast. The number of slices between the fiducial and the lesion is counted and multiplied by the slice thickness. This gives the location in the x (horizontal) axis. The distance from the lesion to the fiducial reference line determines the y axis (vertical) location. The pillar is then moved to these coordinates, the fiducial moved, and the patient rescanned to be certain that the location is correct. The depth of the lesion is then measured from the skin surface to determine the z position.

Local Anesthesia

Premedication with an oral anxiolytic agent is not usually necessary but can be helpful for particularly anxious patients. Local anesthesia, typically 1% Lidocaine without epinephrine, is administered with a 25-gauge needle to raise a skin wheal. Buffering the lidocaine with sodium bicarbonate will neutralize the acidic pH to decrease the initial stinging sensation. Depending on lesion depth, deeper anesthesia can be administered before inserting the biopsy needle. Some biopsy devices have the capability of delivering local anesthetic simultaneously with tissue acquisition. Lidocaine (1%) with epinephrine is often used for this deeper anesthesia unless there is a relative contraindication to the use of epinephrine, such as heart disease or arrhythmia.

Tissue Acquisition

Once the lesion is targeted, the appropriate grid and needle-guide opening determined, and local anesthesia delivered, a skin nick can be made with a scalpel to facilitate needle insertion. The introducer used with biopsy kits is so sharp that it can be placed in the breast without a skin nick, but this results in a circular wound rather than the linear one created by a scalpel and can result in a more visible scar.

When a nick in made with a scalpel and the grid device used, the tip of the introducer should be placed in the nick before the needle guide is popped into the grid to ensure that the needle does not make a separate wound (Figure 12.7). The introducer is then placed to the predetermined depth and replaced by the nonmetallic obturator to allow scanning to determine accuracy of positioning.

Different needle devices have obturators of different lengths. Some obturators mark the center of the sampling trough. For these needles, the scan done when the sheath and obturator are in place should ideally show the signal void from the obturator end in the center of the lesion (Figure 12.8). Other obturators actually show the location of the sampling trough, and for these, imaging done with the obturator in place should show the trough adjacent to the lesion (Figure 12.9) .

The number of cores that should be obtained has not been validated in the literature, but our experience with stereotactic and ultrasound biopsies indicates generally six to twelve cores are taken. One approach to sampling is to acquire six cores in a clock-face pattern and then reimage to be sure the lesion was appropriately sampled. Care should be taken to ensure that the needle remains sterile after the initial tissue acquisition and during the repeat scanning. If the scan shows that the lesion is still present or if there is any question as to adequacy of sampling, additional cores can be obtained and another postacquisition scan can be performed (Figure 12.10).

After sampling is completed, a tissue marker should be placed. Obtaining a sequence after marker placement is not often useful because the postbiopsy changes can obscure

LESION LOCALIZER CHART

	Vit. E	Lesion A	Difference	Clip
LR				
AP				
SI				

	Vit. E	Lesion A	Difference	Clip
LR				
AP				
SI				

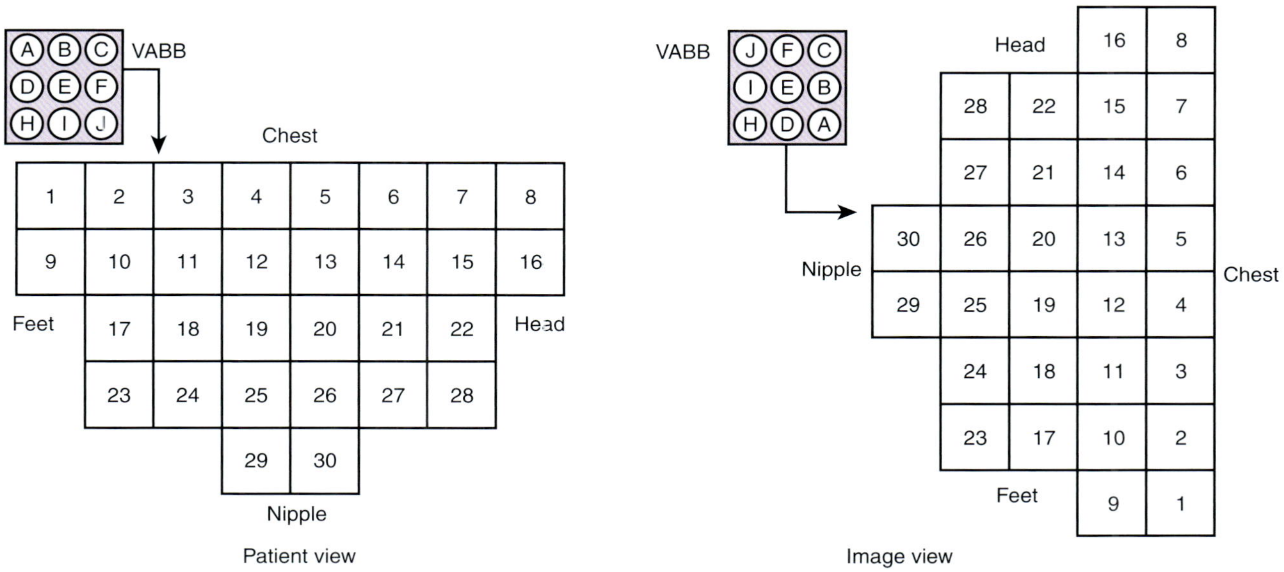

FIGURE 12.6 Diagram for marking appropriate grid opening based on the workstation image and rotating in the magnet room to reflect the patient's position.

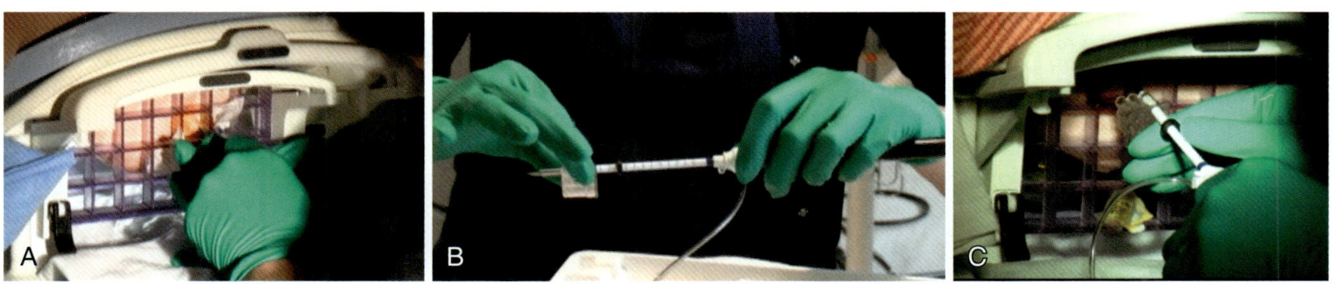

FIGURE 12.7 Placing the needle sheath. **A,** Once the location of the lesion has been determined, the skin cleansed, and local anesthesia administered, a skin nick is made with a scalpel. **B,** The lesion depth is set on the sheath, and a sharp introducer is placed through the sheath. **C,** The tip of the needle is placed in the skin nick before the needle guide is positioned to be sure the introducer enters the nick.

visualization of the marker. Doing a postbiopsy mammogram, however, is essential to document clip placement.

Challenges, Pitfalls, and Technical Tips

The performance of MRI-guided core biopsies is similar in many respects to stereotactic biopsies. This modality has unique challenges, however, and there are a number of tips and techniques that can be used to address them.[20]

Lesion Nonvisualization

Studies of MRI-guided biopsy procedures have reported that in a small proportion of cases, the lesion seen on the diagnostic study will not enhance at the time of the biopsy.[1] Hefler and colleagues[21] reported that 37 of 291 (13%) scheduled MRI-guided biopsies were canceled because of lesion nonvisualization. This occurred in 74 of 911 (8%) lesions reported by Brennan and coworkers[22] and in 52 (12.5%) in the multicenter study by Perlet and colleagues.[6] In the series by Brennan and coworkers[22] lesions occurring in breasts that were heterogeneously or extremely dense were more likely to be canceled that those in fatty or scattered fibroglandular breasts, and lesions in breasts with moderate or marked background enhancement were more likely to be canceled than those with minimal or mild enhancement. There was no significant difference in cancellation based on lesion type, mass or nonmass.

If the lesion is not seen, several steps can be taken. First, delayed scanning should be performed. Because of the compression from the biopsy grid, enhancement can be delayed and may not be apparent on the first postcontrast sequence. If the lesion is still not seen after several sequences, obtaining subtraction images might be helpful. Finally, loosening compression and rescanning may reveal the lesion. If, after all of these steps, the lesion still cannot be seen, the biopsy can be performed using landmarks. Usually, however, the procedure is canceled because accurate targeting cannot be ensured and also most lesions that do not enhance at the time of attempted biopsy will not reappear on follow-up.[6,21,22] In the series of 74 lesions not seen at the time of biopsy reported by Brennan and colleagues,[22] follow-up MRI was performed in 58 and lesions were reidentified in 17 (29%) of them. None of these proved to be malignant on further follow-up or biopsy, but an additional case went on to mastectomy and ductal carcinoma in situ (DCIS) was found in the same quadrant of the breast in which the original MRI lesion was seen. In the series by Hefler and coworkers,[21] 30 canceled cases underwent follow-up imaging and the lesion was reidentified in 5 (17%). Of these, four were seen on the initial follow-up examination and one on a subsequent MRI, but not on the first follow-up examination. All five of these cases underwent biopsy, and two (40%) were malignant.[21] Perlet and colleagues[6] reported that three (6.5%) of 46 lesions reappeared on follow-up. It is clear from these reports that follow-up of lesions not seen at the time of attempted biopsy must be performed to confirm the absence of a malignancy. The timing of the follow-up in these reports was variable. In the series by Brennan and coworkers, the median time of the follow-up was 12 months (range 0-58 months). Hefler and colleagues recommend performing the follow-up without compression as soon as 4 hours after the attempted biopsy or during the next day. Perlet and coworkers did the follow-up in 1 to 4 days.

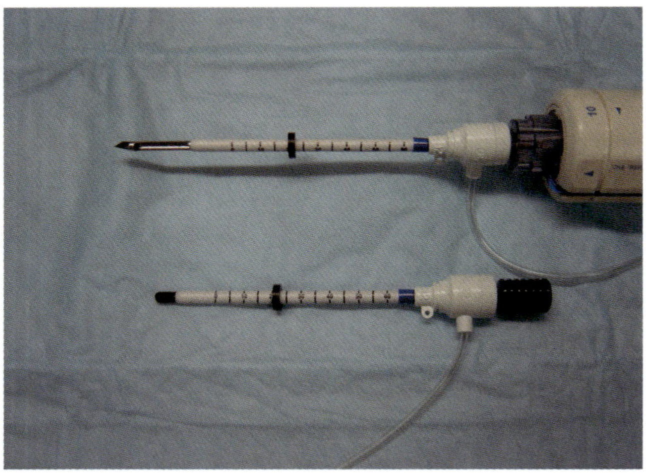

FIGURE 12.8 An obturator marks the center of the sampling trough. Once the sheath is placed to the appropriate depth, the introducer is removed and replaced with an obturator such as is shown here to allow scanning to determine the position of the sheath.

Posterior Lesions

As with stereotactic biopsy, some lesion locations in the breast are difficult to access. These include those that are close to the chest wall or in the axillary tail. To include these lesions in the biopsy grid, the patient can be obliqued to include more posterior tissue from the lateral or from the medial breast. Breast coils are equipped with padding and this can be removed to allow more tissue to be included. Finally, the needle can be positioned close to the anterior aspect of the mass, and sampling with the vacuum device can be preferentially directed to the posterior aspect of the breast rather than circumferentially, to draw the lesion into the sampling trough. There are some posterior lesions, however, that are simply not accessible with MRI-guided core

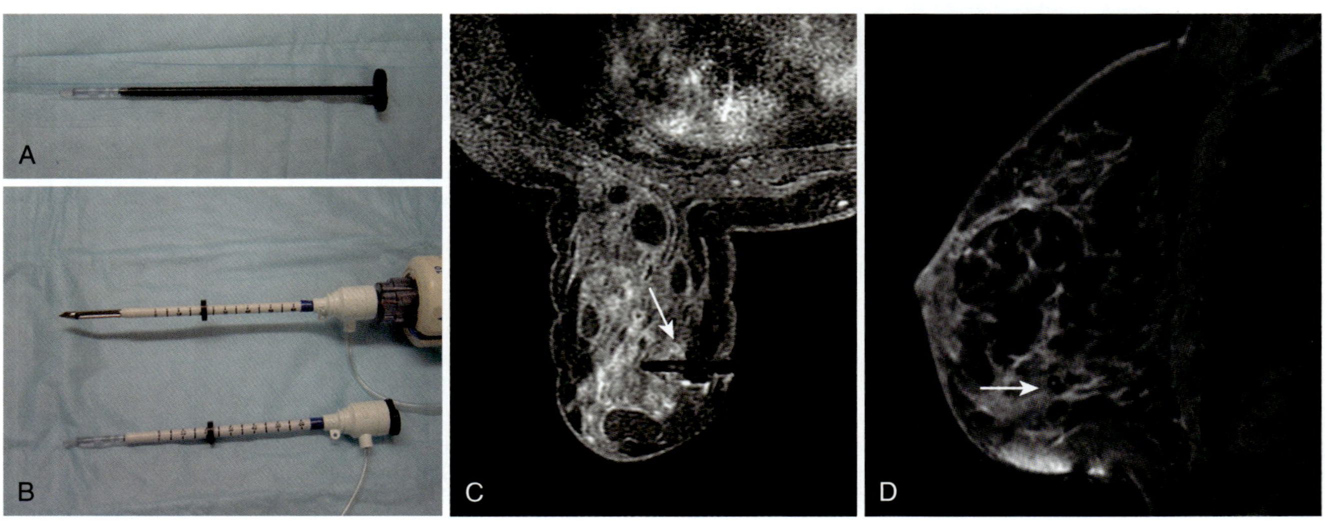

FIGURE 12.9 Obturator showing the length of the sampling trough. **A,** This obturator contains gadolinium in the tip. **B,** Comparison of obturator and sampling needle showing that the gadolinium in the tip indicates the entire length of the sampling trough. **C,** An MRI scan in the axial plane shows the sampling trough as indicated by the gadolinium to be adjacent to the lesion to be sampled (*arrow*). **D,** Imaged with MRI in the sagittal plane, the end of the obturator appears as a bull's eye with the bright gadolinium surrounded by a signal void (*arrow*). This indicates the location of the sampling trough on sequential sagittal images.

biopsy. If all attempts at including the lesion in the grid fail, MRI-guided wire localization followed by surgical excision can usually be performed because the localization needle can often be placed free-hand posterior to the localizing grid.

Medial Lesions

The design of some of the MRI biopsy grids limits access to medial lesions, and lesions in the posterior medial breast may not be accessible. There are several possible solutions to this situation. First, the patient can be obliqued and padding removed from the coil as with posterior lesions. If the patient is thin enough, the breast that is to undergo biopsy from a medial approach can be placed in the opposite breast coil. For example, if the right breast is to be biopsied, it can be placed in the left breast coil, making the medial surface of the breast readily accessible (Figure 12.11).The problem with this technique is that the positioning is awkward and often uncomfortable for the patient, and many women cannot physically fit into the magnet if they are positioned this way. Also, care must be taken by the technologist during image acquisition to specify that the contralateral coil is being used. Finally, if all else fails, a medial lesion can be biopsied using a lateral approach. If this is done, care must be taken to ensure that there is enough tissue beyond the lesion to accommodate the entire sampling trough and end of the biopsy needle.

Thin Breasts

Breasts that are very thin when compressed pose a challenge in performing MRI-guided biopsies. Vacuum-assisted biopsy devices generally have sampling troughs that are nearly 2 cm long, and in general at least 2.5 cm of tissue is needed in order to accommodate the needle. There are needles with shorter sampling troughs and blunt tips that can be used in thin breasts without running the risk of piercing the skin on the opposite side of the breast (Figure 12.12). These can also be employed when using a lateral approach for a medial lesion if there is not enough tissue beyond the lesion to accommodate a regular-size needle. Other helpful tips for biopsy of lesions in thin breasts include using as little compression as possible to immobilize the breast to allow as much thickness as possible and using fenestrated grids both medially and laterally as well as a blunt-tipped needle. This allows the needle to be buried in the tissue and can result in successful sampling of the lesion. As with stereotactic biopsies, however, there are some breasts that are so thin that MRI-guided needle biopsies are not technically feasible.

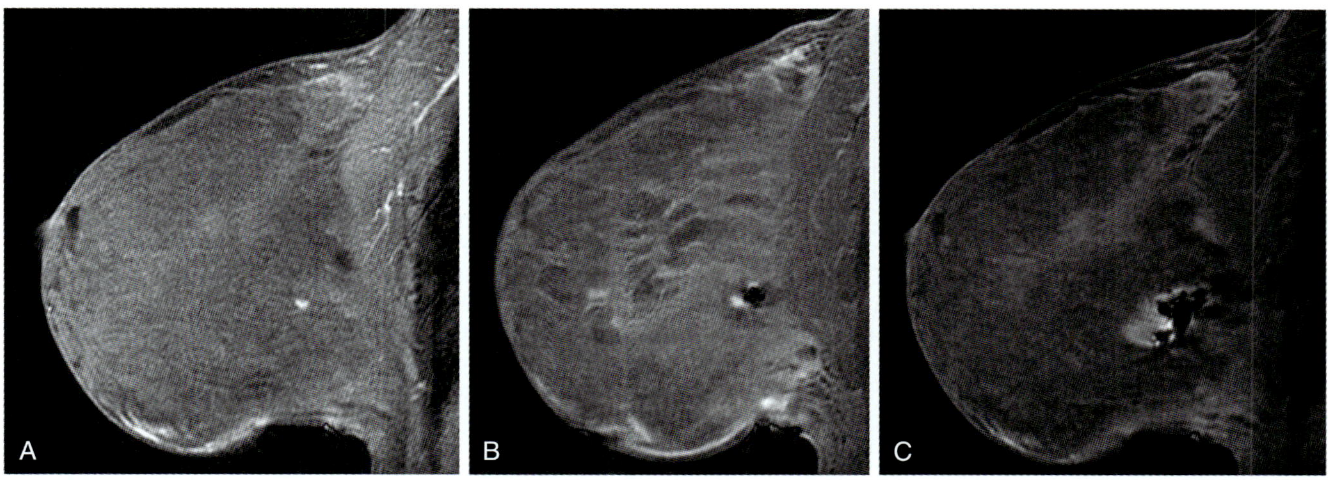

FIGURE 12.10 A lesion is still present in this image after sampling. **A,** An enhancing mass was targeted for MRI-guided core biopsy. **B,** After six cores were obtained, the patient was rescanned and the lesion is still present proximal to biopsy-site changes, indicating that the needle was too deep. **C,** After repositioning the needle and acquiring additional cores, scanning indicates that the lesion appears to have been sampled.

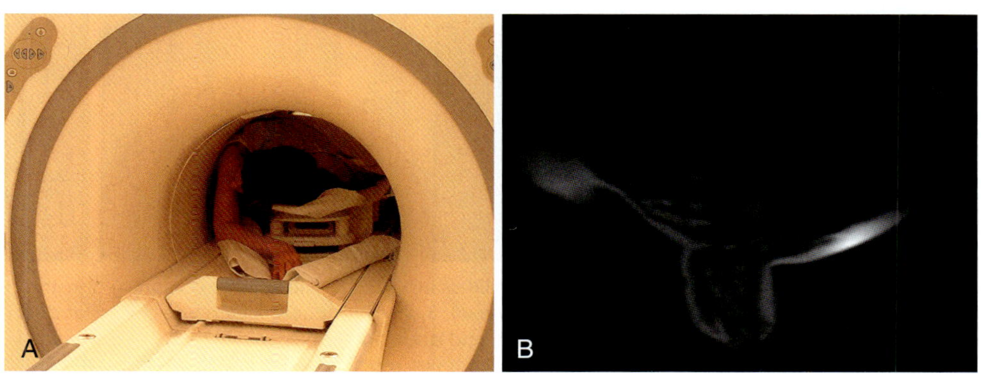

FIGURE 12.11 Access to a medial lesion is illustrated. **A,** If regular positioning does not allow access to a medial lesion, the breast with the lesion can be placed in the contralateral breast coil opening. **B,** Appearance of the localizer when the right breast is placed in the left coil.

Superficial Lesions

When lesions are located close to the skin, there is a danger of taking pieces of skin with each core. This can be a particular problem with MRI-guided biopsies done with the grid device, because once the needle guide block is placed in the grid, direct visualization of the needle entrance site is not possible. If skin is taken with the cores, a large skin wound that can leave a relatively large scar or that can require stitches for closure may result.

In targeting for MRI biopsies, the calculated depth marks the center of the sampling trough, which means that some of the trough is superficial to the lesion and can include the skin surface. To prevent this, the depth of the lesion should be at least 1 cm. Care must be taken to keep from tenting the skin when placing the introducer. This can be accomplished by pushing the introducer beyond the calculated depth, then withdrawing to the appropriate position. Twisting the sheath once it is in place can also allow the skin to surround the sheath. An indication that the sampling trough is not completely in the breast is a sucking sound when the vacuum is on and samples are obtained. If this occurs, sampling should be stopped and the needle repositioned deeper in the breast.

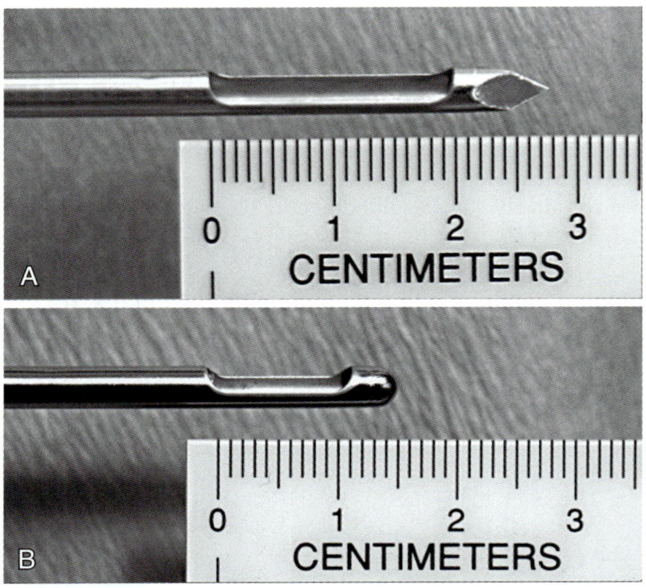

FIGURE 12.12 Sampling devices are shown. **A,** Regular sampling devices with sharp-tipped needle. **B,** Blunt-tipped sampling device with shorter sampling trough. This is used when the breast is thin in compression and cannot accommodate the regular device.

Lesion Displacement

The needles used for MRI-guided vacuum-assisted biopsies do not fire as they do for stereotactic or ultrasound procedures. Therefore there is more of a chance that the lesion will be displaced by the needle (the snowplow effect). Also, scanning to confirm accurate positioning is done with an obturator and there is a possibility that the actual sampling needle will not end up in appropriate position, even if the confirmatory obturator scan shows correct positioning. Lesions can be displaced in the *x*, *y*, or *z* axis, and careful review of the prebiopsy scans is necessary to determine if the lesion has been displaced (Figure 12.13). Inserting the introducer with a twisting motion rather than a direct thrust can be helpful. If the lesion is slightly displaced, preferential sampling in the direction of the lesion rather than in an around-the-clock-face pattern can sometimes result in successful sampling (Figure 12.14).

Implants

The presence of implants does not automatically preclude the possibility of performing an MRI-guided biopsy. As with stereotactic biopsies or mammographically guided needle localizations, the implant can often be displaced outside of the grid device, allowing the lesion to be biopsied without danger of rupturing the implant (Figure 12.15). In some cases, however, the lesion is located so close to the implant that the biopsy cannot be performed without a high likelihood of implant rupture. In those cases, MRI-guided needle

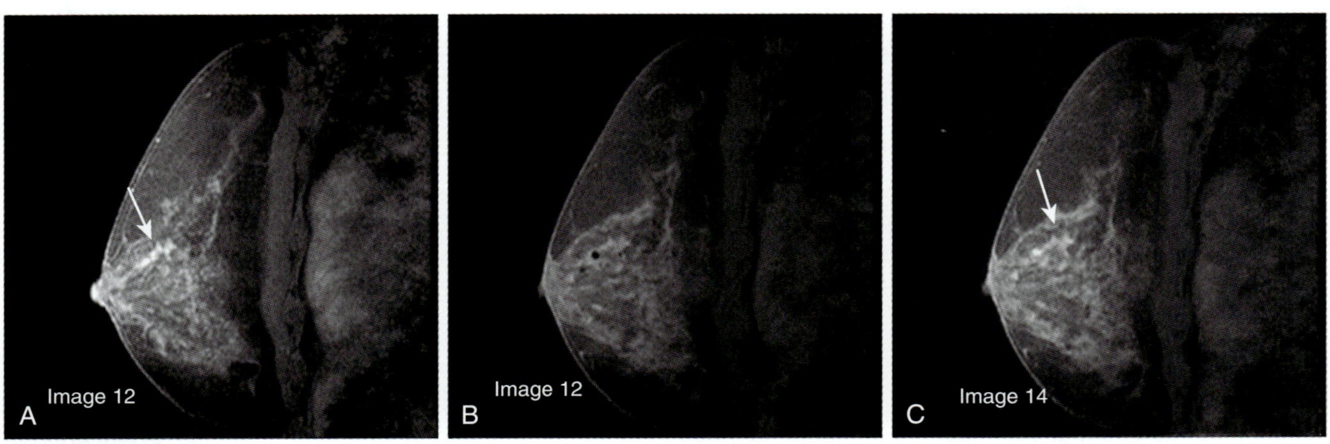

FIGURE 12.13 Lesion displacement is shown on MRI scans. **A,** The patient was compressed in the breast coil. Nonmass enhancement to undergo MRI core biopsy was seen on image 12 (*arrow*). **B,** The introducer sheath was placed, and scanning showed the tip of the obturator to be at image 12. However, the lesion was not seen, and landmarks appeared different. **C,** The lesion was seen on image 14 (*arrow*), indicating that it had been displaced by the introducer. The sheath was repositioned deeper in the breast.

localization can often be successfully performed by placing the needle in front of the lesion, away from the implant.

Post-Biopsy Management

Tissue Marker Placement

As a final step after adequate sampling has been ascertained, a tissue marker should always be placed at the biopsy site. Not only will the marker help guide subsequent excision should that be necessary, but in addition, if pathology results are benign and concordant, the marker will help indicate on future MRI examinations the site that was biopsied. If more than one lesion is biopsied in one breast, markers of different shapes should be placed to avoid confusion. It should be made very clear in the description of the procedure which marker was placed at which lesion location. A postprocedure mammogram should always be obtained to document the location of the marker in relation to the biopsy site, and this should be noted in the report. If biopsy changes are not evident, the location of the marker on the mammogram relative to the expected location based on the MRI lesion location should be noted. If the marker appears displaced relative to the biopsy site changes and/or the expected location of the lesion on the mammogram, the approximate amount and direction of the displacement should be mentioned in the procedure report (Figure 12.16).

Concordance Determination

The pathology report should be reviewed by the radiologist who did the MRI-guided biopsy, and a determination as to whether the histologic finding explains the MRI finding should be made. Determining concordance for MRI-guided procedures can be more challenging than for other image-guided biopsies because of the large number of benign entities that can enhance on MRI, including normal parenchyma. Additionally, unlike stereotactic or ultrasound-guided

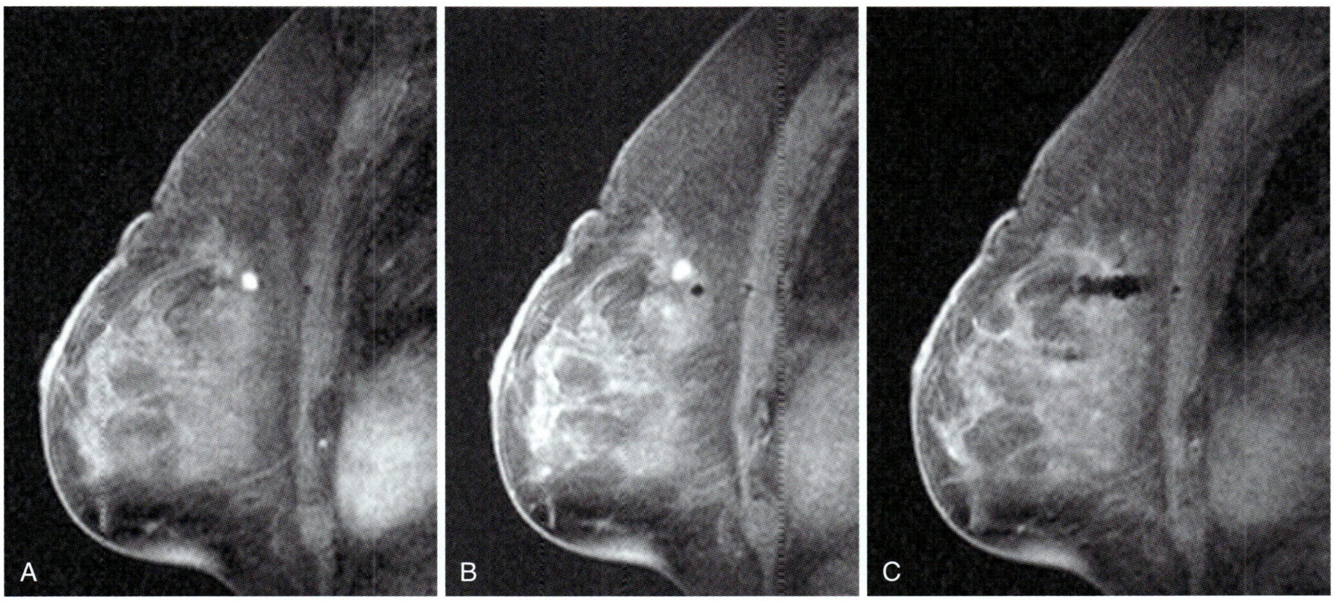

FIGURE 12.14 Preferential sampling is illustrated in MRI scans. A, Small enhancing mass that will undergo MRI-guided biopsy. B, Scanning after placement of the introducer sheath shows signal void from the obturator posterior to the mass. All samples were obtained in the direction of the mass rather than in an around-the-clock-face pattern. C, Image following tissue acquisition shows the mass has been sampled.

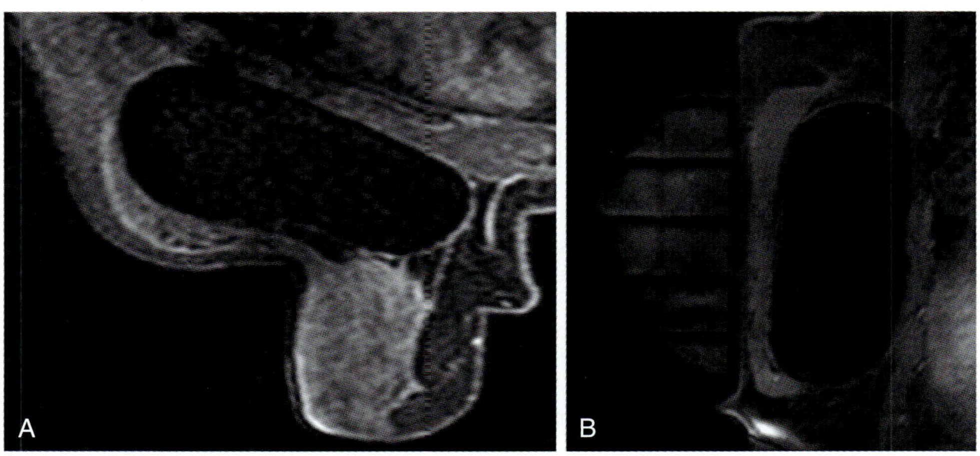

FIGURE 12.15 MRI-guided core biopsy in a woman with implants is shown. A, Axial image showing the implant displaced from the breast tissue. B, Sagittal imaging showing the localizer grid over the breast tissue with the implant displaced.

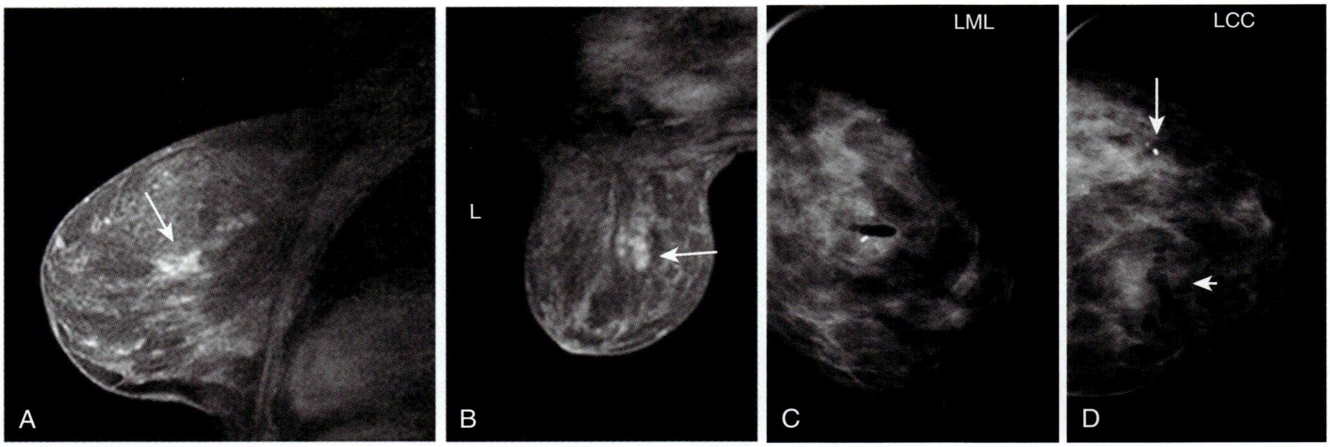

FIGURE 12.16 A postbiopsy mammogram shows clip position. **A,** Sagittal postcontrast T1-weighted MRI scan shows nonmass enhancement (*arrow*) for which MRI-guided core biopsy was performed. **B,** Axial postcontrast T1-weighted image showing the lesion slightly medial to the nipple line (*arrow*). **C,** Postbiopsy mediolateral view mammogram shows biopsy changes, and the clip appears to be in accurate position. **D,** Postbiopsy craniocaudal view mammogram, however, shows biopsy-site changes medially (*arrowhead*) and clip displaced laterally (*arrow*).

biopsies, there are no specimen images or real-time visualization of the biopsy to confirm that the lesion was indeed adequately sampled.

Discordant results at MRI-guided biopsy have been reported to occur in 7% of cases, with an upgrade to malignancy in 30% of discordant cases undergoing excision.[23] Both the rate of discordance and the upgrade rate for MRI-guided biopsies are higher than those reported for ultrasound and stereotactic-guided core biopsies.[24-26]

High-Risk Lesions

Because MRI-guided biopsy is a relatively new technique, published data on high-risk lesions encountered on MRI biopsy are not as extensive as information on high-risk lesions on stereotactic or ultrasound-guided procedures. The histopathologic entities considered to be high-risk lesions on MRI-guided biopsies are the same as those encountered with any image-guided core biopsy, and management is generally similar. High-risk lesions include atypical ductal hyperplasia (ADH), lobular neoplasia including atypical lobular neoplasia and lobular carcinoma in situ (LCIS), papillomas and papillary lesions, and radial scars. The reported frequency of these lesions on MRI-guided core biopsy varies in the literature from 3% to 21%.[9,27-29] As with other image guided procedures, ADH is the most commonly encountered high-risk lesion on MRI-guided core biopsies. In a European multi-institutional study reported by Perlet and colleagues,[6] ADH was encountered in 3% (17/517) of lesions biopsied with an 11-gauge vacuum-assisted device. Liberman and coworkers reported ADH in 6% (15/237) of MRI-detected lesions in which biopsy was performed with a 9-gauge vacuum probe.[29]

Overall, ADH accounts for approximately 50% of the total number of high-risk lesions found on MRI-guided biopsy.[27,29] The second most frequently encountered high-risk lesion is lobular neoplasia, comprising both atypical lobular hyperplasia (ALH) and LCIS.[27]

The rate at which high-risk lesions on MRI core biopsy are upgraded to malignancy varies from 13% to 57% across a number of reported series.[2-9,27-29] The upgrade rate associated with ADH is the highest among all high-risk lesions encountered on MRI biopsy, on the order of 30% to 40%.[27-29] This upgrade rate of ADH on MRI-guided core biopsies is higher than the upgrade of ADH found on stereotactic biopsy, which is about 20% for biopsies done with an 11-gauge vacuum assisted device.[24,26,28] Most cases of upgrade of ADH on MRI core biopsy have been to DCIS, though there have been some upgrades to invasive cancer.[27]

The data on upgrade of high-risk lesions other than ADH are very sparse. To date, no upgrades of radial scar to malignancy have been reported, though the numbers are quite small. The upgrade rate of lobular neoplasia in one study was reported to be 50% (4 of 8).[29]

The most appropriate management of benign papillomas encountered on any image-guided core biopsy, including those done with MRI, is still a matter of debate. A study by Brennan and coworkers[30] that specifically addressed papillomas found at 9-gauge vacuum-assisted MRI-guided biopsy reported that papillomas with and without atypia were encountered in 5% of cases. The upgrade was 9% for papillomas with atypia and 5% for papillomas without atypia. They concluded that papillomas encountered on MRI-guided biopsy should be excised.

No clinical or imaging features have been found that are helpful in predicting which high-risk lesions are likely to be upgraded to malignancy.[29,31] The frequency of high-risk lesions and upgrade rates are summarized in Table 12.1.

Follow-Up After Magnetic Resonance–Guided Biopsy

For cases in which malignancy, atypia, or discordant results are obtained at MRI-guided core biopsy, surgical excision is recommended. For benign, concordant results, however, the best management is less clear-cut. Studies of follow-up after stereotactic or ultrasound-guided biopsies have reported lesion progression requiring repeat biopsy, as well as cases of missed cancers.[32,33] This also has been shown for MRI-guided biopsies. A study by Li and colleagues[34] found that 9.6% (17/177) of lesions with benign concordant results at MRI biopsy underwent repeat biopsy after follow-up MRI imaging,

Table 12.1 Frequency and Upgrade of High-Risk Lesions on MRI-Guided Biopsy

Study	Year	Number	Needle	Number of cores	High Risk	Upgrade
Rauch et al.[8]	2012	218	9-gauge vacuum	6-12	37 (17%)	5/37 (14%)
Crystal et al.[29]	2011	161	9-gauge vacuum	NA	31 (19%)	13/26 (50%)
Han et al.[9]	2008	150	9-gaute, 10-gauge vacuum	4-10	21 (14%)	4 /21 (19%)
Liberman et al.[28]	2007	237	9-gauge vacuum	9	15 (6%)	5/13 (38%)
Orel et al.[3]	2006	85	9-gauge vacuum	NA	18 (21%)	2/18 (11%)
Perlet et al.[6]	2006	517	11-gauge vacuum	≥20	17 (3%)	5/17 (29%)
Liberman et al.[28]	2005	98	9-gauge vacuum	NA	10 (11%)	3/9 (33%)

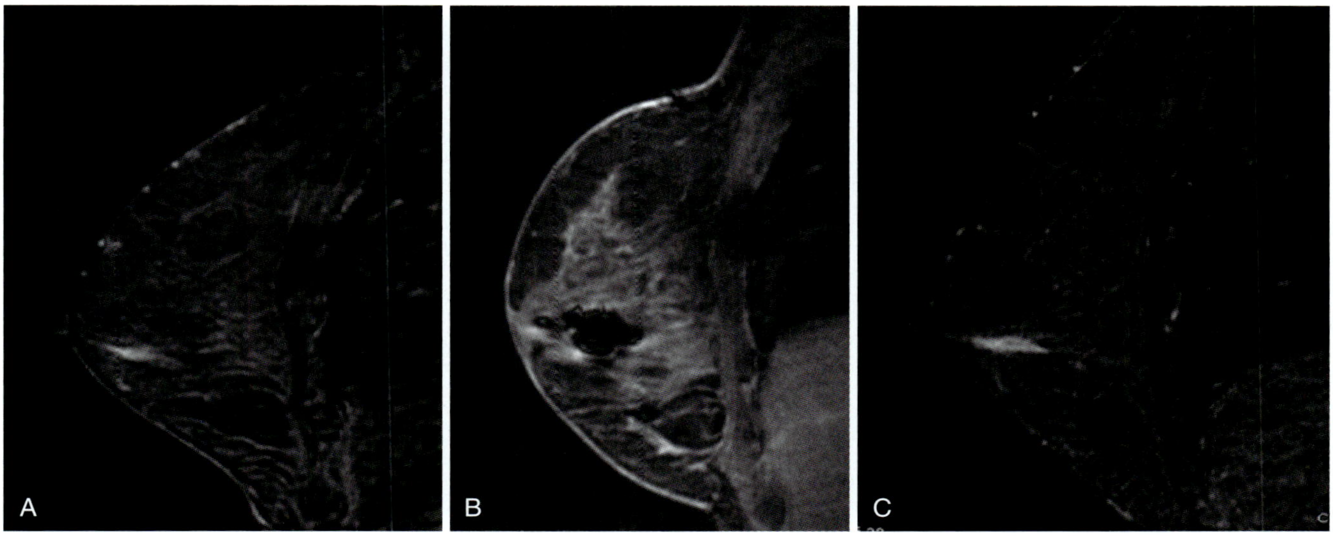

FIGURE 12.17 An unsuspected, missed lesion at MRI-guided core biopsy is shown. **A,** Sagittal T1-weighted postcontrast subtraction image showing nonmass enhancement behind the nipple that underwent MRI-guided core biopsy. **B,** Postbiopsy image showing biopsy site changes. The lesion is no longer seen. Pathology revealed sclerosing adenosis and fibrocystic change but no evidence of atypia or malignancy. **C,** Sagittal T1-weighted postcontrast subtraction image done 6 months later shows the nonmass enhancement is still present and slightly larger than on the prior study. Repeat biopsy revealed DCIS.

and four of these were malignant (Figure 12.17). They also found that doing the follow-up MRI before 6 months did not contribute to detecting false-negative biopsies and suggested that for all benign concordant MRI-guided biopsies, follow-up MRI scan be performed routinely at 6 months.

False-Negative Magnetic Resonance–Guided Biopsies

False-negative results have been reported for MRI-guided biopsies, as they have with other image-guided interventions. Hauth and coworkers[35] reported that MRI 24 hours after core biopsy showed that 14% (4 of 29) of lesions were actually missed by the biopsy. Perlet and colleagues[6] reported no false negatives among 316 women who had benign MRI cores biopsies and subsequent MRI follow-up. In the series by Li and coworkers,[34] however, four cancers were subsequently found among 177 lesions that had initially yielded benign results on MRI core biopsy. Raher and colleagues[36] reported that 4 of 69 (4.5%) patients had cancer diagnosed on follow-up imaging, and Friedlander and coworkers[37] reported a 2.5% false-negative MRI biopsy rate. Unlike stereotactic biopsy, in which a specimen radiograph can confirm successful sampling, or ultrasound-guided core biopsy, in which real-time imaging can show accurate tissue acquisition, MRI-guided procedures require follow-up imaging for definite confirmation of adequate sampling.

Conclusion

For facilities that perform breast MRI, the ability to also offer MRI-guided biopsy is crucial for providing optimal patient care. There are many factors that contribute to the successful completion of MRI-guided core biopsies, including appropriate lesion and equipment selection, careful attention to technique, correlation of pathology results with imaging features, and a standard follow-up protocol. When these elements are optimized, outcomes for patients who undergo these procedures are similarly improved.

References

1. Breast MRI Accreditation. Available at: www.ACR.org/Quality-Safety/Accreditation/BreastMRI
2. Liberman L, Bracero N, Morris E, Thornton CM, VanZee KJ, Tan LK: MRI-guided vacuum-assisted breast biopsy: initial experience, *AJR Am J Roentgenol* 181:1283–1293, 2003.

3. Orel SG, Rosen M, Mies C, Schnall MD: MR imaging-guided 9-gauge vacuum-assisted core-needle breast biopsy: initial experience, *Radiology* 238:54–61, 2006.
4. Lehman CD, Deperi ER, Peacock S, McDonough MD, Demartini WB, Shook J: Clinical experience with MRI-guided vacuum-assisted breast biopsy, *AJR Am J Roentgenol* 184:1782–1787, 2005.
5. Liberman L, Bracero N, Morris E, Thornton C, Dershaw DD: MRI-guided 9-gauge vacuum-assisted breast biopsy: initial clinical experience, *AJR Am J Roentgenol* 185:183–193, 2005.
6. Perlet C, Heywang-Kobrunner SH, Heinig A, et al: Magnetic resonance-guided, vacuum-assisted breast biopsy: results from a European multicenter study of 538 lesions, *Cancer* 106:982–990, 2006.
7. Mahoney MC: Initial clinical experience with a new MRI vacuum-assisted breast biopsy device, *J Magn Reson Imaging* 28:900–905, 2008.
8. Rauch GMDogan BE, SmithB, Liu P, Yang WT: Outcome analysis of 9-gauge MRI-guided vacuum-assisted core needle breast biopsies, *AJR Am J Roentgenol* 198:292–299, 2012.
9. Han B-K, Schnall MD, Orel SG, Rosen M: Outcome of MRI-guided breast biopsy, *AJR Am J Roentgenol* 191:1798–1804, 2008.
10. Abe H, Schmidt RA, Shah RN, et al: MR directed ("second look") ultrasound examination for breast lesions detected initially on MRI: MR and sonographic findings, *AJR Am J Roentgenol* 194:370–377, 2010.
11. Meissnitzer M, Dersahw DD, Lee CH, Morris EA: Targeted ultrasound of the breast in women with abnormal MRI findings for whom biopsy has been recommended, *AJR Am J Roentgenol* 193:1025–1029, 2009.
12. Morris EA, Liberman L, Dershaw DD, et al: Pre-operative MR imaging-guided needle localization of breast lesions, *AJR Am J Roentgenol* 178:1211–1220, 2002.
13. Melotti MK, Berg WA: Core needle biopsy in patients undergoing anticoagulation therapy: Preliminary results, *AJR Am J Roentgenol* 174: 245–249, 2000.
14. Somerville P, Seifert PJ, Destounis SV, Murphy PF, Young W: Anticoagulation and bleeding risk after core needle biopsy, *AJR Am J Roentgenol* 191:1194–1197, 2008.
15. Kettritz U, Rotter K, Schreer I, et al: Stereotactic vacuum-assisted breast biopsy in 2874 patients: a multicenter study, *Cancer* 100: 245–251, 2004.
16. Simon JR, Kalbhen CL, Cooper RA, Flisak ME: Accuracy and complication rates of US-guided vacuum-assisted core breast biopsy: initial results, *Radiology* 215:694–697, 2000.
17. Meeuwis C, Veltman J, van Hall HN, et al: MR-guided breast biopsy at 3T: diagnostic yield of large core needle biopsy compared with vacuum-assisted biopsy, *Eur Radiol* 22:341–349, 2012.
18. Lehman CD, DePeri ER, Peacock S, McDonough MD, DeMartini WB, Shook J: Clinical experience with MRI-guided vacuum-assisted breast biopsy, *AJR Am J Roentgenol* 184:1782–1787, 2005.
19. Noroozian M, Gombos EC, Chikarmane S, et al: Factors that impact the duration of MRI-guided core needle biopsy, *AJR Am J Roentgenol* 194:W150–W157, 2010.
20. Price ER, Morris EA: Magnetic resonance imaging-guided breast biopsies: tips and tricks, *Can Assoc Radiol J* 62:15–21, 2011.
21. Hefler L, Casselman J, Amaya B, et al: Follow-up of breast lesions detected by MRI not biopsied due to absent enhancement of contrast medium, *Eur Radiol* 13:344–346, 2003.
22. Brennan SB, Sung JS, Dershaw DD, Liberman L, Morris EA: Cancellation of MR imaging-guided breast biopsy due to lesion nonvisualization: frequency and follow-up, *Radiology* 261:92–99, 2011.
23. Lee J-M, Kaplan JB, Murray MP, et al: Imaging-histologic discordance at MRI-guided 9-gauge vacuum-assisted breast biopsy, *AJR Am J Roentgenol* 189:852–859, 2007.
24. Philpotts LE, Shaheen NA, Carter D, Lange RC, Lee CH: Comparison of rebiopsy rates after stereotactic core needle biopsy of the breast with 11-gauge vacuum suction probe versus 14-gauge needle and automatic gun, *AJR Am J Roentgenol* 172:683–687, 1999.
25. Liberman L, Drotman MB, Morris EA, et al: Imaging-histologic discordance at percutaneous breast biopsy, *Cancer* 89:2538–2546, 2000.
26. Philpotts LE, Hooley RJ, Lee CH: Comparison of automated versus vacuum-assisted biopsy methods for sonographically guided core biopsy of the breast, *AJR Am J Roentgenol* 180:717–720, 2003.
27. Heller SL, Moy L: Imaging features and management of high-risk lesions on contrast-enhanced dynamic breast MRI, *AJR Am J Roentgenol* 198:249–255, 2012.
28. Liberman L, Holland AE, Marjan D, et al: Underestimation of atypical ductal hyperplasia at MRI-guided 9-gauge vacuum-assisted breast biopsy, *AJR Am J Roentgenol* 188:684–690, 2007.
29. Crystal P, Sadaf A, Bukhanov K, McCready D, O'Malley F, Helbich TH: High-risk lesions diagnosed at MRI-guided vacuum-assisted breast biopsy: can underestimation be predicted? *Eur Radiol* 21:582–589, 2011.
30. Brennan SB, Corben A, Liberman L, et al: Papilloma diagnosed at MRI-guided vacuum-assisted breast biopsy: is surgical excision still warranted? *AJR Am J Roentgenol* 199:W512–W519, 2012.
31. Strigel RM, Eby PR, DeMartini WB, et al: Frequency, upgrade rates, and characteristics of high-risk lesions initially identified with breast MRI, *AJR Am J Roentgenol* 195:792–798, 2010.
32. Jackman RJ, Marsoni FA Jr, Rosenberg J: False-negative diagnoses at stereotactic vacuum-assisted needle breast biopsy: long-term follow-up of 1,280 lesions and review of the literature, *AJR Am J Roentgenol* 192:341–351, 2009.
33. Youk JH, Jung I, Kim E-K, et al: US follow-up protocol in concordant benign result after US-guided 14-gauge core needle breast biopsy, *Breast Cancer Res Treat* 132:1089–1097, 2012.
34. Li J, Dershaw DD, Lee CH, Kaplan J, Morris EA: MRI follow-up after concordant, histologically benign diagnosis of breast lesions sampled by MRI-guided biopsy, *AJR Am J Roentgenol* 193:850–855, 2009.
35. Hauth EA, Jaeger HJ, Lubman J, et al: MR-guided vacuum-assisted breast biopsy with a handheld biopsy system: clinical experience and results in postinterventional MR mammography after 24 h, *Eur Radiol* 18:168–176, 2008.
36. Raher L, Wisner D, Chang B, Esserman L, Hylton N, Joe B: *False negatives found on follow-up MRI after benign concordant MRI-guided breast biopsies (abstr)*, Chicago, IL, 2011, RSNA.
37. Friedlander L, Lee C, Comstock D, Morris E, Dershaw DD: *Frequency of unsuspected missed lesions and false-negative rate at MRI-guided core biopsy (abstr)*, Chicago, IL, 2011, RSNA.

Index

A

B

Page numbers followed by f indicate figures; t, tables; b, boxes.

N

O

P

U

V

W

Z